Rare Diseases of the Immune System

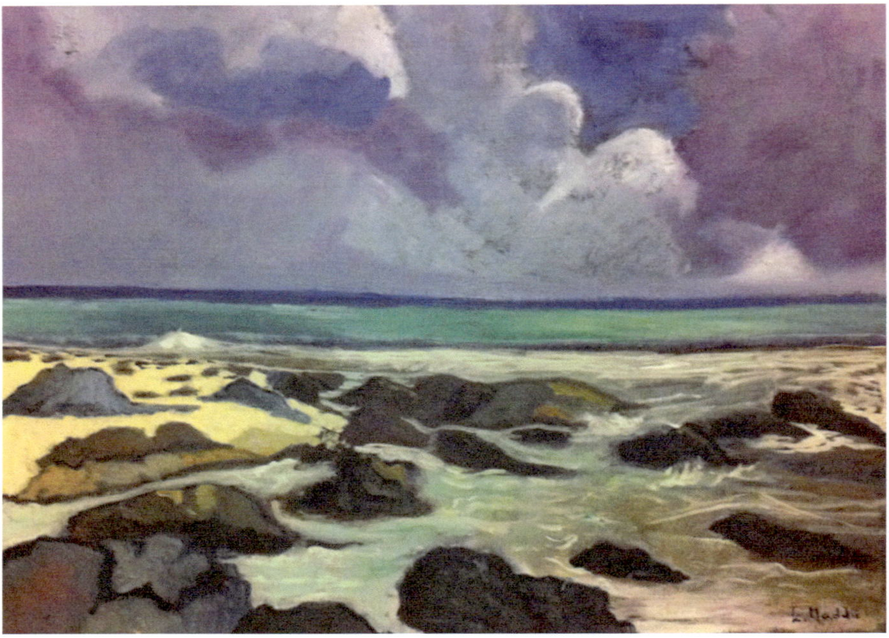

Nuvole sul mare, Laura Maddii Emmi (Private collection)

Renato Alberto Sinico • Loïc Guillevin
Editors

Anti-Neutrophil Cytoplasmic Antibody (ANCA) Associated Vasculitis

Springer

Editors
Renato Alberto Sinico
Department of Medicine and Surgery
University of Milano-Bicocca
Monza
Monza e Brianza
Italy

Loïc Guillevin
Department of Medicine
Paris Descartes University Hospital Cochin
Paris
France

ISSN 2282-6505 ISSN 2283-6403 (electronic)
Rare Diseases of the Immune System
ISBN 978-3-030-02238-9 ISBN 978-3-030-02239-6 (eBook)
https://doi.org/10.1007/978-3-030-02239-6

This Springer imprint is published by the registered company Springer Nature Switzerland AG
The registered company address is: Gewerbestrasse 11, 6330 Cham, Switzerland

Dedicated to my family.

Acknowledgements

We would like to thank all the prestigious colleagues and researches from around the world and from different disciplines for the invaluable contribution to this book. Without their help this book would not have been possible.

Contents

Part I

ANCA-Associated Vasculitis

Introduction: Nomenclature and Classification

1

J. Charles Jennette and Ronald J. Falk

1.1 AAV Pathologic Features

Vasculitis is inflammation in blood vessel walls. Antineutrophil cytoplasmic antibody (ANCA)-associated vasculitis (AAV) is vasculitis accompanied by circulating ANCAs, or phenotypically identical disease without detectable ANCA (ANCA-negative AAV). AAV is a necrotizing vasculitis with few or no immune deposits that affects predominantly small vessels (i.e., capillaries, venules, arterioles, and small arteries) (Table 1.1) [1–3].

An understanding of the pathologic features of AAV is required to understand the historical and contemporary nomenclature and classification of AAV. Acute AAV lesions in blood vessels are characterized by segmental neutrophil-rich inflammation and necrosis (Fig. 1.1). Vessel wall necrosis allows plasma constituents, including coagulation factors, to spill from vessels into perivascular tissue or adjacent spaces, for example, the urinary space adjacent to glomerular capillaries (Fig. 1.1a) and the air space adjacent to alveolar capillaries (Fig. 1.2a). In perivascular tissue, the coagulation factors contact thrombogenic substances (e.g., tissue factor) and form fibrin. The accumulation of fibrin at sites of vascular necrosis is called fibrinoid necrosis (Fig. 1.1a, b). The infiltrating neutrophils and other leukocytes undergo nuclear fragmentation (leukocytoclasia) as a result of cell death producing a pattern of injury called leukocytoclastic vasculitis, which is seen most often

J. C. Jennette (✉)
Department of Pathology and Laboratory Medicine, School of Medicine,
University of North Carolina at Chapel Hill, Chapel Hill, NC, USA
e-mail: jcj@med.unc.edu

R. J. Falk
Department of Medicine, School of Medicine, University of North Carolina at Chapel Hill,
Chapel Hill, NC, USA
e-mail: ronald_falk@med.unc.edu

R. A. Sinico, L. Guillevin (eds.), *Anti-Neutrophil Cytoplasmic Antibody (ANCA) Associated Vasculitis*, Rare Diseases of the Immune System,
https://doi.org/10.1007/978-3-030-02239-6_1

Table 1.1 Vasculitis names adopted by the 2012 International Chapel Hill Consensus Conference on the Nomenclature of Vasculitides (2012 CHCC) [1]

Large-vessel vasculitis (LVV)
Takayasu arteritis (TAK)
Giant cell arteritis (GCA)
Medium-vessel vasculitis (MVV)
Polyarteritis nodosa (PAN)
Kawasaki disease (KD)
Small-vessel vasculitis (SVV)
Antineutrophil cytoplasmic antibody (ANCA)–associated vasculitis (AAV)
Microscopic polyangiitis (MPA)
Granulomatosis with polyangiitis (Wegener's) (GPA)
Eosinophilic granulomatosis with polyangiitis (Churg-Strauss) (EGPA)
Immune complex SVV
Anti-glomerular basement membrane (anti-GBM) disease
Cryoglobulinemic vasculitis (CV)
IgA vasculitis (Henoch-Schönlein) (IgAV)
Hypocomplementemic urticarial vasculitis (HUV) (anti-C1q vasculitis)
Variable vessel vasculitis (VVV)
Behcet's disease (BD)
Cogan's syndrome (CS)
Single-organ vasculitis (SOV)
Cutaneous leukocytoclastic angiitis
Cutaneous arteritis
Primary central nervous system vasculitis - Isolated aortitis
Others
Vasculitis associated with systemic disease
Lupus vasculitis
Rheumatoid vasculitis
Sarcoid vasculitis
Others
Vasculitis associated with probable etiology
Hepatitis C virus–associated cryoglobulinemic vasculitis
Hepatitis B virus–associated vasculitis
Syphilis-associated aortitis
Drug-associated immune complex vasculitis
Drug-associated ANCA-associated vasculitis
Cancer-associated vasculitis
Others

in inflamed venules and arterioles (Fig. 1.1c). At a given site of inflammation, the acute necrotizing lesions evolve within several days or weeks into chronic inflammatory lesions with a predominance of lymphocytes and monocytes, followed by progressive scarring. In patients with active disease, there is ongoing onset of new self-limited acute lesions concurrent with the evolution of chronic lesions. This is

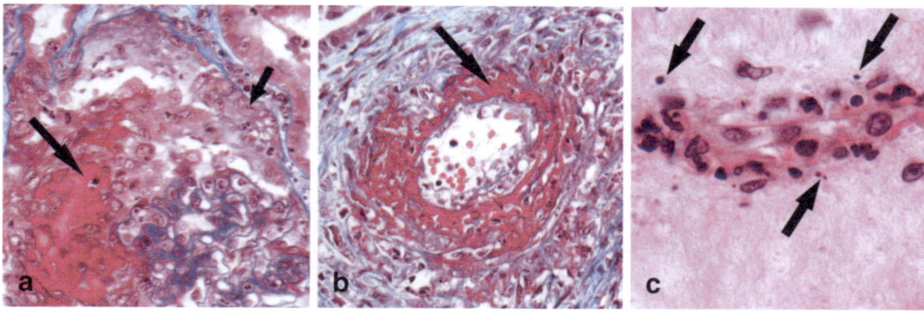

Fig. 1.1 Necrotizing small-vessel vasculitis in patients with AAV. (**a**) Glomerulus with necrotizing and crescentic glomerulonephritis with segmental fibrinoid necrosis (long arrow) and cellular crescent formation (short arrow) (Masson trichrome stain). (**b**) Necrotizing arteritis with circumferential fibrinoid necrosis (arrow) and associated infiltration by leukocytes (Masson trichrome stain). (**c**) Leukocytoclastic angiitis in the renal medulla with transmural accumulation of leukocytes, including neutrophils, and multiple nuclear fragments (arrows) indicative of leukocytoclasia (hematoxylin and eosin stain)

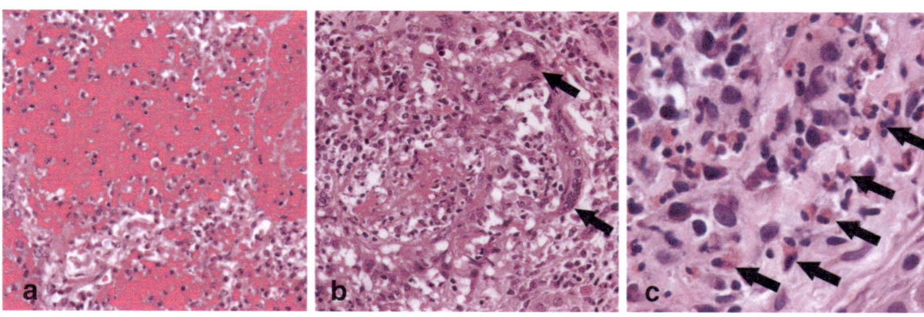

Fig. 1.2 Pulmonary inflammation in patients with AAV. (**a**) Hemorrhagic capillaritis with alveolar air spaces filled with blood (hematoxylin and eosin stain). (**b**) Necrotizing granulomatous inflammation in a GPA patient with infiltrating neutrophils, lymphocytes, monocytes, and macrophages, including multinucleated giant cells (arrows) (hematoxylin and eosin stain). (**c**) Inflammatory infiltrate in an EGPA patient showing conspicuous eosinophils (arrows) (hematoxylin and eosin stain)

observed in renal biopsy specimens that have different glomeruli with necrotizing, mixed necrotizing and sclerotic, or purely sclerotic lesions.

Because AAV can affect vessels in every organ and tissue of the body, the clinical manifestations of disease are extremely variable. These are classified into one of several clinicopathologic categories, including microscopic polyangiitis (MPA), granulomatosis with polyangiitis (GPA) (formerly Wegener's granulomatosis), eosinophilic granulomatosis with polyangiitis (EGPA) (formerly Churg-Strauss syndrome), and organ limited AAV (e.g., renal limited vasculitis, RLV) [1].

MPA has AAV with no granulomatous inflammation, whereas GPA and EGPA have necrotizing granulomatous inflammation, which is most frequent in the respiratory tract (Table 1.1) [1]. Only EGPA is associated with asthma and blood eosinophilia [1]. Pathologically indistinguishable vasculitis and glomerulonephritis occurs in MPA, GPA, and EGPA (Fig. 1.1).

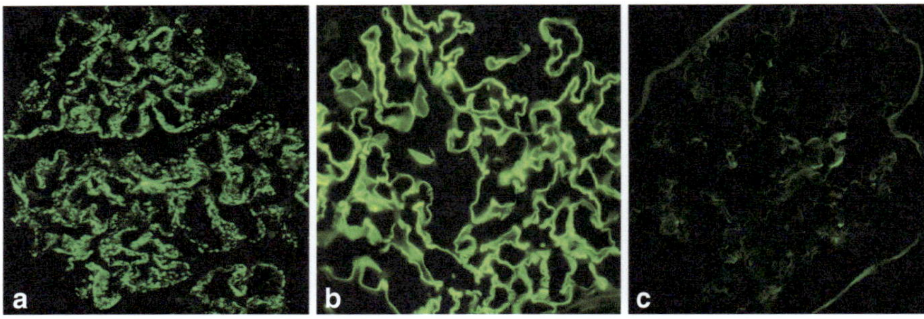

Fig. 1.3 Patterns of glomerular staining for IgG indicative of immune complex glomerulonephritis (**a**), anti-GBM glomerulonephritis (**b**), and pauci-immune ANCA glomerulonephritis (**c**) (FITC anti-IgG stain)

Lung lesions exemplify the diversity of AAV inflammatory lesions. MPA, GPA, and EGPA all can have hemorrhagic capillaritis (Fig. 1.2a), which evolves to interstitial fibrosis. GPA and EGPA can have pulmonary granulomatous inflammation (Fig. 1.2b) that begins as neutrophil-rich necrotizing lesions. These lesions have progressive replacement of neutrophils by lymphocytes, monocytes, and macrophages (including multinucleated giant cells), often surrounding a central zone of necrosis. These lesions may form cavities and may become fibrotic with minimal or no residual inflammation. Vasculitis and granulomatosis in EGPA typically have numerous eosinophils and neutrophils in active inflammatory lesions (Fig. 1.2c).

AAV is characterized immunopathologically by few or no immune deposits of immunoglobulin and complement in vessel walls, which distinguishes AAV from immune complex-mediated vasculitis and anti-glomerular basement membrane antibody (anti-GBM)-mediated vasculitis (Fig. 1.3) [1].

AAV also can be classified based on ANCA antigen specificity, for example, ANCA specific for proteinase 3 (PR3-ANCA AAV) or myeloperoxidase (MPO-ANCA AAV) or with negative serology for ANCA (ANCA-negative AAV) [1, 4, 5]. ANCA-negative AAV has clinical and pathologic features identical to those in ANCA-positive AAV. The most informative classification and diagnosis of AAV include both the clinicopathologic phenotype and the serotype [1]. The correlation of ANCA serotypes with clinicopathologic variants and clinical outcomes is reviewed later in this chapter.

1.2 Historical Background

The investigation of two different manifestations of vasculitis, which eventually intersected, led to the discovery of AAV (Fig. 1.4). These two manifestations are skin purpura caused by inflammation in small vessel in the dermis and segmental inflammation of arteries (arteritis).

Purpura (purple spots on the skin) is caused by segmental inflammation of small vessels in the skin resulting in localized hemorrhage. Robert Willian, a

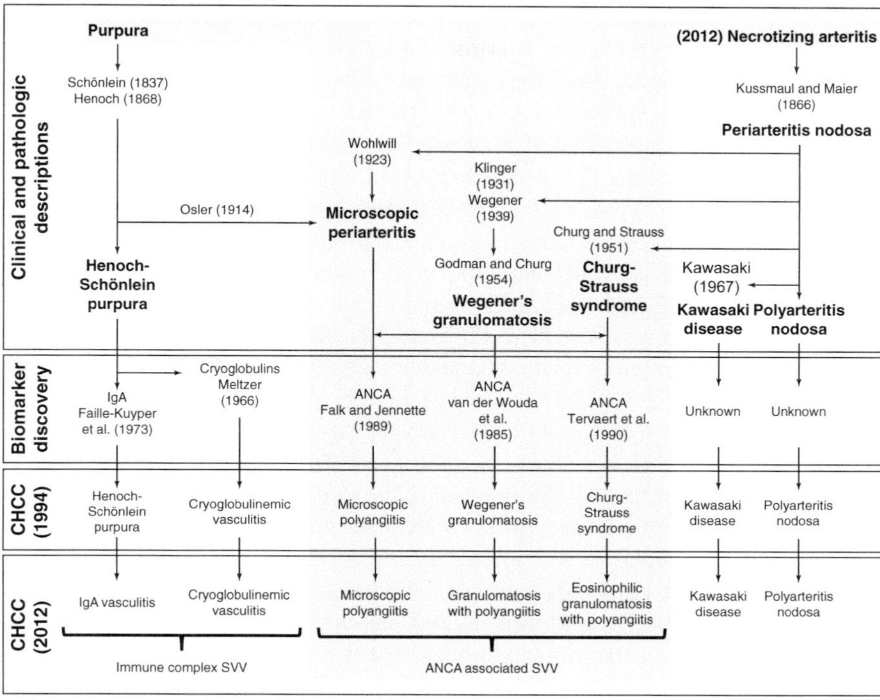

Fig. 1.4 Historical sequence of advances in the recognition and classification of vasculitides that cause purpura and/or necrotizing arteritis. These two pathways of discovery intersect and overlap with AAV (shaded area) because AAV causes both purpura and necrotizing arteritis

dermatologist, reported in 1808 that purpura could be associated with systemic manifestation, such as pain in the extremities and in the abdomen, suggesting that the pathologic process causing purpura in the skin was also causing injury in other organs [6]. The pediatricians, Johann Schönlein and Eduard Henoch, collectively reported the association of purpura with arthralgias, abdominal pain and bleeding, and nephritis [7–9]. The children seen by Schönlein and Henoch most likely had IgA vasculitis (Henoch-Schönlein purpura) rather than AAV, because IgA vasculitis occurs most often in children and AAV occurs most often in adults. On the other hand, the internist William Osler described adults with purpura that was associated with arthritis, peripheral neuropathy, abdominal pain, pulmonary hemorrhage, epistaxis, iritis, and nephritis [10, 11]. Many of his patients had nephritis and some had rapid progression of uremia, and at autopsy had glomeruli "compressed" by "crescentic" masses of cells in Bowman's space [11]. Undoubtedly, some of Osler's patients had AAV.

In 1919, the pathologist Ernest Goodpasture reported the results of an autopsy on a patient who died of pulmonary hemorrhage and rapidly progressive glomerulonephritis [11]. He observed vasculitis affecting small arteries in the spleen, arterioles in the gut, and capillaries in the pulmonary alveoli and glomeruli. Because of this report, his name became associated with pulmonary–renal syndrome caused by anti-GBM, although the presence of arteritis in his patient is not consistent with anti-GBM disease and indicates that the patient probably had AAV, most likely MPA.

At the same time, Schönlein and Henoch were investigating purpura caused by small-vessel vasculitis, Adolf Kussmaul (an internist) and Rudolf Maier (a pathologist) published the first detailed report of a patient with systemic necrotizing arteritis [12]. They coined the name periarteritis nodosa because of the grossly visible focal nodular lesions along medium-sized arteries caused by inflammation extending through vessel walls and into the perivascular tissue [12]. The preferred diagnostic term later became polyarteritis nodosa because the inflammation is transmural rather than perivascular [13]. For over 50 years, virtually any patient who was found to have arteritis was lumped under a diagnosis of periarteritis nodosa or polyarteritis nodosa.

In 1923, Friedrich Wohlwill described two patients with a "microscopic form" of periarteritis nodosa [14]. His observations were confirmed and extended by Davson [15, 16]. This recognition that arteritis can occur along with small-vessel vasculitis began to link studies of arteritis [14–19] with studies of small-vessel vasculitis with purpura, glomerulonephritis, and pulmonary capillaritis [6–11] (Fig. 1.4).

From the 1920s to the 1960s, multiple variants of vasculitis were identified that had arteritis resembling polyarteritis nodosa, but also had distinctive features that warranted specific diagnoses, including microscopic polyarteritis [14], Wegener's granulomatosis [17, 18], Churg-Strauss syndrome [19], and Kawasaki disease [20, 21]. The recognition of specific variants of arteritis resembling polyarteritis nodosa is ongoing (e.g., the discovery of adenosine deaminase-2 deficiency vasculitis) [22].

In 1954, Gabriel Godman and Jacob Churg published a breakthrough article that astutely concluded that "microscopic periarteritis," Wegener's granulomatosis, and Churg-Strauss syndrome were related and were distinct from polyarteritis nodosa [23]. They also suggested that these three variants are probably related pathogenetically. This was a harbinger of the discovery of ANCA, which confirmed the relatedness of ANCA-positive MPA, GPA, and EGPA, and their distinctiveness from ANCA-negative polyarteritis nodosa [24].

Multiple biomarkers related to specific pathogenic mechanisms that cause vasculitis facilitated the classification and diagnosis of vasculitis based on laboratory results, such as vessel wall IgA-dominant immune deposits in Henoch-Schönlein purpura (IgA vasculitis) [25], cryoglobulins in the circulation in cryoglobulinemic vasculitis [26], and circulating ANCA in what is now called MPA, GPA, and EGPA (Fig. 1.4) [27–29] (Fig. 1.4). This set the stage for establishing consensus names and definitions for systemic vasculitides, including AAV [1, 30].

1.3 Vasculitis Nomenclature and Classification

Nomenclature, classification, and diagnosis of vasculitis is difficult because of the broad spectrum of types and locations of vessels affected, multiple patterns of injury, diverse known etiologies and pathogenic mechanisms, absence of known etiologies and pathogenic mechanisms in some forms of vasculitis, and the myriad overlapping and nonspecific signs and symptoms caused by vasculitides.

A nomenclature system provides names and definitions for diseases. A classification system organizes patients into well-defined groups (classes). Classification allows selection of standardized patient groups (classes) to study disease characteristics or perform clinical trials. A diagnostic system uses validated criteria to make a clinically actionable diagnosis in an individual patient. As stated by Hasan Yazici, "diagnosis is nothing different than classification in the individual patient" [31].

Classification criteria are observations or data used to place groups of patients into standardized classes. Diagnostic criteria are observations or data used to confidently predict the presence of the defining features of a disease in a specific patient. Diagnostic criteria allow diagnosing (classifying) a single patient in a specific class.

If useful, names and definitions can remain the same indefinitely. Classification criteria and diagnostic criteria evolve more quickly, driven in part by advances in diagnostic technologies and development of new clinical laboratory tests that were not available when earlier criteria were established.

The goals of nomenclature, classification, and diagnostic systems are to enable effective communication among biomedical investigators and healthcare providers, guide clinical and basic research on well-defined cohorts (classes) of patients, and, most importantly, facilitate diagnosis and effective treatment of individual patients. Nomenclature, classification, and diagnostic systems should be under constant scrutiny and adjusted as new knowledge emerges. Homer Smith, a nephrologist, warns us that "Though we name the things we know, we do not necessarily know them because we name them" [32].

Two overarching etiologic categories of vasculitis are infectious vasculitis caused by proliferation of microorganisms in vessel walls and noninfectious vasculitis not caused by proliferation of microorganisms in vessel walls. The latter nevertheless may be caused indirectly by an infection that initiates a sequence of event that results in vascular inflammation, for example, hepatitis C virus infection secondarily causing cryoglobulinemic vasculitis.

A widely used approach to classifying vasculitis uses three categories based on the types of vessel that are involved, that is, large-vessel vasculitis, medium-vessel vasculitis, and small-vessel vasculitis. This approach was adopted in 1994 at an international consensus conference on the nomenclature of systemic vasculitides [30] and revised in 2012 by at a second consensus conference [1]. These Chapel Hill Consensus Conferences (1994 CHCC and 2012 CHCC) provide standardized names and definitions for different classes of vasculitis (Tables 1.1 and 1.2) (Fig. 1.5), but do not provide validated criteria for classifying cohorts of patients into these classes, or for diagnosing (classifying) individual patients.

According to 2012 CHCC, large-vessel vasculitis (LVV) is vasculitis affecting large arteries more often than other vasculitides [1]. Large arteries are the aorta and its major branches. Any size artery may be affected. Medium-vessel vasculitis (MVV) is vasculitis predominantly affecting medium arteries defined as the main visceral arteries and their branches [1]. Any size artery may be affected. Inflammatory aneurysms and stenoses are common. Small-vessel vasculitis (SVV)

Table 1.2 AAV and AAV variant definitions from the 2012 International Chapel Hill Consensus Conference on the Nomenclature of Vasculitides (2012 CHCC) [1]

2012 CHCC name	2012 CHCC definition
ANCA-associated vasculitis (AAV)	Necrotizing vasculitis, with few or no immune deposits, predominantly affecting small vessels (i.e., capillaries, venules, arterioles, and small arteries), associated with myeloperoxidase (MPO) ANCA or proteinase 3 (PR3) ANCA. Not all patients have ANCA. Add a prefix indicating ANCA reactivity, e.g., MPO-ANCA, PR3-ANCA, ANCA-negative
Microscopic polyangiitis (MPA)	Necrotizing vasculitis, with few or no immune deposits, predominantly affecting small vessels (i.e., capillaries, venules, or arterioles). Necrotizing arteritis involving small and medium arteries may be present. Necrotizing glomerulonephritis is very common. Pulmonary capillaritis often occurs. Granulomatous inflammation is absent
Granulomatosis with polyangiitis (GPA)	Necrotizing granulomatous inflammation usually involving the upper and lower respiratory tract, and necrotizing vasculitis affecting predominantly small to medium vessels (e.g., capillaries, venules, arterioles, arteries, and veins). Necrotizing glomerulonephritis is common
Eosinophilic granulomatosis with polyangiitis (EGPA)	Eosinophil-rich and necrotizing granulomatous inflammation often involving the respiratory tract, and necrotizing vasculitis predominantly affecting small to medium vessels, and associated with asthma and eosinophilia. ANCA is more frequent when glomerulonephritis is present

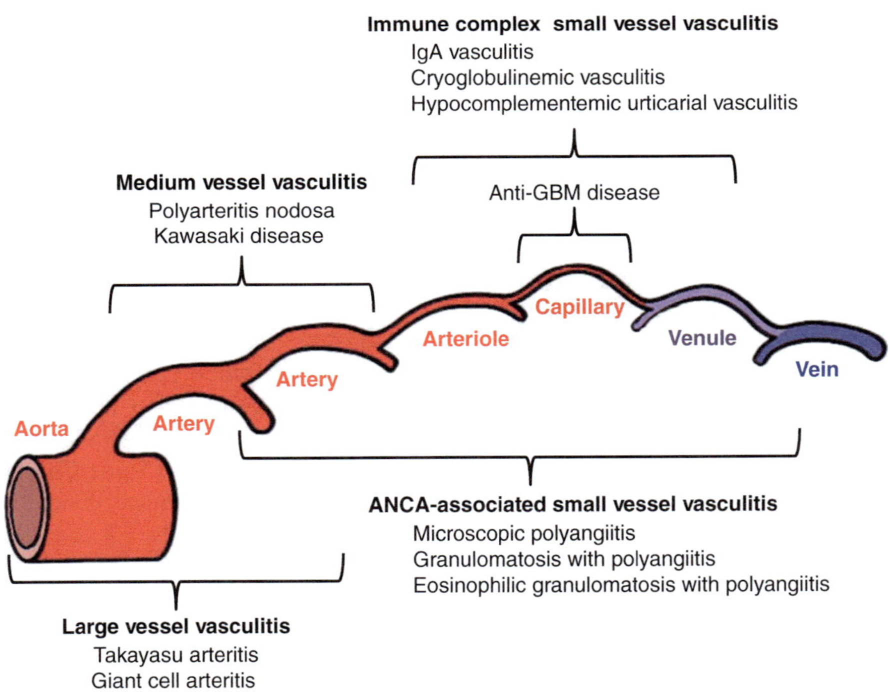

Fig. 1.5 Diagram depicting the predominant vessel involvement by large-vessel vasculitis, medium-vessel vasculitis, and small-vessel vasculitis. Note that AAV is a form of SVV that has a greater diversity of vessel involvement than SVV caused by immune complex disease or anti-GBM disease. Also note that arteritis caused by AAV overlaps with arteritis caused by medium-vessel vasculitis. Reproduced with permission from [1]

is vasculitis predominantly affecting small vessels, defined as small intraparenchymal arteries, arterioles, capillaries, and venules [1]. Medium arteries and veins may be affected. The two pathogenic categories of SVV are immune complex SVV and ANCA-associated SVV (AAV).

1.4 Classification and Diagnosis of AAV

The current names for the three major categories of AAV are microscopic polyangiitis (MPA), granulomatosis with polyangiitis (GPA), and eosinophilic granulomatosis with polyangiitis (EGPA) (Table 1.2) [1]. The descriptive names GPA and EGPA were adopted by 2012 CHCC and replaced the names Wegener's granulomatosis and eosinophilic granulomatosis that were used in 1994 CHCC.

Except for the preposition (i.e., with), all of the words in the names for MPA, GPA, and EGPA refer to pathologic features. However, importantly, this does not mean that direct histopathologic observation of pathologic features is required for diagnosis or classification. Histopathologic observations may not be practicable or necessary if validated noninvasive surrogate criteria are available. For example, in an appropriate clinical context, destructive nodular or cavitary pulmonary lesions, or destructive lesions in nasal cartilage or bone, can suffice to reasonably conclude that an ANCA-positive patient with pauci-immune necrotizing and crescentic glomerulonephritis should be classified or diagnosed as GPA rather than MPA.

Clinical evidence for SVV that raises the possibility of AAV includes skin purpura, petechiae, or small ulcers; glomerulonephritis with dysmorphic erythrocyturia, erythrocyte cylindruria, or proteinuria >1 g/day; pulmonary hemorrhage, radiographic consolidation, or hemoptysis; or ocular scleritis, uveitis, or ulcerative keratitis. Pathologic findings that confirm SVV include dermal venulitis, necrotizing glomerulonephritis (Fig. 1.1a), renal medullary angiitis (Fig. 1.1c), and pulmonary capillaritis (Fig. 1.2a). Immunohistologic identification of few or no immune deposits in vessel walls supports a diagnosis of AAV (Fig. 1.3c). However, immunohistologic identification of moderate to marked vessel wall deposits of immunoglobulin and/or complement does not rule out AAV, because AAV can be concurrent with anti-GBM disease or immune complex disease [33]. Positive serology for ANCA has strong positive predictive value for AAV, but a negative result does not rule out AAV because a minority of patients with a clinical and pathologic phenotype that is identical to ANCA-positive AAV are ANCA-negative (i.e., ANCA-negative AAV). For example, at least 10% of patients with pauci-immune crescentic glomerulonephritis are ANCA-negative [34].

AAV patients may have arteritis (Fig. 1.1b), but this alone does not distinguish between medium-vessel vasculitis (e.g., polyarteritis nodosa and Kawasaki disease) and SVV with arterial involvement. Clinical evidence for arteritis includes skin erythematous nodules or ulcers >1 cm; peripheral neuropathy (mononeuritis multiplex or asymmetrical polyneuropathy); or imaging showing arterial aneurysms, visceral infarcts, or gut perforation.

Importantly, classification or diagnosis of AAV clinicopathologic variants requires consideration of both inclusion criteria and exclusion criteria. For example, classification or diagnosis of RLV and MPA requires exclusion of evidence for GPA and EGPA (i.e., no evidence of granulomatous inflammation, blood eosinophilia, or asthma). A patient can have every possible positive (inclusion) classification or diagnostic criterion for MPA, but these criteria alone will not be sufficient for classification or diagnosis unless they are paired with negative (exclusion) criteria to rule out other diseases that share the positive criteria, for example, absence of evidence for granulomatous inflammation to rule out GPA.

Classification or diagnosis of GPA and EGPA requires clinical or pathologic evidence for granulomatous inflammation (Fig. 1.2b). Clinical evidence for granulomatous inflammation includes pulmonary nodules or cavities, or destructive bone or cartilage lesions in the upper respiratory tract. Pathologic confirmation of granulomatous inflammation includes identification of either active necrotizing granulomatous inflammation (especially in the respiratory tract) or chronic changes consistent with earlier necrotizing granulomatous inflammation. EGPA is distinguished from GPA by the presence of asthma and blood eosinophilia. The vasculitic and granulomatous lesions of EGPA typically contain conspicuous eosinophils (Fig. 1.2c); however, this is not specific for EGPA because MPA and GPA, as well as polyarteritis nodosa, may have numerous eosinophils in inflammatory lesions.

To our knowledge, there are no widely accepted, well validated, classification or diagnostic criteria for AAV and its variants. However, a major effort is underway to remedy this deficiency. The Diagnostic and Classification Criteria in Vasculitis Study (DCVAS) is an international, multicenter, observational study that has collected data on over 1000 AAV patients from more than 100 sites, as well as data from patients with other forms of vasculitis and patients with diseases that mimic vasculitis [35, 36]. The DCVS goal is to develop and validate diagnostic and classification criteria for systemic vasculitides, including AAV [35].

1.5 Both Serotype and Phenotype Are Useful for Classification and Diagnosis

2012 CHCC requires that the name (diagnosis) of AAV should include a prefix indicating ANCA serotype, for example, MPO-ANCA, PR3-ANCA, and ANCA-negative [1]. This is because both the clinicopathologic phenotype and the serotype are useful for classification, diagnosis, and patient management. Classifying or diagnosing a patient as only MPO-ANCA AAV or only GPA is less informative and less valuable than classifying or diagnosing a patient as MPO-ANCA GPA. Undoubtedly, identifying the serotype is much easier than confidently identifying the clinicopathologic phenotype; and the phenotype may change over time as more data are available or as the disease process evolves in a given patient.

Classifying patients based on PR3-ANCA versus MPO-ANCA serotype correlates with clinical and pathologic features, and with clinical course and outcome [4, 5, 37, 38], thus ANCA serotype is important component of an AAV diagnosis. Figure 1.6 shows data from an inception cohort of ANCA-positive AAV patients from the Southeastern USA (excluding EGPA patients) patients [37]. The relative frequency of MPO-ANCA and PR3-ANCA varies based on the clinicopathologic phenotype (Fig. 1.6). For example, renal-limited vasculitis (RLV) patients have the highest frequency of MPO-ANCA, whereas patients with pulmonary nodules, nasal mucosal ulcers, and inflammatory destruction of nasal cartilage causing saddle nose deformity have a predominance of PR3-ANCA. This relationship indicates that ANCA antigen specificity modulates the targets and nature of pathogenic events. However, the serotype is not specific for a given clinicopathologic phenotype.

Table 1.3 shows data from the same patient cohort used in Fig. 1.6 [4, 37]. In the Southeastern USA, 81% of ANCA-positive RLV patients have MPO-ANCA, whereas 74% of GPA patients have PR3-ANCA. MPA patients have a more equal distribution of serotypes. However, even though PR3-ANCA is more frequent in GPA patients, because of the higher frequency of MPO-ANCA in this region, PR3-ANCA patients more often have MPA (50%) than GPA (40%) (Table 1.3) [4].

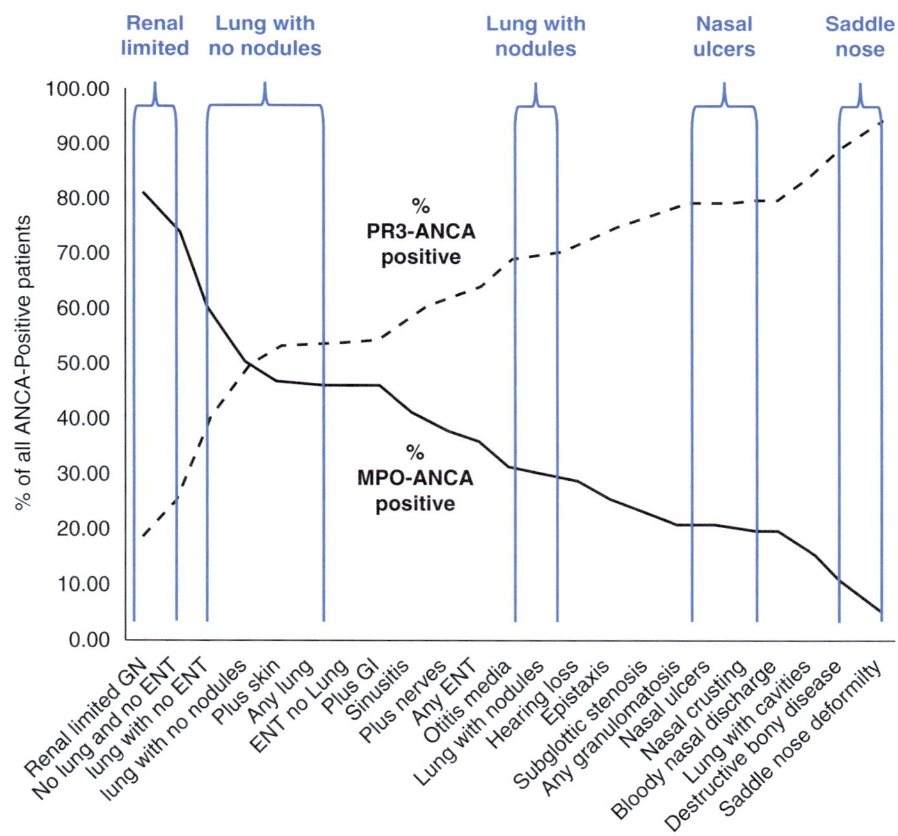

Fig. 1.6 Correlation between serotype and clinical phenotype in an inception cohort of ANCA-positive AAV patients from the Southeastern USA evaluated at the UNC Kidney Center (excluding EGPA patients). Reproduced with permission from [4, 38]

Table 1.3 ANCA serotype (MPO-ANCA+ versus PR3-ANCA+) and clinicopathologic phenotype (RLV, MPA, GPA) of an inception cohort of ANCA-positive vasculitis patients with high-frequency renal disease evaluated at the UNC Kidney Center (excluding EGPA patients)

Phenotype	MPO-ANCA+ (%)	PR3-ANCA+ (%)
RLV (*n* = 121)	81	19
MPA (*n* = 264)	59	41
GPA (*n* = 117)	26	74

Serotype	RLV (%)	MPA (%)	GPA (%)
All ANCA+ (*n* = 502)	24	53	23
MPO-ANCA+ (*n* = 283)	35	55	11
PR3-ANCA+ (*n* = 219)	10	50	40

Additional features of this cohort were published in refs. [4, 38]

The relative association of serotype with phenotype in a classification or diagnostic system for AAV varies based on geography and ethnicity. This will impact the positive and negative predictive value of a serotype for a given phenotype in a given location or ethnic group. An interim analysis of DCVAS AAV patient data indicates that PR3-ANCA AAV is the predominant type of vasculitis in patients with Northern Europeans, Middle Eastern/Turkish and Indian subcontinent ethnicity, whereas MPO-ANCA AAV is the predominant serotype of vasculitis in Japanese and Chinese populations [36]. MPO-AAV is more common in Caucasian Americans and Southern Europeans than in Northern Europeans.

ANCA-positive patients with EGPA usually have MPO-ANCA; however, less than 50% of patients with EGPA have ANCA [39–42]. Patients with clinical features of EGPA, such as asthma and blood eosinophilia, who are ANCA-positive, are more likely to have phenotypic features of vasculitis including glomerulonephritis, skin lesions, alveolar capillaritis, and peripheral neuropathy [42]. ANCA-positive EGPA appears to be a subset of patients with asthma and eosinophilia, which may be a separate disease process, or a distinct variant that develops over time in some but not all patients.

Table 1.4 uses the same 502 AAV patient cohort shown in Table 1.3 and Fig. 1.6 to compare the correlation of three different classification systems for AAV with clinical outcomes [4, 37]. The three classification approaches are as follows: (1) classification based on the 2012 CHCC names and definitions [1]; (2) the 2007 European Medicines Agency (EMA) classification system [43], which blends elements of the 1990 American College of Rheumatology classification system [44], 1994 CHCC definitions [30], and ANCA serotypes; and (3) classification based on serotype alone. The clinical outcomes are the result of different treatment regimens from 1985 to 2007, and thus, the responses are not in line with current optimum therapy; however, all classes of patients were treated similarly. Additional outcome correlations are in the publication by Lionaki et al. [37]. Table 1.4 indicates that

Table 1.4 ANCA vasculitis outcomes based on different classification systems evaluated in the same cohort by Lionaki et al. [37] shown in Table 1.3 and Fig. 1.6

	Treatment resistance (*N* = 109/483)	Relapse (*N* = 147/374)	ESKD (*N* = 161/502)	Death (*N* = 139/502)
Classification based on CHCC 2012 definitions				
GPA	20/117 (17%)	58/97 (60%)	24/117 (21%)	20/117 (17%)
MPA	56/255 (22%)	74/199 (37%)	80/264 (30%)	79/264 (30%)
RLV	33/111 (30%)	15/78 (19%)	57/121 (47%)	40/121 (33%)
P value	0.0711	<0.0001	<0.0001	0.0091
Classification based on the European medicines agency system				
GPA	68/317 (22%)	110/249 (44%)	92/324 (28%)	84/324 (26%)
MPA	41/166 (25%)	37/125 (30%)	69/178 (39%)	55/178 (31%)
P value	0.4244	0.0071	0.0214	0.2520
Classification based on ANCA specificity in ANCA-positive patients				
PR3 ANCA	37/213 (17%)	90/176 (51%)	56/219 (26%)	50/219 (23%)
MPO ANCA	72/270 (27%)	57/198 (29%)	105/283 (37%)	89/283 (31%)
P value	0.0160	<0.0001	0.0069	0.034

Treatment Resistance = persistence or new appearance of extrarenal manifestations and/or progressive decline in renal function with active urine sediment in spite of immunosuppressive therapy. Relapse = reactivation of vasculitis in any organ after initial response to treatment. ESKD = chronic need for dialysis or transplantation. Death = death from any cause

classification based on phenotype as well as classification based on serotype correlate with disease outcomes.

1.6 Concluding Remarks

As noted earlier in this chapter, the goals of classification and diagnostic systems are to enable effective communication among biomedical investigators and healthcare providers, guide clinical and basic research on well-defined cohorts (classes) of patients, and, most importantly, facilitate diagnosis and effective treatment of individual patients. Physicians and scientists have made many advances in the classification and diagnosis of vasculitides since the early seminal observational studies of Schönlein and Henoch [7, 8], Kusmal and Maier [12], and Godman and Churg [23], but validated and widely applied classification criteria and diagnostic criteria that are sufficiently accurate and precise for clinical research and patient care, respectively, remain elusive.

We agree with Homer Smith that "Though we name the things we know, we do not necessarily know them because we name them" [32]. But we also believe that being able to accurately name (i.e., diagnose) the disease in a patient will help us know the disease better and provide better care to the patient.

References

1. Jennette JC, Falk RJ, Bacon PA, et al. 2012 revised international Chapel Hill consensus conference nomenclature of vasculitides. Arthritis Rheum. 2013;65:1–11.
2. Jennette JC, Falk RJ. Pathologic classification of vasculitis. Pathol Case Rev. 2007;12:179–85.
3. Jennette JC, Thomas DB. Pauci-immune and antineutrophil cytoplasmic autoantibody glomerulonephritis and vasculitis. In: Jennette JC, Olson JL, Silva FG, D'Agati V, editors. Heptinstall's pathology of the kidney. 7th ed. Philadelphia: Wolters Kluwer; 2015, Chapter 16. p. 685–714.
4. Jennette JC, Nachman PH. ANCA glomerulonephritis and vasculitis. Clin J Am Soc Nephrol. 2017;12:1680–91.
5. Cornec D, Cornec-Le Gall E, Fervenza FC, Specks U. ANCA-associated vasculitis - clinical utility of using ANCA specificity to classify patients. Nat Rev Rheumatol. 2016;12:570–9.
6. Willan R. On cutaneous diseases, vol. I. London: J. Johnson; 1808.
7. Schönlein JL. Allegemeine und specielle Pathologie und Therapie, vol. 2. 3rd ed. Herisau: Literatur-Comptoir; 1837. p. 48.
8. Henoch E. Uber den zusammenhang von purpura und intestinal-stoerungen. Berl Klin Wochenschur. 1868;5:517–9.
9. Henoch E. Lectures on diseases of children: a handbook for physicians and students. New York: W. Wood and Co; 1882.
10. Osler W. The visceral lesions of purpura and allied conditions. Br Med J. 1914;1:517–25.
11. Goodpasture WE. The significance of certain pulmonary lesions in relation to the etiology of influenza. Am J Med Sci. 1919;158:863–70.
12. Kussmaul A, Maier R. Über eine bisher nicht beschreibene eigenthümliche Arterienerkrankung (Periarteriitis nodosa), die mit Morbus Brightii und rapid fortschreitender allgemeiner Muskellähmung einhergeht. Dtsch Arch Klin Med. 1866;1:484–518.
13. Dickson W. Polyarteritis acuta nodosa and periarteritis nodosa. J Pathol Bacteriol. 1908;12:31–57.
14. Wohlwill F. Uber die mur mikroskopisch erkenbarre form der periarteritis nodosa. Arch Pathol Anat. 1923;246:377–411.
15. Davson J, Ball M, Platt R. The kidney in periarteritis nodosa. QJM. 1948;17:175–202.
16. Wainwright J, Davson J. The renal appearance in the microscopic form of periarteritis nodosa. J Pathol Bacteriol. 1950;62:189–96.
17. Klinger H. Grenzformen der Periarteriitis nodosa. Frankf Ztschr Pathol. 1931;42:455–80.
18. Wegener F. Über eine eigenartige rhinogene Granulomatose mit besonderer Beteiligung des Arteriensystems unter den Nieren. Beitr Pathol Anat. 1939;102:36–68.
19. Churg J, Strauss L. Allergic granulomatosis, allergic angiitis, and periarteritis nodosa. Am J Pathol. 1951;27:277–94.
20. Kawasaki T. MLNS showing particular skin desquamation from the finger and toe in infants. Allergy. 1967;16:178–89.
21. Tanaka N, Naoe S, Kawasaki T. Pathological study on autopsy cases of mucocutaneous lymph node syndrome. J Jpn Red Cross Central Hosp. 1971;2:85–94.
22. Karadag O, Jayne DJ. Polyarteritis nodosa revisited: a review of historical approaches, subphenotypes and a research agenda. Clin Exp Rheumatol. 2018;36 Suppl 111(2):135–42.
23. Godman G, Churg J. Wegener's granulomatosis. Pathology and review of the literature. Arch Pathol Lab Med. 1954;58:533–53.
24. Guillevin L1, Lhote F, Amouroux J, Gherardi R, Callard P, Casassus P. Antineutrophil cytoplasmic antibodies, abnormal angiograms and pathological findings in polyarteritis nodosa and Churg-Strauss syndrome: indications for the classification of vasculitides of the polyarteritis Nodosa group. Br J Rheumatol. 1996;35:958–64.
25. Faille-Kuyber EH, Kater L, Kooiker CJ, Dorhout Mees EJ. IgA-deposits in cutaneous bloodvessel walls and mesangium in Henoch-Schönlein syndrome. Lancet. 1973;1:892–3.

26. Meltzer M, Franklin EC, Elias K, McCluskey RT, Cooper N. Cryoglobulinemia-a clinical and laboratory study. II. Cryoglobulins with rheumatoid factor activity. Am J Med. 1966;40:837–56.
27. van der Woude FJ, Rasmussen N, Lobatto S, et al. Autoantibodies against neutrophils and monocytes: tool for diagnosis and marker of disease activity in Wegener's granulomatosis. Lancet. 1985;1:425–9.
28. Falk RJ, Jennette JC. Anti-neutrophil cytoplasmic autoantibodies with specificity for myeloperoxidase in patients with systemic vasculitis and idiopathic necrotizing and crescentic glomerulonephritis. N Engl J Med. 1988;318:1651–7.
29. Tervaert JW, Elema JD, Kallenberg CG. Clinical and histopathological association of 29kD-ANCA and MPO-ANCA. APMIS Suppl. 1990;19:35.
30. Jennette JC, Falk RJ, Andrassy K, et al. Nomenclature of systemic vasculitides: the proposal of an international consensus conference. Arthritis Rheum. 1994;37:187–92.
31. Yazici H. Diagnostic versus classification criteria - a continuum. Bull NYU Hosp Jt Dis. 2009;67:206–8.
32. Smith HW. Renal physiology. In: Fishman AP, Richards DW, editors. Circulation of the blood: men and ideas. New York: Springer; 1982, Chapter 9. p. 581.
33. Jennette JC. Rapidly progressive and crescentic glomerulonephritis. Kidney Int. 2003;63:1164–72.
34. Chen M, Kallenberg CG, Zhao MH. ANCA-negative pauci-immune crescentic glomerulonephritis. Nat Rev Nephrol. 2009;5:313–8.
35. Craven A, Robson J, Ponte C, et al. ACR/EULAR-endorsed study to develop diagnostic and classification criteria for vasculitis (DCVAS). Clin Exp Nephrol. 2013;17:619–21.
36. Pearce FA, Craven A, Merkel PA, et al. Global ethnic and geographic differences in the clinical presentations of anti-neutrophil cytoplasm antibody-associated vasculitis. Rheumatology. 2017;56:1962–9.
37. Lionaki S, Blyth ER, Hogan SL, et al. Classification of antineutrophil cytoplasmic autoantibody vasculitides: the role of antineutrophil cytoplasmic autoantibody specificity for myeloperoxidase or proteinase 3 in disease recognition and prognosis. Arthritis Rheum. 2012;64:3452–62.
38. Yates M, Watts R. ANCA-associated vasculitis. Clin Med (Lond). 2017;17:60–4.
39. Scott DG, Watts RA. Epidemiology and clinical features of systemic vasculitis. Clin Exp Nephrol. 2013;17:607–10.
40. Sinico RA, Di Toma L, Maggiore U, et al. Prevalence and clinical significance of antineutrophil cytoplasmic antibodies in Churg-Strauss syndrome. Arthritis Rheum. 2005;52:2926–35.
41. Sokolowska BM, Szczeklik WK, Wludarczyk AA, et al. ANCA-positive and ANCA-negative phenotypes of eosinophilic granulomatosis with polyangiitis (EGPA): outcome and long-term follow-up of 50 patients from a single Polish center. Clin Exp Rheumatol. 2014;32:S41–7.
42. Cottin V, Bel E, Bottero P, et al. Revisiting the systemic vasculitis in eosinophilic granulomatosis with polyangiitis (Churg-Strauss): a study of 157 patients by the Groupe d'Etudes et de Recherche sur les Maladies Orphelines Pulmonaires and the European Respiratory Society Taskforce on eosinophilic granulomatosis with polyangiitis (Churg-Strauss). Autoimmun Rev. 2017;16:1–9.
43. Watts R, Lane S, Hanslik T, Hauser T, et al. Development and validation of a consensus methodology for the classification of the ANCA-associated vasculitides and polyarteritis nodosa for epidemiological studies. Ann Rheum Dis. 2007;66:222–7.
44. Fries JF, Hunder GG, Bloch DA, et al. The American College of Rheumatology 1990 criteria for the classification of vasculitis. Summary. Arthritis Rheum. 1990;33:1135–6.

Genetics of ANCA-Associated Vasculitis

2

Federico Alberici, Paul Anthony Lyons,
and Davide Martorana

2.1 Introduction

2.1.1 Why Study the Genetics of AAV

Antineutrophil cytoplasmic antibody (ANCA)-associated vasculitis (AAV) is a multisystem inflammatory-autoimmune disease including granulomatosis with polyangiitis (GPA) (formerly Wegener's granulomatosis), microscopic polyangiitis (MPA), and eosinophilic granulomatosis with polyangiitis (EGPA, formerly Churg-Strauss syndrome) [1].

AAV pathogenesis is complex with a proposed role for environmental and infectious factors as well as dysregulation of the immune system; rare familial cases also suggested a potential role for genetic predisposition supporting further the theory of a multifactorial nature for the disease [2]. Such diseases are usually defined as "complex" meaning that both genetic and environmental factors contribute to the risk of their development.

Several families with GPA have been described although the increased risk for the development of disease in relatives of patients with GPA has been shown to be low compared to other autoimmune disorders [3], such as systemic lupus

F. Alberici
Nephrology and Immunology Unit, ASST Santi Paolo e Carlo, San Carlo Borromeo Hospital, Milan, Italy

P. A. Lyons
Department of Medicine, University of Cambridge School of Clinical Medicine, Cambridge, UK
e-mail: pal34@cam.ac.uk

D. Martorana (✉)
Unit of Medical Genetics, University Hospital of Parma, Parma, Italy
e-mail: dmartorana@ao.pr.it

R. A. Sinico, L. Guillevin (eds.), *Anti-Neutrophil Cytoplasmic Antibody (ANCA) Associated Vasculitis*, Rare Diseases of the Immune System,
https://doi.org/10.1007/978-3-030-02239-6_2

erythematosus (SLE), inflammatory bowel disease (IBD), and multiple sclerosis (MS). Of interest, in a family containing a father with EGPA and a son with GPA, a shared HLA haplotype known to be a marker of autoimmunity was detected in the two affected [4]; other studies have explored the role of genetic predisposition in familial cases of AAV although results have been mainly negative probably due to the genotyping approaches employed.

While these studies were not conclusive, and in some cases contradictory, they provided a rational for exploring further the possible role of genetic factors in the development of AAV.

2.2 Molecular Genetic Approaches

Genetic studies in complex diseases require large numbers of subjects from which to estimate the prevalence of a disease in the population. However, many complex diseases are rare; thus, scientists must rely on case-controlled studies comparing a group of patients who harbor the disease in question with a nonaffected patient group to identify factors that may contribute to the disease. In complex diseases, the most commonly investigated genetic markers are single-nucleotide polymorphisms (SNPs). SNPs are variants in the genome that if located in the coding space may impact directly on gene function or if located in the noncoding space gene expression may be involved in gene expression; despite their causal role differences in allele or genotype, frequencies between patients with a given disease and controls may suggest that they may be associated with the disease itself.

Despite SNPs being the most widely tested markers in case–control association studies, they are not the only ones used. In recent years, copy-number variants (CNVs) have also been investigated, with a number of studies demonstrating their potential to underlie susceptibility to complex diseases [5]. CNVs are areas of the human genome that may be repeated a variable number of times potentially impacting on gene expression and on the amount of protein produced.

Irrespective of the genetic marker studied, what is usually investigated is the relative frequency of a genetic variant in cases and controls or its association with disease. It should be noted that the concept of association does not necessarily mean "causality" with the latter requiring more complex follow-up studies in order to be assumed as true. As discussed previously, we should keep in mind that these are "complex" diseases, and therefore, several genetic variants are expected to contribute to the disease itself with each variant only playing a small effect on the final phenotype.

Several genotyping techniques may be employed; noninclusive approaches are ones testing a specific hypothesis; in other words, they explore the association between a gene thought to play a role in the pathogenesis of a disease and the disease itself. Inclusive approaches are techniques that enable the exploration of common variation across the whole genome or at least a very big proportion of it. These are hypothesis free studies and are, therefore, able to identify novel, unexpected associations. The downside of the latter approach is the easy identification of spurious associations and hence the requirement for a strict p-value threshold to control for this.

The candidate gene approach is the hallmark of noninclusive approaches, usually it investigates genetic variants belonging to a specific biological pathway; in this case, the threshold of significance from the statistical point of view is usually represented by the p value of 0.05 (the one usually employed in any statistical analysis). In order to reduce the risk of associations identified by chance, a correction is strongly suggested with the Bonferroni one being the most commonly used.

Genome-wide association studies (GWASs) are the most used and the hallmark nowadays of possible inclusive approaches; these use a simple case–control design but rely on genotyping techniques able to investigate millions of SNPs usually tagging 90% of the human genome. In order to avoid spurious associations, a very high level of statistical significance ($p < 5 \times 10^{-8}$) is required for an association to be considered true. Although very robust, such studies have limitations as well, for example, large sample sizes are generally required; the number of identified associations is in fact proportional to the cohort dimension, and therefore, the bigger the study, the higher the probability of obtaining useful information, and this may be problematic in the field of rare diseases.

In both candidate gene and GWAS studies, replication in independent cohorts plays a central role to ensure the finding is robust; this is a key step to avoid findings that, for some reason, may be restricted only to the population initially explored. Irrespective of the genetic approach employed, the study design stage is of great importance in order to maximize the probability for a successful study; in particular, the cases should represent a well-defined phenotype of disease and controls should be matched for age, gender, and geographical area.

Other examples of inclusive genetics approaches are whole-exome/genome sequencing; these are approaches not yet routinely employed in the field of genetics of AAV but may have a big potential especially in the investigation of familial cases or clusters of extreme phenotypes; the employment of such approaches to large cohorts is still not clear, but the potential is significant allowing the exploration of the whole genome.

A genetic design halfway between inclusive and noninclusive approaches may relay on the use of chips exploring a big set of SNPs identified a priori as of potential interest. The main example in the field of rare immunological diseases is the Immunochip that investigates SNPs and CNVs previously found as associated with inflammatory and autoimmune diseases [6] including a dense coverage of the HLA area. Due to relatively lower costs compared to conventional GWAS chips, this is a feasible and economically sustainable approach able to provide useful information probably more meaningful than candidate gene approach studies but yet lacking the wide exploratory nature of the ones provided by GWASs.

Genetic studies in the field of AAV have so far mainly been restricted to candidate gene approaches, with only a few GWAS carried out; we will critically discuss the results of such studies performed so far.

2.3 Genetics of GPA and MPA

Rare diseases genetics is always a balance between the reliability of the information obtained and the challenges in performing the studies themselves. The size of the cohorts analyzed impacts significantly on the findings and on the analytical methods that may be employed. Only large cohorts of patients may be studied with inclusive genetic methods to obtain solid results with the bigger the population studied, the higher the probability of finding associations with small effect sizes. On the other hand, due to the rarity of some diseases, the cohorts available may not always allow identification of associations employing inclusive genetic methods of analysis, and in these cases, a candidate gene approach may be required. In the field of AAV, three GWAS studies [7–9] have provided four strong biologically plausible associations; in addition, some focused candidate gene studies have also identified other associations of potential interest but, with the exception of one, the level of evidence underpinning the result is lower and this should be taken into account when these studies are considered.

The first piece of information that genetics has provided to the field of AAV confirms the autoimmune nature of the disease. Several genetic studies have described an association with the HLA Class II region even in relatively small cohorts [7]. Of interest, the HLA association with GPA and MPA is different being respectively *HLA-DP* and the *HLA-DQ*. The association is stronger when the population is stratified according to ANCA specificity rather than clinical syndrome with *HLA-DP* being restricted to patients with PR3-ANCA and *HLA-DQ* restricted to patients with MPO-ANCA [7]. The mechanisms by which a predisposing HLA may facilitate the development of autoimmunity are several and may include abnormal antigen presentation, positive selection of autoreactive T cells, or prevention of their negative selection [10]. A further mechanism recently described in Japanese MPA patients carrying the HLA–DRB1∗09:01, which is in strong linkage disequilibrium with HLA-DQ, is the ability to process and present the antigen MPO at the cell surface; this complex appears to be recognized by MPO-ANCA providing an important pathogenetic insight [11].

In the case of MPA, GWASs have not been able to so far identify other genetic associations largely due to the small samples size of the cohorts analyzed; further studies with larger samples will be required to shed further light on the genetic architecture of MPA. On the other hand, in case of GPA, the larger sample sizes have allowed the identification of three further associations at *PRTN3, SERPINA1*, and *PTPN22*.

PRTN3 encodes the serum protease PR3, the fact that patients with GPA are more often PR3-ANCA positive already pointed toward this enzyme playing a central in the pathogenesis. PR3 is expressed on the surface of a proportion of neutrophils, and it has been described that only this membrane bound form is able to interact with ANCA facilitating neutrophil activation. In addition, PR3 may mediate direct tissue damage once it is released by the neutrophils [12]. Of interest, the SNP associated with GPA has been found to be linked to the levels of PR3 expression with the carriers of the susceptibility genotype characterized by higher expression of the protein [9]. This is in keeping with studies that had previously described that neutrophils with high expression of membrane bound PR3 were found more frequently in GPA patients compared to controls [13] and suggest that higher levels of PR3 is an important step in the pathogenesis of the disease.

SERPINA1 encodes alpha-1 antitrypsin which is a protease inhibitor, with PR3 being one of its targets. The SNP associated with the risk of developing GPA has been identified as one encoding a variant of the enzyme with null activity (the so-called Z allele) [9]. The importance of reduced activity of alpha-1 antitrypsin in the pathogenesis of AAV had been already suggested by studies from the pre-GWAS era; in a cohort of 433 GPA cases and 421 controls, the presence of two of the alleles with null or reduced enzymatic activity ("Z" and "S" allele) increased the probability of developing disease with an odds-ratio of 14.58 [14].

PTPN22 is a genetic hallmark of autoimmunity, and it encodes the lymphoid tyrosine phosphatase (Lyp) which may be aberrant in the form encoded by the genetic variant associated with autoimmunity, causing abnormal CD4 T-cell (T_{reg}) activity, increased humoral activity, and enhanced neutrophil functions [15–17]. Interestingly, *Ptpn22* knock-out mice have higher IgG levels, further supporting the significant impact of this gene on the B-cell compartment [18]. The central role of B cells in the pathogenesis of AAV is now well established as confirmed by the therapeutic efficacy of the anti-CD20 monoclonal antibody rituximab [19], providing a further biological rationale for the important role of this gene in AAV. Some candidate gene studies in well-replicated cohorts have suggested a role for the 620W variant in the development of GPA. Importantly, recently this has been further confirmed at the level of GWAS significance. Of interest, this association was observed after combining GPA and MPA cases while, when stratifying the cohort according to the diagnoses, the magnitude of the association was similar in both GPA and MPA, but with lower level of significance probably due to the reduction of case numbers when analyzing subgroups; this suggests that, differently from *PRTN3* and *SERPINA1*, *PTPN22* might actually be a shared association between GPA and MPA [9].

Although still lacking confirmation at genome-wide significance, *CTLA4* is likely to play a central role in the pathogenesis of AAV as well as other autoimmune diseases. The inhibitory glycoprotein encoded by this gene is expressed on activated T cells and competes with the co-stimulatory molecule CD28 for the binding of CD80 and CD86 preventing the stimulatory drive induced by CD28 itself. The central role in the immunological response of this immune checkpoint is nicely demonstrated by the fact that the CTLA4 inhibitors are now in use in the field of oncology to enhance immune system activity while a fusion protein CTLA4-Ig (abatacept) is now in use in autoimmune diseases, including GPA with nonsevere manifestations, aiming to achieve the opposite result. So far, several candidate gene studies have proposed a role for this gene as risk factor in AAV [20, 21]; however, bigger cohorts will be required to confirm its association at genome-wide significance. Table 2.1 summarizes the genes robustly described as associated with GPA and/or MPA.

Several other genes have been identified as potentially associated with GPA and/or MPA by smaller genetic studies. These relied on a candidate gene approach design, meaning that some genes thought a priori to be involved in the disease have been explored. The threshold of the association required to be considered significant is lower than that of GWAS; on one hand, this allows easier identification of associations; on the other hand, it may increase the rate of spurious ones. Findings obtained by such studies may be of potential interest but should be considered preliminary as long as confirmation in bigger cohorts is lacking. Among these associations, the most potentially significant are reported in Table 2.2.

The genetics of GPA and MPA is still at a relative early stage of development compared to other diseases. However, it has already contributed in a significant way to improving our understanding of the disease. First of all, it has provided significant insight into a better classification of AAV which will be discussed below. Second, it has confirmed and provided further rational for potential therapeutic targets: the confirmation of the central role of B-cell hyperactivity as well as of the

Table 2.1 Genes robustly associated with the risk of developing AAV

Gene	Disease	Phenotype resulting from the variant associated with the disease
HLA-DPB1	GPA	Abnormal antigen presentation
HLA-DQ	MPA	Abnormal antigen presentation
PRTN3	GPA	Increased expression of PR3 on neutrophils surface
SERPINA1	GPA	Reduced activity of alpha1-antitrypsine, main inhibitor of PR3 activity
PTPN22	GPA	Abnormal T_{reg} function, increase B cells and neutrophils function
CTLA4	GPA	Increased T-cell activity

GPA granulomatosis with polyangiitis, *MPA* microscopic polyangiitis, *PR3* proteinase 3

Table 2.2 Genes proposed as associated with the risk of developing AAV with a high degree of uncertainty

Gene	Disease	Limitation	Role of the protein encoded by the gene
IL10 [22, 23]	GPA-MPA	Not robustly replicated	Anti-inflammatory activity
IL2RA [21]	AAV	Weak association, not replicated	Immune system function
CD226 [24]	GPA	Not replicated	NK- and T-cell stimulation
FCGRs [25–28]	AAV	Not replicated	Binding of the FC portion of the immunoglobulins on cells surface
IRF5 [29, 30]	AAV	Not robustly replicated	Interferon-alpha regulatory factor
TLR9 [31]	AAV	Not robustly replicated	Recognition of microbiological structures and activation of the immune response
DEFB4 [32]	GPA	Not replicated	Proteins with antimicrobial activity
ETS1 [33]	GPA	Not replicated	Regulation of immune system activity

GPA granulomatosis with polyangiitis, *MPA* microscopic polyangiitis, FCGRs Fc gamma receptors

immune checkpoint CTLA4 supports, respectively, the use of B-cell depleting strategies and abatacept among the treatment armamentarium of the disease.

Another important contribution of genetics is an increased understanding of the underlying pathogenesis. The central role of an HLA association has been the definitive confirmation of the autoimmune nature of the disease. Moreover in GPA, increased PR3 expression or activity has been recognized as key. As expected in a disease with a multifactorial pathogenesis, other factors play a role such as an abnormal and increased function of the T- and B-cell compartments as supported by the associations with *PTPN22* and *CTLA4*.

However, what we know so far is still the tip of the iceberg; bigger studies and combined analyses of the studies performed so far will provide further insight on this topic and contributing to an even deeper understanding of AAV.

2.4 Genetics of EGPA

The challenges of performing genetic studies in EGPA are even more striking than in GPA and MPA mainly due to the lower frequency of the disease as well as difficulties from the classification point of view. ANCA-positive EGPA is more often characterized by vasculitic manifestations, such as lung hemorrhage, neuropathy, glomerulonephritis, and purpura, and is the subset of EGPA most easy to diagnose having a clear-cut clinical presentation and frequently relying on a biomarker such as ANCA. In the ANCA-negative cases, the diagnostic challenges have more significant difficulties in terms of differential diagnoses with other immunological diseases such as allergy/atopy or hypereosinophilic syndrome. These difficulties have been the major obstacles to the running of genetics studies with an inclusive approach in EGPA; so far, in fact, no GWAS has been published in this disease, although one is now ongoing by the European Vasculitis Genetic Consortium (EVGC).

What data exist in terms of the genetics of EGPA come from relatively small candidate gene studies; however, despite providing some insight, these data are probably still insufficient in order to draw firm conclusions.

The first set of candidate genes that were chosen to be explored were within the HLA area: two studies identified a robust association with the genes DRB4 and DRB3 [34, 35]; of interest, the likelihood of having this association increased with the increasing of the number of vasculitic manifestation. The identification of an association in the HLA area pointed also in EGPA toward an autoimmune nature of the disease, providing an important step forward in the understanding of the disease.

Unfortunately, these findings have been the most robust so far in EGPA; other small studies have been performed with, however, relatively inconsistent results. One of them regarded the gene encoding IL10; IL-10 is a cytokine produced by the T-helper cells characterized by anti-inflammatory properties, including the inhibition of immune mediator secretion, antigen presentation, and phagocytosis. A polymorphism in this gene has been found to be associated with EGPA, although this association was restricted to the ANCA-positive subtype [23].

CNVs represent a significant source of genetic heterogeneity in addition to SNPs; CNVs refer to the intrinsic characteristics of some genes being potentially represented in a variable number of copies; this may induce phenotypic heterogeneity influencing protein expression. In patients with autoimmune diseases, CNVs involving Fcγ receptor (FcγR) genes have reported an association of CNVs of the Fcγ-receptor 3B (*FCGR3B*) with systemic lupus erythematosus (SLE). Since carriers of low copies of the *FCGR3B* were shown to express lower protein levels, the pathogenetic mechanism proposed for this association was a reduced ability to clear immune complexes in subjects at risk [36]. The role of CNVs of *FCGR3B* has been investigated also in EGPA, and it has been found that being carrier of one copy of *FCGR3B* was a risk factor for the disease; this is relatively surprising since the role of immune complexes in the pathogenesis of the disease may not be considered as relevant as in SLE. However, of interest, this association was stronger in the subgroup of patients showing vasculitic manifestations, the subgroup more likely to be ANCA positive, suggesting that in some way an altered interaction with the autoantibody ANCA might be the explanation for this association.

Data on genetics in EGPA are still scanty; what we may so far conclude is a likely autoimmune nature for the disease and a possible different genetic background between subsets of the disease with and without vasculitic manifestations; these conclusions are, however, preliminary and the results of the ongoing GWAS run by the EVGC might be able to provide further insight.

2.5 Contribution of Genetics to Better AAV Classification

AAV has been historically classified into three different clinical entities: GPA, MPA, and EGPA. Significant overlap exists between these leading to difficulties in clinical classification, which may impact on the therapeutic approach and disease monitoring with important consequences for the single patient. Of interest, ANCAs are a shared biomarker, and this, together with the important clinical overlap, may suggest a pathogenetic overlap between GPA, MPA, and EGPA. Of note, only 40% of EGPA cases are ANCA-positive and the ANCA-negative subgroup is more frequently represented by a variant of the disease usually without vasculitic manifestations and more often characterized by clinical characteristics that arise as a consequence of hypereosinophilia. In this context of clinical uncertainty, genetics has played a big role in improving our understanding of AAV classification.

First of all, the GWASs in GPA and MPA provided the insight that the genetic background is more clearly associated with the ANCA specificity rather than the clinical diagnoses. The associations were in fact stronger when the population was stratified according to the ANCA specificity rather that the clinical phenotype. This provides the rational for the suggestion of the probable need of re-think GPA and MPA more as PR3+ and MPO+ AAV. The idea that ANCA specificity might be more robustly able to differentiate disease subtypes rather than clinical syndrome was not new, and some clinical observations already pointed toward this direction; the contribution of genetics has been to confirm that giving a very strong rational to the observation. Table 2.3 reports the clinical and genetic characteristics supporting

Table 2.3 Proposed reclassification of GPA and MPA in PR3+ and MPO+ AAV as supported by clinical phenotype and genetic evidence [37]

Variable	PR3+ AAV	MPO+ AAV
Mean age at onset	56–59	62–65
Male gender	66%	48%
ENT involvement	77%	23%
Eye involvement	40%	15%
Kidney-limited disease	2%	31%
Interstitial lung disease	0%	7.2%
Relapse (HR of PR3+ vs MPO+)	1.89 (95% CI 1.33–2.69)	
Relapse free patients 5 years after diagnoses	32%	60%
Cardiovascular risk (patients with at least one event over 5 years of follow-up)	6.6%	19.2%
Genetics associations	*HLA-DP* *PRTN3* *SERPINA1*	*HLA-DQ*
	PTPN22	

ENT ear, nose, and throat involvement, *HR* hazard ratio

a re-classification of GPA and MPA according to ANCA specificity rather than the clinical characteristics [37].

However, it is common experience of physicians used to dealing with vasculitis that even a classification based on ANCA specificity may not reflect everyday life in our clinics. MPO positivity in vasculitis is more frequent in certain geographical areas, such as south Europe or East Asia, and this may reflect, as well demonstrated in the Japanese population, a higher prevalence of the HLA-DQ risk allele. Of interest, despite the lower prevalence of PR3 positivity, clinical phenotypes resembling GPA and the clinical characteristics of PR3+ AAV are indeed still detected also in MPO-positive patients. This overlap suggests that, although convenient, the classification according to ANCA specificity has some limitations as well, and there must therefore be also likely shared genetics variants associated with both syndromes; *PTPN22* is at the moment a strong candidate, but others may well be detected by better powered studies. Future studies will need to be able to identify these associations in order to provide improvement in the understanding of disease pathogenesis as well as identifying new potential therapeutic targets.

In terms of EGPA genetics, data so far are very weak and the conclusions that we may draw are partial. The first thing of interest is a signal suggesting that the subtype of EGPA showing vasculitic manifestations (the group of patients more likely to be ANCA positive) may have differences in terms of genetic background compared to the subtype without vasculitic manifestations. Of great interest is also the association of EGPA with *HLA-DR*, due to its strong LD with the *HLA-DQ;* this may raise the idea of some potential shared genetic background with MPO+ AAV; this would provide a nice justification to the observation that *HLA-DR* was more represented in the subgroups of EGPA cases with vasculitic manifestation and increases as these increase. Furthermore, we should underline how, in the subgroup

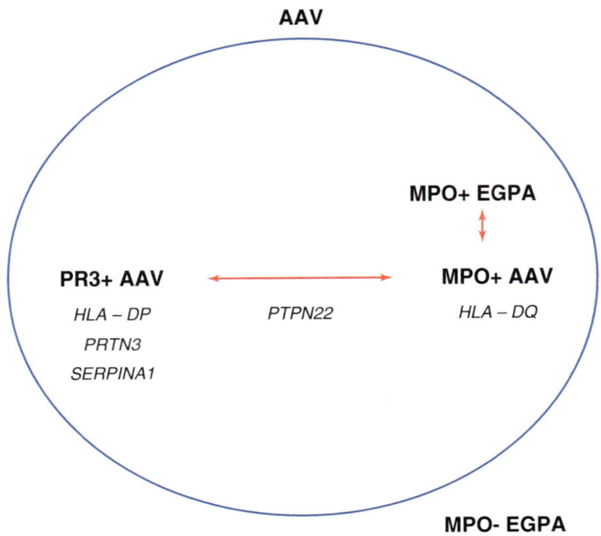

Fig. 2.1 Proposed classification of AAV according to the genetics information provided by the studies so far published integrated by AAV clinical phenotypes characteristics. In Italics are reported the genes associated with the different disease entities

of ANCA-positive EGPA, roughly in 90% of the cases the ANCA specificity is directed to MPO. Another important justification would be the clinical observation of quite strikingly overlapping phenotypes between MPO+ AAV and ANCA-positive EGPA with frequently challenging differential diagnoses.

We are, therefore, heading toward the direction of a likely need to reclassify AAV: on one hand, we may have PR3+ and MPO+ AAV with indeed two clinical extremes well differentiated and then some forms with overlapping characteristics. Genetic results available so far and preliminary results of the GWAS in EGPA might suggest that, while ANCA-positive EGPA should really be considered in close link with MPO+ AAV, ANCA-negative EGPA may be a variant with a less clear relationship with the rest of AAV and might eventually need to be reclassified under a different umbrella (Fig. 2.1).

In conclusion, although genetic data in AAV are still scanty compared to other diseases characterized by higher prevalence, their interpretation in light of our clinical knowledge has so far provided significant insight in terms of improving disease classification. This eventually may allow not only better understanding of the disease but also a huge rational for changes in disease management and monitoring as well as for trial design and eventually to therapeutic approach. Further studies are still needed to expand our understanding in the field, and the completion of a GWAS in EGPA will be of great help in confirming some of this speculation.

2.6 Genetics and Prognosis

In the end, genetic studies are mainly case–control studies looking for associations of genes with the diseases. We have discussed how this may improve our understanding of the disease pathogenesis, and classification as well as contributing to the identification of potential therapeutic targets and biomarkers. Interest has recently moved to the potential use of genetics as a way to better define prognosis. As clinicians, what we are eventually interested in is understanding how the disease is going to behave in an individual patient, if it is going to have a chronic relapsing course, or if it is going to have a benign outcome and genetics may contribute to that as well. Recently, a prognostic GWAS has been carried out in the field of inflammatory bowel disease showing that the genes associated with outcome, despite having a significant biological rational, were not overlapping with the ones associated with the risk of developing the disease itself, suggesting in some way that the biology of prognosis may not necessarily overlap with the biology of disease susceptibility [38]. In designing such studies, great effort should be directed to careful patient selection as well as long-term outcome definitions in terms of remission and relapse; such studies are designed as case–case ones where two groups of patients with different outcomes will be compared with no need of healthy controls. Genetic studies in AAV are still at early stage, and very few such studies have been performed so far; a prognostic GWAS has been planned by the EVGC but results are not available at the moment.

Epigenetics explores the regulation of gene expression via modification of the DNA structure itself; DNA methylation and acetylation are markers frequently explored. A recent study has shown that methylation of *PRTN3* and *MPO* correlates with protein expression and patients with decrease *PRTN3* methylation had a greater risk of relapse identifying a subgroup that may need a more intense immunosuppressive approach.

Pharmacogenetics explores association of SNPs and response to treatment or risk of side effects to a specific drug. Three studies of pharmacogenetics have so far been performed in the field of AAV all exploring the role of some candidate genes and response to therapy. One of them identified a SNP in the regulatory region of the B-cell activating factor (BAFF) associated with a poor outcome after rituximab treatment; interestingly, the carriers of the unfavorable genotype showed signs for increased B-cell activity, such as a higher proportion of detectable B cells and a smaller IgM reduction 6 months after therapy [39]. BAFF has already been identified as central in AAV pathogenesis, and a rebound of its levels after rituximab treatment has been considered as a risk factor for treatment failures [19] at the point that trials exploring a combined approach of anti-CD20 and anti-BAFF drugs are ongoing; this genetic study provides a further rational for identifying a potential biomarker. The second study identified, in a cohort of patients enrolled for a clinical trial comparing the use of rituximab and cyclophosphamide as induction therapy in AAV, a SNP in the *FCGR2A* gene as associated with quicker remission; this may also play an important role as biomarker since as far as we know, the quicker remission is induced, the lower the probability of developing serious damage induced by AAV [40]. The third identified a role for a SNP in cytochrome P450 in predicting response of AAV patients treated with cyclophosphamide [41].

All these studies, despite of interest, are characterized by several limitations and need further replication or follow-up studies in order to have their findings confirmed. However, they represent good examples of what genetics can do in order to contribute to better defining disease prognosis.

2.7 Conclusion

Despite three GWASs in AAV have been performed so far and one in EGPA is currently on-going, the field of genetics in AAV is still at an early stage of development. Few robust associations have been so far identified although those found have significantly contributed to our understanding of disease pathogenesis and classification. Some studies have also started to point their focus toward the role of genetics in defining prognosis with further needed in order to fully develop this interesting branch of genetics.

References

1. Jennette JC, Falk RJ, Andrassy K, et al. Nomenclature of systemic vasculitides. Proposal of an international consensus conference. Arthritis Rheum. 1994;37:187–92.
2. Chen M, Kallenberg CG. The environment, geoepidemiology and ANCA-associated vasculitides. Autoimmun Rev. 2010;9:A293–8.
3. Knight A, Sandin S, Askling J. Risks and relative risks of Wegener's granulomatosis among close relatives of patients with the disease. Arthritis Rheum. 2008;58:302–7.
4. Manganelli P, Giacosa R, Fietta P, Zanetti A, Neri TM. Familial vasculitides: Churg-Strauss syndrome and Wegener's granulomatosis in 2 first-degree relatives. J Rheumatol. 2003;30:618–21.
5. Diabetes Genetics Initiative of Broad Institute of Harvard and MIT, Lund University, and Novartis Institutes of BioMedical Research, et al. Genome-wide association analysis identifies loci for type 2 diabetes and triglyceride levels. Science. 2007;316:1331–6.
6. Cortes A, Brown MA. Promise and pitfalls of the Immunochip. Arthritis Res Ther. 2011;13:101.
7. Lyons PA, Rayner TF, Trivedi S, et al. Genetically distinct subsets within ANCA-associated vasculitis. N Engl J Med. 2012;367:214–23.
8. Xie G, Roshandel D, Sherva R, et al. Association of granulomatosis with polyangiitis (Wegener's) with HLA-DPB1∗04 and SEMA6A gene variants: evidence from genome-wide analysis. Arthritis Rheum. 2013;65:2457–68.
9. Merkel PA, Xie G, Monach PA, et al. Identification of functional and expression polymorphisms associated with risk for antineutrophil cytoplasmic autoantibody-associated vasculitis. Arthritis Rheumatol. 2017;69:1054–66.
10. Taneja V, Behrens M, Basal E, et al. Delineating the role of the HLA-DR4 "shared epitope" in susceptibility versus resistance to develop arthritis. J Immunol. 2008;181:2869–77.
11. Hiwa R, Ohmura K, Arase N, et al. Myeloperoxidase/HLA class II complexes recognized by autoantibodies in microscopic polyangiitis. Arthritis Rheumatol. 2017;69:2069–80.
12. Campbell EJ, Campbell MA, Owen CA. Bioactive proteinase 3 on the cell surface of human neutrophils: quantification, catalytic activity, and susceptibility to inhibition. J Immunol. 2000;165:3366–74.
13. Schreiber A, Busjahn A, Luft FC, Kettritz R. Membrane expression of proteinase 3 is genetically determined. J Am Soc Nephrol. 2003;14:68–75.
14. Mahr AD, Edberg JC, Stone JH, et al. Alpha(1)-antitrypsin deficiency-related alleles Z and S and the risk of Wegener's granulomatosis. Arthritis Rheum. 2010;62:3760–7.
15. Maine CJ, Hamilton-Williams EE, Cheung J, et al. PTPN22 alters the development of regulatory T cells in the thymus. J Immunol. 2012;188:5267–75.
16. Bayley R, Kite KA, McGettrick HM, et al. The autoimmune-associated genetic variant PTPN22 R620W enhances neutrophil activation and function in patients with rheumatoid arthritis and healthy individuals. Ann Rheum Dis. 2015;74(8):1588–95.

17. Zhang J, Zahir N, Jiang Q, et al. The autoimmune disease-associated PTPN22 variant promotes calpain-mediated Lyp/Pep degradation associated with lymphocyte and dendritic cell hyperresponsiveness. Nat Genet. 2011;43:902–7.
18. Hasegawa K, Martin F, Huang G, Tumas D, Diehl L, Chan AC. PEST domain-enriched tyrosine phosphatase (PEP) regulation of effector/memory T cells. Science. 2004;303:685–9.
19. Alberici F, Jayne DR. Impact of rituximab trials on the treatment of ANCA-associated vasculitis. Nephrol Dial Transplant. 2014;29:1151–9.
20. Kamesh L, Heward JM, Williams JM, et al. CT60 and +49 polymorphisms of CTLA 4 are associated with ANCA-positive small vessel vasculitis. Rheumatology (Oxford). 2009;48:1502–5.
21. Carr EJ, Niederer HA, Williams J, et al. Confirmation of the genetic association of CTLA4 and PTPN22 with ANCA-associated vasculitis. BMC Med Genet. 2009;10:121.
22. Bartfai Z, Gaede KI, Russell KA, Murakozy G, Muller-Quernheim J, Specks U. Different gender-associated genotype risks of Wegener's granulomatosis and microscopic polyangiitis. Clin Immunol. 2003;109:330–7.
23. Wieczorek S, Hellmich B, Arning L, et al. Functionally relevant variations of the interleukin-10 gene associated with antineutrophil cytoplasmic antibody-negative Churg-Strauss syndrome, but not with Wegener's granulomatosis. Arthritis Rheum. 2008;58:1839–48.
24. Wieczorek S, Hoffjan S, Chan A, et al. Novel association of the CD226 (DNAM-1) Gly307Ser polymorphism in Wegener's granulomatosis and confirmation for multiple sclerosis in German patients. Genes Immun. 2009;10:591–5.
25. Fanciulli M, Norsworthy PJ, Petretto E, et al. FCGR3B copy number variation is associated with susceptibility to systemic, but not organ-specific, autoimmunity. Nat Genet. 2007;39:721–3.
26. Smith KG, Clatworthy MR. FcgammaRIIB in autoimmunity and infection: evolutionary and therapeutic implications. Nat Rev Immunol. 2010;10:328–43.
27. Dijstelbloem HM, Scheepers RH, Oost WW, et al. Fcgamma receptor polymorphisms in Wegener's granulomatosis: risk factors for disease relapse. Arthritis Rheum. 1999;42:1823–7.
28. Tse WY, Abadeh S, McTiernan A, Jefferis R, Savage CO, Adu D. No association between neutrophil FcgammaRIIa allelic polymorphism and anti-neutrophil cytoplasmic antibody (ANCA)-positive systemic vasculitis. Clin Exp Immunol. 1999;117:198–205.
29. Wieczorek S, Holle JU, Muller S, Fricke H, Gross WL, Epplen JT. A functionally relevant IRF5 haplotype is associated with reduced risk to Wegener's granulomatosis. J Mol Med (Berl). 2010;88:413–21.
30. Kawasaki A, Inoue N, Ajimi C, et al. Association of IRF5 polymorphism with MPO-ANCA-positive vasculitis in a Japanese population. Genes Immun. 2013;14:527–9.
31. Husmann CA, Holle JU, Moosig F, et al. Genetics of toll like receptor 9 in ANCA associated vasculitides. Ann Rheum Dis. 2014;73:890–6.
32. Zhou XJ, Cheng FJ, Lv JC, et al. Higher DEFB4 genomic copy number in SLE and ANCA-associated small vasculitis. Rheumatology (Oxford). 2012;51:992–5.
33. Kawasaki A, Yamashita K, Hirano F, et al. Association of ETS1 polymorphism with granulomatosis with polyangiitis and proteinase 3-anti-neutrophil cytoplasmic antibody positive vasculitis in a Japanese population. J Hum Genet. 2018;63:55–62.
34. Vaglio A, Martorana D, Maggiore U, et al. HLA-DRB4 as a genetic risk factor for Churg-Strauss syndrome. Arthritis Rheum. 2007;56:3159–66.
35. Wieczorek S, Hellmich B, Gross WL, Epplen JT. Associations of Churg-Strauss syndrome with the HLA-DRB1 locus, and relationship to the genetics of antineutrophil cytoplasmic antibody-associated vasculitides: comment on the article by Vaglio et al. Arthritis Rheum. 2008;58:329–30.
36. Willcocks LC, Lyons PA, Clatworthy MR, et al. Copy number of FCGR3B, which is associated with systemic lupus erythematosus, correlates with protein expression and immune complex uptake. J Exp Med. 2008;205:1573–82.
37. Alberici F, Martorana D, Vaglio A. Genetic aspects of anti-neutrophil cytoplasmic antibody-associated vasculitis. Nephrol Dial Transplant. 2015;30(Suppl 1):i37–45.

38. Lee JC, Biasci D, Roberts R, et al. Genome-wide association study identifies distinct genetic contributions to prognosis and susceptibility in Crohn's disease. Nat Genet. 2017;49:262–8.
39. Alberici F, Smith RM, Fonseca M, et al. Association of a TNFSF13B (BAFF) regulatory region single nucleotide polymorphism with response to rituximab in antineutrophil cytoplasmic antibody-associated vasculitis. J Allergy Clin Immunol. 2017;139:1684–7 e10.
40. Cartin-Ceba R, Indrakanti D, Specks U, et al. The Pharmacogenomic association of Fcgamma receptors and cytochrome P450 enzymes with response to rituximab or cyclophosphamide treatment in antineutrophil cytoplasmic antibody-associated vasculitis. Arthritis Rheumatol. 2017;69:169–75.
41. Schirmer JH, Bremer JP, Moosig F, et al. Cyclophosphamide treatment-induced leukopenia rates in ANCA-associated vasculitis are influenced by variant CYP450 2C9 genotypes. Pharmacogenomics. 2016;17:367–74.

3 Etiopathogenesis of ANCA-Associated Vasculitis

Delphine Sterlin, Alexis Mathian, and Makoto Miyara

3.1 Introduction

ANCA-associated vasculitides (AAVs) are characterized by the inflammation of small vessels leading to organ damages due to the pathogenic role of ANCA. Those autoantibodies recognize either myeloperoxidase or proteinase 3 that are present in neutrophils granules [1]. Accumulating experimental evidence indicate that AAVs are autoimmune conditions since all the mechanistic criteria required for a disease to be considered autoimmune are observed in patients or animal models. All autoimmune diseases are defined by the presence of autoimmune immune cells, either T cells and B cells or both, the presence of autoantibodies that can be pathogenic or not, and the observation that the disease can be transferred in animal models or in individuals [2]. In this chapter, we discuss the etiopathogenesis of autoimmune responses in AAV and the ensuing molecular processes that are responsible for tissue lesions.

D. Sterlin · M. Miyara (✉)
Sorbonne Université, Inserm, Centre d'Immunologie et des Maladies Infectieuses (CIMI-Paris), AP-HP Hôpital Pitié-Salpêtrière, Paris, France

Immunology Department, AP-HP Hôpital Pitié-Salpêtrière, Paris, France
e-mail: makoto.miyara@aphp.fr

A. Mathian
Centre d'Immunologie et des Maladies Infectieuses (CIMI-Paris), AP-HP Hôpital Pitié-Salpêtrière, INSERM, Sorbonne Université, Paris, France

Internal Medicine Department, French National Reference Center for Rare Systemic Autoimmune Diseases, AP-HP Hôpital Pitié-Salpêtrière, Paris, France
e-mail: alexis.mathian@aphp.fr

R. A. Sinico, L. Guillevin (eds.), *Anti-Neutrophil Cytoplasmic Antibody (ANCA) Associated Vasculitis*, Rare Diseases of the Immune System,
https://doi.org/10.1007/978-3-030-02239-6_3

3.2 Genesis of the ANCA Autoimmune Response

Original events leading to a breakdown of tolerance and generation of autoantibodies are still poorly understood. The exposure of the main target antigens MPO and PR3 to the immune system is greatly limited. Indeed, both are localized in cytoplasmic granules of neutrophils and are quickly inhibited after degranulation by specific inhibitors: ceruloplasmin for MPO [3] and α1-antitrypsin for PR3 [4]. Several factors may play a role in revealing these antigens to the immune system and enhancing the development of autoantibodies. Evidence for a genetic contribution to AAV susceptibility has been extensively reviewed in previous chapter. It includes *HLA* variants and *SERPINA1* that encodes for α1-antitrypsin [5]. A variety of microbial agents such as *Staphylococcus aureus, Ross River virus,* and *Entamoeba histolytica* have also been implicated in the pathogenic autoimmune response of AAV [6], suggesting that ANCA autoimmunity is likely multifactorial and may vary among individuals. Here, we focus on three key hypotheses that dominate the current understanding of ANCA generation (Fig. 3.1).

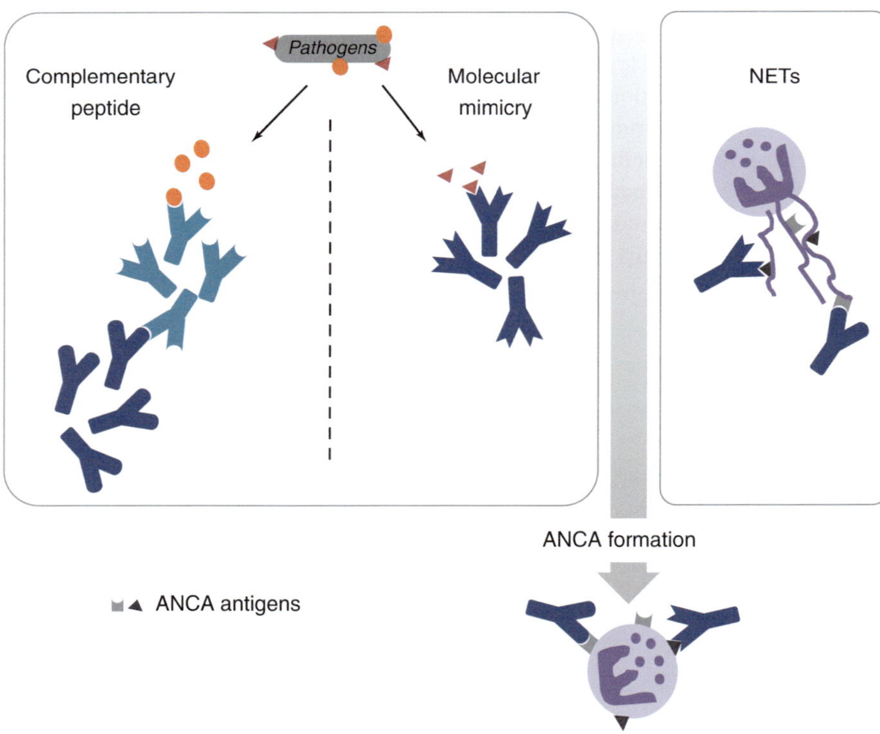

Fig. 3.1 Putative events in the genesis of ANCA autoimmune response. A first theory suggests that initial immune response could target complementary peptides of PR3 expressed by a range of microbes, which initiates anti-idiotypic antibodies reacting as a consequence to PR3. A second hypothesis proposed that microbe antigens could mimic autoantigen and induce pathogenic autoantibodies. Finally, an alternative mechanism involves neutrophils extracellular traps (NETs) that expose danger signals and facilitate breakdown of tolerance

3.2.1 Molecular Mimicry Theory

The molecular mimicry theory points out the protein lysosome-associated membrane protein 2 (LAMP2) as a possible autoantigen. LAMP2 belongs to a family of membrane glycoproteins mostly expressed in lysosomes and cell surface that have essential roles in maintaining cellular homeostasis and shuttling polysaccharides from lysosomes to the cell surface of neutrophils [7]. Kain et al. demonstrated the presence of antibodies against LAMP2 in 80–90% of AAV patients with active glomerulonephritis regardless of their ANCA status. These autoantibodies decrease much more rapidly than other ANCA after immunosuppression-induced remission and so may reflect disease activity [8]. The pathogenicity of anti-LAMP2 antibodies has been shown in a rodent adoptive immunization model. Indeed, rats injected with high titers of rabbit IgG anti-hLAMP2 (which cross-react with rat LAMP2) developed a glomerulonephritis with proteinuria, hematuria, and focal necrotizing crescents in about 25% of glomeruli. Furthermore, a monoclonal antibody to hLAMP activates primed neutrophils and induces apoptosis of human endothelial cells in vitro. While the most common LAMP2 epitope in human shows 100% homology to a bacterial adhesin FimH, immunization with FimH causes both LAMP-2 IgG and a pauci-immune glomerulonephritis in rats [9]. Theoretically, an infection by fimbriated FimH-expressing bacteria such as *E. coli* could lead to a pathogenic immune response that cross-react with LAMP2 through molecular mimicry, resulting in the induction of AAV. However, the low prevalence of systemic vasculitis compared to the high frequency of such infections suggests that individual susceptibility factors likely take part in the development of AAV. Importantly, other studies using different assays for anti-LAMP2 detection highlight difficulties in replicating these findings and reach contrasting results [10, 11].

3.2.2 Complementary Peptides

The complementary PR3 (cPR3) and anti-idiotype antibodies hypothesis is supported by the presence of antibodies to cPR3 peptide (generated from antisense DNA strand of PR3) in PR3-ANCA AAV patients [6]. In addition to anti-cPR3 antibodies, these patients also harbor specific anti-cPR3 CD4+ T cells, which are not found in MPO-ANCA AAV patients [12]. Pendergraft and colleagues, therefore, postulated that anti-PR3 response could be developed through an immune response against a peptide complementary to the original autoantigen, which in turn initiates anti-idiotypic antibodies that react not only with the idiotype but also with the epitope on the sense PR3. Indeed, immunization of naïve mice with cPR3 resulted in the production of both anti-cPR3 and anti-PR3 antibodies. Interestingly, cPR3 sequence shares partial homology with sequences carried by a range of microbes such as *S. aureus, Entamoeba histolytica,* and *Ross River virus* making them capable of inducing the ANCA autoimmune response [6]. While chronic nasal carriage of *S. aureus* has been shown as an independent risk factor for GPA relapses, rodents immunized with these bacteria do no develop AAV [13, 14]. Besides, no study to date has demonstrated that anti-cPR3 antibodies also recognize *S. aureus*. Thus, further work is necessary to translate the concept of anti-idiotypic antibodies in the pathogenesis of AAV in vivo.

3.2.3 NETosis

Neutrophils extracellular traps (NETs) are fibrous structures released by activated neutrophils that contain double-stranded DNA, citrullinated peptides, and an array of antimicrobial peptides such as MPO and PR3. Initially described as a mechanism to trap and kill extracellular microorganisms, NETs have been found in a wide variety of conditions, including malignancy, atherosclerosis, and autoimmune diseases [15]. In addition to MPO and PR3, NETs also expose danger signals that could facilitate breakdown of tolerance [16]. Nevertheless, the most persuasive clues that NETs present autoantigens leading to a pathogenic immune response in AAV arise from reports on drug-induced vasculitis. First, combined immunization of anti-thyroid drug propylthiouracil (PTU) and phorbol 12-myristate 13-acetate (PMA) resulted in the formation of NETs which enhanced the production of MPO-ANCA in mice [17]. Another group demonstrated that cocaine and levamisole, its common adulterant, induced NETs that may be an important source of autoantigens. Notably, patients with cocaine-associated vasculitis possess autoantibodies against NET components, including neutrophil elastase, PR3, MPO which in turn contribute to NETosis which likely create a vicious circle in these patients [18]. *S. aureus* is also known as a strong inducer of NETs. This pathway could provide another explanation for the relationship between *S. aureus* carriage and increased relapse risk discussed above. Altogether, these findings proposed NETs as a bridge between innate and adaptive immune systems in the pathogenesis of AAV.

3.2.4 T-Cell Dysregulation and MPO/PR3 Autoimmunity

Autoreactive CD4+ T cells play a major in the pathogenesis of most autoimmune diseases as they provide co-activation signals for B cells to produce autoantibodies [2]. CD3+ T lymphocytes specific for MPO or PR3 peptides have been described in murine models of AAV [19, 20] and in patients [21, 22]. An important pathway in the pathogenesis of AAV involved the autoimmune response directed against the complementary peptides of PR3 (cPR3). This includes the production of anti-cPR3 autoantibodies, described in details above, and the presence of cPR3-specific T cells [12]. Autoreactive T cells with pathogenic potential can theoretically be found in every individual [23]. Those cells are permanently controlled by a key mechanism of maintenance of tolerance to self-antigens, that is, dominant peripheral tolerance mediated by transcription factor FOXP3 expressing CD4+ regulatory T (Treg) cells [24]. Treg cells play a crucial role in the prevention of autoimmune disease [25]. The preventive role of Treg cells against autoimmune responses directed against the MPO protein has been demonstrated in mice [26] and in humans [21]. Deficiencies in the number and/or in the function of Treg cells have been observed in humans, accounting for the lack of immune suppression of ANCA-specific autoreactive T cells [27–30].

Th17 cells are a subset of effector CD4+ T cells that promote responses toward fungi and some bacteria by stimulating neutrophils [31]. Those cells, increased in patients with granulomatosis with polyangiitis, are also involved in autoimmune reaction [20]. Indeed, T cells escaping Treg cells control in AAV have been shown to be, in part, Th17 cells [32]. Thus, the activation of Th17 cells and their uncontrolled effector function can also lead to vessels and tissue damages [33]. Beyond Th17 cells, CD4+ T cells demonstrated a skewed Th2 (IL-4, IL-5) and Th9 (IL-9) polarization in PR3 microenvironment [20].

3.3 Evidence for the Pathogenic Role of ANCAs

While AAV is characterized by a "pauci-immune" vascular inflammation, in which only scarce immunoglobulin and complement deposition can be detected, there is in vitro and in vivo human and animal evidence that ANCAs are pathogenic (Fig. 3.2).

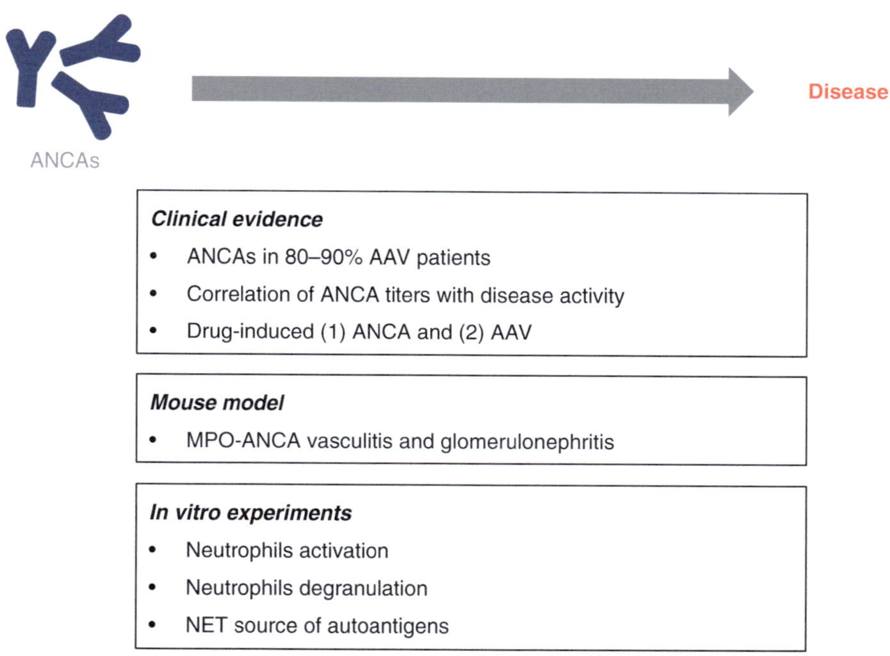

Fig. 3.2 Evidence for the pathogenic role of ANCAs. In addition to clinical studies, numerous in vitro and in vivo experiments readily documented that ANCA can mediate inflammatory processes and induce vasculitis. Antineutrophil cytoplasmic antibodies (ANCA), ANCA-associated vasculitis (AAV)

3.3.1 Clinical Support for ANCA Pathogenicity

The presence of ANCAs in about 80–90% of AAV patients is consistent with the possibility that ANCA may cause the disease but also may accompany the disease without driving it. More convincing is the temporal relationship between the development of AAV and the administration of specific drugs such as hydralazine, allopurinol, propylthiouracil, and levamisole, which may contaminate illicit cocaine. The clinical manifestations of drug-induced AAV are similar to those of primary AAV, and the prognosis of patients is good after the offending drug is discontinued [34]. The correlation of ANCA titers with disease activity or with response to treatment also supports their pathogenicity [35]. However, ANCA-negative vasculitis and the persistence of ANCA in some remitting patients sustain controversy [36]. Roth et al. suggested that the immunological assays used routinely might be partly responsible for these inconsistent correlations. Indeed, using sensitive mass spectrometry and epitope excision approaches, they identified autoantibody diversity in ANCAs with some epitope specificities that only occur in active patients, whereas others were found in active patients as well as in patients in remission. Among over 20 different epitopes, they further separated pathogenic autoantibodies as showed by their ability to induce nephritis in mice and non-pathogenic ones. They also observed that current laboratory tests could not detect some pathogenic MPO epitopes because of the presence in serum of ceruloplasmin, which play a role of confounder for serological detection [37].

Another clinical observation that strongly supports ANCA pathogenicity is the development of renal and pulmonary disease in a neonate who acquired maternal MPO-ANCA by transplacental transfer [38]. Finally, the efficacy of targeted B-cell therapy (e.g., rituximab) and plasma exchanges, which reduce ANCA levels in serum, suggests an antibody-mediated process [39–41].

3.3.2 In Vitro Support for ANCA Pathogenicity

Compelling in vitro experiments showed that ANCA could activate neutrophils and cause small-vessels damage, resulting in vasculitis. Indeed, incubation of normal human neutrophils with PR3-ANCA or MPO-ANCA IgG leads not only to toxic oxygen radicals and destructive enzymes release but also to NETs formation that induce tissue injury and facilitate autoimmune response [42–44]. In line with these observations, NETs have been reported in kidney biopsies and skin specimens from AAV patients [45, 46]. NETs can damage the vasculature both directly and indirectly. Directly, NETs release toxic substances such as enzymes and histones that induce endothelial cells apoptosis and vascular leakage. Indirectly, NETs activate the alternative complement pathway which causes necrotizing crescentic glomerulonephritis in AAV mouse model [47, 48]. As noted earlier, ANCA IgG from patients with active AAV harbors different epitope specificities than those from patients in remission, resulting in variant efficiency levels in activating neutrophils in vitro. Thereby, ANCA from active patients activates more neutrophils in vitro than does ANCA from remitting patients.

An increase of MPO and PR3 expression that can facilitate interactions between ANCA and their targets has been demonstrated in AAV patients. While MPO and PR3 expression is tightly regulated during neutrophils maturation process, AAV patients have perturbed epigenetic modifications associated with gene silencing which contribute to an elevated neutrophil membrane expression of both enzymes [49, 50]. Inflammatory factors such as cytokines (e.g., tumor necrosis factor alpha, TNFα) or microbial products (e.g., lipopolysaccharides) activate neutrophils and raise the exposure of ANCA target antigens at the cell surface or in the microenvironment where they can interact with autoantibodies [51, 52]. Neutrophil activation by ANCA involves both Fab'2 -mediated antigen binding and Fc receptors engagement, but the latter mechanism is likely predominant [53, 54]. ANCA also binds to MPO and PR3 that have been adsorbed onto endothelial cells or expressed by monocytes in the inflammatory environment [55, 56].

3.3.3 Animal Model Supports ANCA Pathogenicity

Animal models readily confirmed in vitro experiments and documented ANCA pathogenicity. A model of MPO-ANCA vasculitis based on injection of mouse anti-MPO antibodies in mice has been reproduced in numerous labs [57]. However, a convincing animal model for PR3-ANCA AAV is still lacking likely because of the differences in the biology of PR3 between humans and mice. Indeed, two main problems stand in this way of progress: (a) primed murine neutrophils exhibit only small amounts of PR3 at their surface [58] and (b) human anti-PR3 antibodies do not react with mouse targets.

MPO-deficient mice immunized with murine MPO generate a robust immune response such that injection of anti-MPO antibodies from these mice into wild-type mice leads to a pauci-immune glomerulonephritis similar to human AAV disease [57]. Interestingly, the genetic background of the mice has a significant effect on the severity of the disease, with more affected glomeruli in 129S6 than in C57BL6J mice [59]. Using $Rag2^{-/-}$ mice that lack B and T lymphocytes and neutrophil-depleting treatment, Xiao et al. also showed that neutrophils, but not lymphocytes, are the main drivers of MPO-ANCA disease [60]. To confirm neutrophils requirement in anti-MPO-induced disease, the same group irradiated immunized MPO-deficient mice and then transferred either MPO-expressing or MPO-deficient hematopoietic cells. Only mice with MPO-expressing cells developed necrotizing glomerulonephritis, which demonstrated that hematopoietic cells are sufficient to induce the disease [61]. Confirming in vitro data, proinflammatory stimuli such as LPS exacerbate the autoimmune response in MPO-disease model via the TNFα signaling [60].

As noted earlier, animal models for PR3-ANCA AAV are encouraging but less convincing. In contrast to MPO-ANCA, no spontaneous vasculitis has been observed after injection of anti-PR3 antibodies [62]. Indeed, in an effort to replicate the MPO-ANCA model, Pfister et al. immunized PR3-deficient mice with murine PR3 and transferred their autoantibodies to LPS-pretreated mice but failed to induce glomerulonephritis or vasculitis. However, they showed a stronger cutaneous inflammation by intradermal injection of TNFα, suggesting an enhanced neutrophil activation [58]. Using autoimmunity-prone nonobese diabetic (NOD) mice, Primo et al. observed high titers of anti-PR3 antibodies after immunization. While these mice did not develop vasculitis, the transfer of their splenocytes into NOD-SCID recipients (which lack T- and B-lymphocytes) led to the development of vasculitis and glomerulonephritis. $Rag^{-/-}$ B6 injected with the same splenocytes did not develop disease, which underlines the role of genetic background in disease susceptibility [49]. More recently, Little et al. generated chimeric mice by injecting human hematopoietic stem cells into irradiated NOD-SCID IL2R KO mice. Following passive transfer of human PR3-ANCA IgG, 39% of treated mice showed hematuria within 6 days. Microscopic examination of lungs and kidneys revealed pulmonary hemorrhage and mild glomerulonephritis [63]. Even though the extent of kidney disease was moderate compared with human AAV, this model may open an encouraging way to further investigate pathogenic mechanisms of PR3-ANCA disease.

3.3.4 Mechanisms of ANCA-Induced Lesions: The Role of Complement

The role of complement activation in AAV has been overlooked initially because deposits of complement and of immune complexes are rarely observed in kidneys with necrotizing crescentic glomerulonephritis. However, when closely analyzing histopathological samples of tissues with vasculitis, some fractions of complement can be detected [64]. Furthermore, a crucial role for the complement alternate activation pathways has been demonstrated in experimental models and confirmed in a recent clinical trial. In transfer models of anti-MPO antibodies, while C4 KO mice develop the disease, C5 knock-out mice do not [65]. The blockade of C5a receptor in mice could prevent the development of vasculitis, while the blockade of C6 did not, indicating that the formation of membrane attack complex was not required to induce vessel lesions [66]. C5a can bind to C5a receptor 1 (C5aR1) that is present on neutrophils. The priming of neutrophils trough their C5a receptor is an additional mechanism for the induction of vasculitis since C5aR1 inhibition prevents the retention of neutrophil and reactive oxygen species burst within glomerular capillaries [67, 68]. Those findings indicate that the neutralization of C5a can be a specific therapeutic target in AAV. This has been verified recently in a clinical trial evaluating the efficacy of avacopan, an oral C5a receptor inhibitor which was shown to be efficient in replacing high-dose glucocorticoids as an induction therapy of vasculitis along with cyclophosphamide or rituximab [69]. Moreover, the use of eculizumab, a monoclonal antibody targeting C5a, has also been shown to be effective in a patient with AAV with complement activation [70].

Altogether, those recent findings highlight the unexpected role for the alternate activation pathway of complement in enhancing neutrophil-induced vasculitis lesions. Of note, it is still unknown how the alternate complement activation pathway is triggered in AAV. An autonomous activation loop by primed neutrophils that would be able to activate the alternate pathways themselves is suspected [71].

3.4 Conclusion: Pathogenic Mechanism Overview

Animal model studies, in vitro experiments, and clinical observations provide a putative sequence of events leading to vascular and tissue injury in AAV (Fig. 3.3). As an initial event, a multifactorial process results in the genesis of pathogenic ANCA. Then, priming factors such as inflammatory cytokines (e.g., TNF-α) or complement factors cause the release of ANCA antigens (e.g., MPO and PR3) on the surface of neutrophils and in their microenvironment. Primed neutrophils, after binding of ANCA to ANCA antigens, undergo activation and degranulation, mostly through Fc receptor engagement. Monocyte activation by ANCA also occurred in parallel, but less importantly. Of note, in PR3-ANCA-associated vasculitis, those monocytes can be involved in the formation of granulomas in the sites of vasculitis [72]. ANCA-activated neutrophils release reactive oxygen species and destructive enzymes that mediate acute endothelial damage [44]. Moreover, activated neutrophils release complement-activating factors resulting in C5a production, which recruits and activates more neutrophils to the site of injury. This amplification loop leads to accumulation and subsequent death of a large number of neutrophils within vessel wall and matrix that is a histologic hallmark of AAV. At sites of endothelium

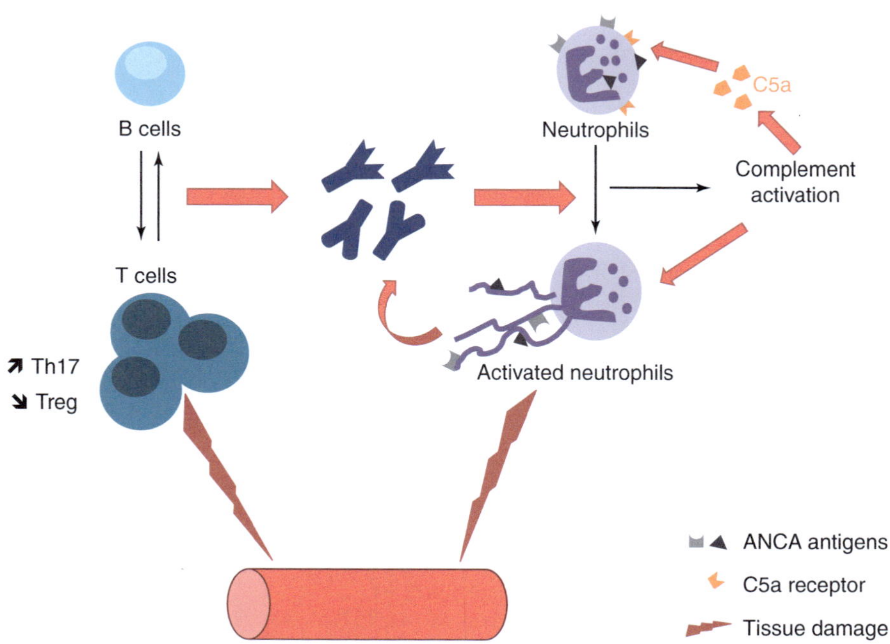

Fig. 3.3 Schematic illustration of the pathogenesis of AAV. Primed neutrophils (e.g., by cytokines) present ANCA antigens at the cell surface and into the microenvironment where they bind ANCA. Activated neutrophils release factors that enhance C5a production through the alternative complement pathway. C5a amplifies the inflammatory loop by recruiting and priming more neutrophils. Activated neutrophils spill into vessel walls and release inflammatory factors resulting in vascular necrosis. Uncontrolled activation of Th17 cells contributes to vessels and tissue damages

injury, leakage of plasma and coagulation factors give rise to fibrinoid necrosis in vessels and crescents in glomeruli. Within a few days, infiltrating macrophages and T lymphocytes replace apoptotic neutrophils and facilitate injury resolution. In case of persistent injury, collagen deposit by fibroblasts and myofibroblasts results in fibrosis/sclerosis of damaged vessels.

The etiopathogeny of AAV vasculitis has been deeply studied since the discovery of ANCA [73, 74], resulting in a rapidly obtained step-by-step precise description of the cellular and molecular processes resulting in vasculitis lesions. Today, those well-defined processes are already targeted by specific therapeutic strategies that have proven efficient.

References

1. Gross WL, Schmitt WH, Csernok E. ANCA and associated diseases: immunodiagnostic and pathogenetic aspects. Clin Exp Immunol. 1993;91(1):1–12.
2. Rose NR, Bona C. Defining criteria for autoimmune diseases (Witebsky's postulates revisited). Immunol Today. 1993;14(9):426–30.
3. Chapman AL, Mocatta TJ, Shiva S, et al. Ceruloplasmin is an endogenous inhibitor of myeloperoxidase. J Biol Chem. 2013;288(9):6465–77.
4. Duranton J, Bieth JG. Inhibition of proteinase 3 by [alpha]1-antitrypsin in vitro predicts very fast inhibition in vivo. Am J Respir Cell Mol Biol. 2003;29(1):57–61.
5. Lyons PA, Rayner TF, Trivedi S, et al. Genetically distinct subsets within ANCA-associated vasculitis. N Engl J Med. 2012;367(3):214–23.
6. Pendergraft WF 3rd, Preston GA, Shah RR, et al. Autoimmunity is triggered by cPR-3(105-201), a protein complementary to human autoantigen proteinase-3. Nat Med. 2004;10(1):72–9.
7. Kain R, Rees AJ. What is the evidence for antibodies to LAMP-2 in the pathogenesis of ANCA associated small vessel vasculitis? Curr Opin Rheumatol. 2013;25(1):26–34.
8. Kain R, Tadema H, McKinney EF, et al. High prevalence of autoantibodies to hLAMP-2 in anti-neutrophil cytoplasmic antibody-associated vasculitis. J Am Soc Nephrol. 2012;23(3):556–66.
9. Kain R, Exner M, Brandes R, et al. Molecular mimicry in pauci-immune focal necrotizing glomerulonephritis. Nat Med. 2008;14(10):1088–96.
10. Roth AJ, Brown MC, Smith RN, et al. Anti-LAMP-2 antibodies are not prevalent in patients with antineutrophil cytoplasmic autoantibody glomerulonephritis. J Am Soc Nephrol. 2012;23(3):545–55.
11. Fervenza FC, Specks U. Vasculitis: will LAMP enlighten us about ANCA-associated vasculitis? Nat Rev Nephrol. 2012;8(6):318–20.
12. Yang J, Bautz DJ, Lionaki S, et al. ANCA patients have T cells responsive to complementary PR-3 antigen. Kidney Int. 2008;74(9):1159–69.
13. Zycinska K, Wardyn KA, Zielonka TM, Demkow U, Traburzynski MS. Chronic crusting, nasal carriage of Staphylococcus aureus and relapse rate in pulmonary Wegener's granulomatosis. J Physiol Pharmacol. 2008;59(Suppl 6):825–31.
14. Savige J, Nassis L, Cooper T, Paspaliaris B, Martinello P, MacGregor D. Antineutrophil cytoplasmic antibody (ANCA)-associated systemic vasculitis after immunisation with bacterial proteins. Clin Exp Rheumatol. 2002;20(6):783–9.
15. Jorch SK, Kubes P. An emerging role for neutrophil extracellular traps in noninfectious disease. Nat Med. 2017;23(3):279–87.
16. Garcia-Romo GS, Caielli S, Vega B, et al. Netting neutrophils are major inducers of type I IFN production in pediatric systemic lupus erythematosus. Sci Transl Med. 2011;3(73):73ra20.

17. Kusunoki Y, Nakazawa D, Shida H, et al. Peptidylarginine deiminase inhibitor suppresses neutrophil extracellular trap formation and MPO-ANCA production. Front Immunol. 2016;7:227.
18. Lood C, Hughes GC. Neutrophil extracellular traps as a potential source of autoantigen in cocaine-associated autoimmunity. Rheumatology (Oxford). 2017;56(4):638–43.
19. Ooi JD, Chang J, Hickey MJ, et al. The immunodominant myeloperoxidase T-cell epitope induces local cell-mediated injury in antimyeloperoxidase glomerulonephritis. Proc Natl Acad Sci U S A. 2012;109(39):E2615–24.
20. Millet A, Martin KR, Bonnefoy F, et al. Proteinase 3 on apoptotic cells disrupts immune silencing in autoimmune vasculitis. J Clin Invest. 2015;125(11):4107–21.
21. Chavele KM, Shukla D, Keteepe-Arachi T, et al. Regulation of myeloperoxidase-specific T cell responses during disease remission in antineutrophil cytoplasmic antibody-associated vasculitis: the role of Treg cells and tryptophan degradation. Arthritis Rheum. 2010;62(5):1539–48.
22. Brouwer E, Stegeman CA, Huitema MG, Limburg PC, Kallenberg CG. T cell reactivity to proteinase 3 and myeloperoxidase in patients with Wegener's granulomatosis (WG). Clin Exp Immunol. 1994;98(3):448–53.
23. Danke NA, Koelle DM, Yee C, Beheray S, Kwok WW. Autoreactive T cells in healthy individuals. J Immunol. 2004;172(10):5967–72.
24. Sakaguchi S, Yamaguchi T, Nomura T, Ono M. Regulatory T cells and immune tolerance. Cell. 2008;133(5):775–87.
25. Miyara M, Gorochov G, Ehrenstein M, Musset L, Sakaguchi S, Amoura Z. Human FoxP3+ regulatory T cells in systemic autoimmune diseases. Autoimmun Rev. 2011;10(12):744–55.
26. Tan DS, Gan PY, O'Sullivan KM, et al. Thymic deletion and regulatory T cells prevent antimyeloperoxidase GN. J Am Soc Nephrol. 2013;24(4):573–85.
27. Rimbert M, Hamidou M, Braudeau C, et al. Decreased numbers of blood dendritic cells and defective function of regulatory T cells in antineutrophil cytoplasmic antibody-associated vasculitis. PLoS One. 2011;6(4):e18734.
28. Morgan MD, Day CJ, Piper KP, et al. Patients with Wegener's granulomatosis demonstrate a relative deficiency and functional impairment of T-regulatory cells. Immunology. 2010;130(1):64–73.
29. Abdulahad WH, Stegeman CA, van der Geld YM, Doornbos-van der Meer B, Limburg PC, Kallenberg CG. Functional defect of circulating regulatory CD4+ T cells in patients with Wegener's granulomatosis in remission. Arthritis Rheum. 2007;56(6):2080–91.
30. Marinaki S, Neumann I, Kalsch AI, et al. Abnormalities of CD4 T cell subpopulations in ANCA-associated vasculitis. Clin Exp Immunol. 2005;140(1):181–91.
31. Korn T, Bettelli E, Oukka M, Kuchroo VK. IL-17 and Th17 cells. Annu Rev Immunol. 2009;27:485–517.
32. Eriksson P, Andersson C, Cassel P, Nystrom S, Ernerudh J. Increase in Th17-associated CCL20 and decrease in Th2-associated CCL22 plasma chemokines in active ANCA-associated vasculitis. Scand J Rheumatol. 2015;44(1):80–3.
33. Gan PY, Steinmetz OM, Tan DS, et al. Th17 cells promote autoimmune anti-myeloperoxidase glomerulonephritis. J Am Soc Nephrol. 2010;21(6):925–31.
34. Gao Y, Zhao MH. Review article: drug-induced anti-neutrophil cytoplasmic antibody-associated vasculitis. Nephrology (Carlton). 2009;14(1):33–41.
35. Boomsma MM, Stegeman CA, van der Leij MJ, et al. Prediction of relapses in Wegener's granulomatosis by measurement of antineutrophil cytoplasmic antibody levels: a prospective study. Arthritis Rheum. 2000;43(9):2025–33.
36. Thai LH, Charles P, Resche-Rigon M, Desseaux K, Guillevin L. Are anti-proteinase-3 ANCA a useful marker of granulomatosis with polyangiitis (Wegener's) relapses? Results of a retrospective study on 126 patients. Autoimmun Rev. 2014;13(3):313–8.
37. Roth AJ, Ooi JD, Hess JJ, et al. Epitope specificity determines pathogenicity and detectability in ANCA-associated vasculitis. J Clin Invest. 2013;123(4):1773–83.
38. Schlieben DJ, Korbet SM, Kimura RE, Schwartz MM, Lewis EJ. Pulmonary-renal syndrome in a newborn with placental transmission of ANCAs. Am J Kidney Dis. 2005;45(4):758–61.

39. Jones RB, Tervaert JW, Hauser T, et al. Rituximab versus cyclophosphamide in ANCA-associated renal vasculitis. N Engl J Med. 2010;363(3):211–20.
40. Stone JH, Merkel PA, Spiera R, et al. Rituximab versus cyclophosphamide for ANCA-associated vasculitis. N Engl J Med. 2010;363(3):221–32.
41. Jayne DR, Gaskin G, Rasmussen N, et al. Randomized trial of plasma exchange or high-dosage methylprednisolone as adjunctive therapy for severe renal vasculitis. J Am Soc Nephrol. 2007;18(7):2180–8.
42. Alpha-antitrypsin-alpha therapeutic corporation. AAT - Alpha Therapeutic Corporation, alpha-1 proteinase inhibitor - Alpha Therapeutic Corporation, alpha-1-antitrypsin - Alpha Therapeutic Corporation, Aralast, Respitin. Drugs R D. 2003;4(2):113–4.
43. Soderberg D, Segelmark M. Neutrophil extracellular traps in vasculitis, friend or foe? Curr Opin Rheumatol. 2018;30(1):16–23.
44. Guilpain P, Servettaz A, Goulvestre C, et al. Pathogenic effects of antimyeloperoxidase antibodies in patients with microscopic polyangiitis. Arthritis Rheum. 2007;56(7):2455–63.
45. Kessenbrock K, Krumbholz M, Schonermarck U, et al. Netting neutrophils in autoimmune small-vessel vasculitis. Nat Med. 2009;15(6):623–5.
46. Carmona-Rivera C, Purmalek MM, Moore E, et al. A role for muscarinic receptors in neutrophil extracellular trap formation and levamisole-induced autoimmunity. JCI Insight. 2017;2(3):e89780.
47. Kumar SV, Kulkarni OP, Mulay SR, et al. Neutrophil extracellular trap-related extracellular histones cause vascular necrosis in severe GN. J Am Soc Nephrol. 2015;26(10):2399–413.
48. Schreiber A, Rousselle A, Becker JU, von Massenhausen A, Linkermann A, Kettritz R. Necroptosis controls NET generation and mediates complement activation, endothelial damage, and autoimmune vasculitis. Proc Natl Acad Sci U S A. 2017;114(45):E9618–E25.
49. Abdgawad M, Gunnarsson L, Bengtsson AA, et al. Elevated neutrophil membrane expression of proteinase 3 is dependent upon CD177 expression. Clin Exp Immunol. 2010;161(1):89–97.
50. Ciavatta DJ, Yang J, Preston GA, et al. Epigenetic basis for aberrant upregulation of autoantigen genes in humans with ANCA vasculitis. J Clin Invest. 2010;120(9):3209–19.
51. Charles LA, Caldas ML, Falk RJ, Terrell RS, Jennette JC. Antibodies against granule proteins activate neutrophils in vitro. J Leukoc Biol. 1991;50(6):539–46.
52. Falk RJ, Terrell RS, Charles LA, Jennette JC. Anti-neutrophil cytoplasmic autoantibodies induce neutrophils to degranulate and produce oxygen radicals in vitro. Proc Natl Acad Sci U S A. 1990;87(11):4115–9.
53. Williams JM, Ben-Smith A, Hewins P, et al. Activation of the G(i) heterotrimeric G protein by ANCA IgG F(ab́) 2 fragments is necessary but not sufficient to stimulate the recruitment of those downstream mediators used by intact ANCA IgG. J Am Soc Nephrol. 2003;14(3):661–9.
54. Porges AJ, Redecha PB, Kimberly WT, Csernok E, Gross WL, Kimberly RP. Anti-neutrophil cytoplasmic antibodies engage and activate human neutrophils via Fc gamma RIIa. J Immunol. 1994;153(3):1271–80.
55. Savage CO, Gaskin G, Pusey CD, Pearson JD. Myeloperoxidase binds to vascular endothelial cells, is recognized by ANCA and can enhance complement dependent cytotoxicity. Adv Exp Med Biol. 1993;336:121–3.
56. Weidner S, Neupert W, Goppelt-Struebe M, Rupprecht HD. Antineutrophil cytoplasmic antibodies induce human monocytes to produce oxygen radicals in vitro. Arthritis Rheum. 2001;44(7):1698–706.
57. Xiao H, Heeringa P, Hu P, et al. Antineutrophil cytoplasmic autoantibodies specific for myeloperoxidase cause glomerulonephritis and vasculitis in mice. J Clin Invest. 2002;110(7):955–63.
58. Pfister H, Ollert M, Frohlich LF, et al. Antineutrophil cytoplasmic autoantibodies against the murine homolog of proteinase 3 (Wegener autoantigen) are pathogenic in vivo. Blood. 2004;104(5):1411–8.
59. Salama AD, Little MA. Animal models of antineutrophil cytoplasm antibody-associated vasculitis. Curr Opin Rheumatol. 2012;24(1):1–7.

60. Huugen D, Xiao H, van Esch A, et al. Aggravation of anti-myeloperoxidase antibody-induced glomerulonephritis by bacterial lipopolysaccharide: role of tumor necrosis factor-alpha. Am J Pathol. 2005;167(1):47–58.
61. Schreiber A, Xiao H, Falk RJ, Jennette JC. Bone marrow-derived cells are sufficient and necessary targets to mediate glomerulonephritis and vasculitis induced by anti-myeloperoxidase antibodies. J Am Soc Nephrol. 2006;17(12):3355–64.
62. van der Geld YM, Hellmark T, Selga D, et al. Rats and mice immunised with chimeric human/mouse proteinase 3 produce autoantibodies to mouse Pr3 and rat granulocytes. Ann Rheum Dis. 2007;66(12):1679–82.
63. Little MA, Al-Ani B, Ren S, Al-Nuaimi H, Leite M Jr, Alpers CE, et al. Anti-proteinase 3 anti-neutrophil cytoplasm autoantibodies recapitulate systemic vasculitis in mice with a humanized immune system. PLoS One. 2012;7(1):e28626.
64. Chen M, Xing GQ, Yu F, Liu G, Zhao MH. Complement deposition in renal histopathology of patients with ANCA-associated pauci-immune glomerulonephritis. Nephrol Dial Transplant. 2009;24(4):1247–52.
65. Xiao H, Schreiber A, Heeringa P, Falk RJ, Jennette JC. Alternative complement pathway in the pathogenesis of disease mediated by anti-neutrophil cytoplasmic autoantibodies. Am J Pathol. 2007;170(1):52–64.
66. Xiao H, Dairaghi DJ, Powers JP, et al. C5a receptor (CD88) blockade protects against MPO-ANCA GN. J Am Soc Nephrol. 2014;25(2):225–31.
67. Schreiber A, Xiao H, Jennette JC, Schneider W, Luft FC, Kettritz R. C5a receptor mediates neutrophil activation and ANCA-induced glomerulonephritis. J Am Soc Nephrol. 2009;20(2):289–98.
68. Dick J, Gan PY, Ford SL, et al. C5a receptor 1 promotes autoimmunity, neutrophil dysfunction and injury in experimental anti-myeloperoxidase glomerulonephritis. Kidney Int. 2018;93(3):615–25.
69. Jayne DRW, Bruchfeld AN, Harper L, et al. Randomized trial of C5a receptor inhibitor avacopan in ANCA-associated vasculitis. J Am Soc Nephrol. 2017;28(9):2756–67.
70. Manenti L, Urban ML, Maritati F, Galetti M, Vaglio A. Complement blockade in ANCA-associated vasculitis: an index case, current concepts and future perspectives. Intern Emerg Med. 2017;12(6):727–31.
71. Shingu M, Nonaka S, Nishimukai H, Nobunaga M, Kitamura H, Tomo-Oka K. Activation of complement in normal serum by hydrogen peroxide and hydrogen peroxide-related oxygen radicals produced by activated neutrophils. Clin Exp Immunol. 1992;90(1):72–8.
72. Hilhorst M, van Paassen P, Tervaert JW. Proteinase 3-ANCA vasculitis versus myeloperoxidase-ANCA vasculitis. J Am Soc Nephrol. 2015;26(10):2314–27.
73. Falk RJ, Jennette JC. Anti-neutrophil cytoplasmic autoantibodies with specificity for myeloperoxidase in patients with systemic vasculitis and idiopathic necrotizing and crescentic glomerulonephritis. N Engl J Med. 1988;318(25):1651–7.
74. Jennette JC, Hoidal JR, Falk RJ. Specificity of anti-neutrophil cytoplasmic autoantibodies for proteinase 3. Blood. 1990;75(11):2263–4.

ANCA: Methods and Clinical Significance

4

Elena Csernok and Antonella Radice

4.1 Introduction

In 1982, Davies and colleagues [1] discovered the association of the *a*nti*n*eutrophil *c*ytoplasmic *a*ntibody (ANCA) in segmental necrotizing glomerulonephritis, and 3 years later, Van der Woude and coworkers [2] characterized their presence as a diagnostic tool and marker of disease in Wegener's granulomatosis. The spectrum of diseases associated with ANCA has since increased [3]. Two ANCA specificities are highly associated markers for the collectively called ANCA-associated vasculitides (AAV), which include granulomatosis with polyangiitis (GPA [Wegener's]), microscopic polyangiitis (MPA), eosinophil granulomatosis with polyangiitis (EGPA [Churg-Strauss syndrome]), and primary pauci-immune crescentic glomerulonephritis, namely proteinase 3 (PR3-ANCA) and myeloperoxidase (MPO-ANCA). By indirect immunofluorescence, two main fluorescence patterns can be recognized, a cytoplasmic fluorescence (C-ANCA), which usually occurs with PR3 specificity, and a perinuclear staining (P-ANCA), largely caused by MPO-ANCA. However, ANCA can be demonstrated in patients with inflammatory bowel disease (IBD), autoimmune liver disease, connective tissue diseases, infections, and drug-induced vasculitis, often with multiple antigen specificities and unclear clinical significance [3–5].

E. Csernok (✉)
Department of Internal Medicine, Rheumatology and Immunology,
Vasculitis-Center South Tübingen-Kirchheim, Medius Klinik Kirchheim, Akademisches Lehrkrankenhaus der Universität Tübingen, Kirchheim unter Teck, Germany
e-mail: e.csernok@medius-kliniken.de

A. Radice
Department of Microbiology and Virology, San Carlo Borromeo Hospital—ASST Santi Paolo e Carlo, Milan, Italy
e-mail: antonella.radice@asst-santipaolocarlo.it

R. A. Sinico, L. Guillevin (eds.), *Anti-Neutrophil Cytoplasmic Antibody (ANCA) Associated Vasculitis*, Rare Diseases of the Immune System,
https://doi.org/10.1007/978-3-030-02239-6_4

Detection of ANCA in vasculitis is based on primary screening by immunofluorescence test (IFT) on ethanol-fixed neutrophils, and positive IIF test should always be followed by a specific PR3-ANCA and MPO-ANCA immunoassays. Ideally, all three tests should be used in each sample [6, 7] Since the establishment of this consensus, many new antigen-specific immunoassays have become available, and this has challenged the position of IFT in the testing algorithm for ANCA in vasculitis [8, 9]. Furthermore, there is a need for screening algorithm including clinical gating policies to guide the flow of analysis in diagnostic laboratories. In the right clinical context, a positive test for PR3-ANCA or MPO-ANCA has high sensitivity and specificity for a diagnosis of AAV. The value of measuring ANCA during follow-up to predict relapse is controversial [10]. Recent studies have shown that the longitudinal ANCA measurements may be useful in patients with renal involvement and patients treated with rituximab [11, 12]. This chapter considers current data on ANCA testing, presents the new international consensus on ANCA testing, and discusses the usefulness of PR3-ANCA and MPO-ANCA in the diagnosing and managing of patients with small-vessel vasculitis.

4.2 Detection of ANCA in Small-Vessel Vasculitis

Standard methods for detection of ANCA include immunofluorescence technique on ethanol-fixed human neutrophils and antigen-specific immunoassays for PR3-ANCA and MPO-ANCA [6]. Three main patterns of fluorescence have been demonstrated with IFT on ethanol-fixed neutrophils. The first is a diffuse, granular cytoplasmic neutrophil fluorescence with central interlobular accentuation ("C-ANCA") so noted overall in 90% of patients with active generalized GPA [3]. The second is perinuclear neutrophil staining pattern often with nuclear extension ("P-ANCA") so noted in those with MPA and EGPA. So-called atypical patterns (A-ANCA) are infrequent comprising a mix of cytoplasmic and perinuclear/nuclear fluorescence, with multiple antigen specificities, for example, in association with drug exposure, inflammatory bowel disease, rheumatoid arthritis, most often in the absence of vasculitis. The perinuclear/nuclear staining pattern actually is an artifact, and really, P-/A-ANCA causes a cytoplasmic staining after formalin fixation. The use of differentially fixed neutrophils (ethanol and formalin) allows differentiation between P- /A-ANCA and ANAs [8]. The alternative to conventional IFT is *image analysis*, which quantifies fluorescence in a single dilution of a patient sample in comparison with the intensity of standardized calibrators. Evaluation of the image analysis for the potential to detect ANCA in a cohort of a consecutive PR3-ANCA-positive GPA patients [13] revealed detectable ANCA levels in 75% of patients at the time of renal relapse, indicating a lower diagnostic sensitivity as compared with IFT and capture ELISA (100%). Quantitative image analysis predicted disease relapse somewhat better than IFT, but was comparable to direct ELISA [14].

Positive immunofluorescence results should be tested subsequently by antigen-specific tests for PR3-ANCA and MPO-ANCA [6]. The most frequently used tests to identify types of ANCA with different specificities are enzyme-linked immunosorbent assay (ELISA). However, a combination of both IFT and antigen-specific assays (PR3-ANCA and MPO-ANCA) was confirmed in several studies to be the best strategy for ANCA detection in vasculitis [15]. In addition to PR3 and MPO, other antigenic specificity for ANCA can be detected by ELISA screening for elastase, cathepsin G, bactericidal increasing protein, lactoferrin, and other. These ANCA specificities have no diagnostic value for patients with AAV.

Although many studies report particular epitopes of PR3 and MPO, routine testing for epitopes of major ANCA antigens has not been accomplished.

Over the last decade, several new developments in the ANCA detection techniques, in particular, PR3-ANCA and MPO-ANCA detection, such as addressable-laser-bead immunoassays (ALBIA), chemiluminescent immunoassays (CLIA), dot-/line-immunoassays, and fluorescent-enzyme immunoassays (FEIA) have been introduced (for review, see [8, 9, 16]). Besides, there have been advances in assay setup (antigen presentation) with development of second- (capture-based) and third- (anchor-based) generation assays. Most often, these novel assays have been clinically evaluated as an isolated entity, and this obviously hampers comparability due to distinct sample selection, study design, and data analysis. The specific applications of these novel techniques could improve and simplify ANCA testing in vasculitis.

Dot blot is a qualitative technique, with antigen coated to a nitrocellulose strip. This assay is especially suitable for examination of a single serum in case of emergency, because it is a single strip preparation. For rapid ANCA testing, a biochip technology has also been developed [17]. In this assay, IFT is combined with a dot blot test for PR3-ANCA and MPO-ANCA. However, the results obtained are only qualitative and should be confirmed and quantified by other ANCA assays.

4.3 Revised 2017 International Consensus on ANCA Testing in Small-Vessel Vasculitis

The emergence of new detection technologies, automated platforms, and laboratory environments has led to updating of the standardization process and a revision of existing ANCA detection strategies. Recent European Vasculitis Study Group (EUVAS) multicenter study has compared the diagnostic performance of manual and automated IIF with various antigen-specific immunoassays for ANCA detection [18–21]. Four international vasculitis centers (Klinikum Bad Bramstedt, Germany; Staten Serum Institute, Denmark; Maastricht University Medical Centre, The Netherlands, and University Hospitals Leuven, Belgium) contributed newly diagnosed GPA (total n = 186) and MPA (total n = 65) patients and relevant diseased controls (total n = 924). The antigen-specific immunoassays evaluated (n = 8) were from seven manufacturers and included first-, second-, and third-generation assays applied on different technological platforms (ALBIA, CLIA, ELISA, and FEIA). For manual IIF, two different approaches were used. The original approach described in 1989 (Copenhagen) used an ethanol-fixed mixture of neutrophils and lymphocytes, whereas the other approach (Bad Bramstedt) used ethanol-fixed neutrophils in combination with additional tests on formalin-fixed neutrophils and HEp-2 cells to better discriminate between MPO-related P-ANCA and ANA reactivity [8, 22].

The results of the study revealed a large variability between IIF methods, and variation in pattern assignment between IIF methods [18]. The area under the curve (AUC, 95% CI) of the receiver operating characteristics (ROC) curve to discriminate AAV from controls considerably differed for the two IIF methods with AUC values of 0.925 (0.904–0.946) and 0.848 (0.821–0.876), respectively. By contrast, PR3-ANCA and MPO-ANCA by immunoassay had a somewhat higher diagnostic performance, with AUCs (95% CI) that only varied between 0.936 (0.912–0.960) and 0.959 (0.941–0.976), except for one immunoassay for which the AUC was 0.919 (0.892–0.945) [19]. This study, which was performed on diagnostic samples obtained from patients without immunosuppressive treatment, did not reveal consistent differences between different assay generations and formats. It should be mentioned that there were some AAV patients that tested negative by both IIF and immunoassay or by either immunoassay or IIF. Thus, a diagnosis of AAV cannot be excluded for ANCA-negative patients as well as the opposite.

New guidelines for ANCA testing have been developed based on these data. According to the revised 2017 international consensus recommendations, testing for ANCA in small-vessel vasculitis can be done by PR3-ANCA and MPO-ANCA immunoassays, without the categorical need for IIF. Thus, IIF can be discarded completely or can be used as confirmation assays instead of as screening test [21]. Finally, these data challenged the role of IIF in the ANCA testing algorithm, and consequently, the earlier international consensus on ANCA detection utilizing dual IIF/antigen-specific immunoassay testing of each sample was revised [21].

4.4 Clinical Usefulness of ANCA Testing

At present, ANCA testing is a noninvasive diagnostic tool widely used by clinicians when considering a diagnosis of AAV. The most relevant clinical issue is accurate identification of all patients with active AAV and avoidance of any misdiagnosis. For patients with inflammatory conditions of unknown origin, it is better to use ANCA tests with high specificity rather than high sensitivity for vasculitis. The highest specificity is obtained by antigen-specific immunoassays [18, 19]. With this strategy, PR3-ANCA or MPO-ANCA is detectable in nearly all patients with active generalized GPA or MPA, but only in approximately 60% of patients with limited ("initial phase") disease [23] and about 40% of patients affected by EGPA [24]. In cases of emergency, such as the pulmo-renal syndrome, several rapid screening assays for ANCA are available [9]. If the results are clearly PR3-ANCA or MPO-ANCA positive, immunosuppressive therapy should be started immediately. However, patients with ANCA should receive a careful workup, because conditions other than vasculitis, such infections or drugs, may be implicated in the presence of ANCA and may be dramatically worsened by immunosuppression. Thus, rapid ANCA tests may be helpful as an adjunct to urgent therapeutic decisions, but they cannot supplant the need for critical appraisal of all findings including the patient's history, clinical and imaging results, as well as other laboratory result. Histological confirmation of vasculitis is still the gold-standard and should be sought in every patient.

Whereas PR3-ANCA and MPO-ANCA have been shown to be highly specific for AAV, their diagnostic value in nonvasculitic conditions is very limited. An overestimation of the diagnostic relevance of a positive ANCA test may erroneously misdirect clinicians and delay adequate treatment. The diagnostic accuracy of ANCA testing in vasculitis should be improved by an increased pretest probability [20].

4.4.1 Gating Policy

Accurate identification of all patients with AAV and the avoidance of misdiagnosis can be achieved by the use of a "gating policy" based on clinical information given to the laboratory at the time of request. This policy limits requests for ANCA testing exclusively to clinical scenarios that may suggest a diagnosis of necrotizing vasculitis [20, 21]. Two studies demonstrated that a "gating policy," based on the consensus statement clinical ordering guidelines for ANCA testing, makes ANCA screening clinically more relevant [25, 26]. Recently, Arnold et al. investigated the impact of a "gating policy" at a single regional center in the year prior to and following the consensus guidelines, and they demonstrated that adherence to a "gating policy" for ANCA testing coupled with close liaison between clinician and laboratory does not result in either a missed or delayed diagnosis of AAV [27].

4.4.2 Utility of ANCA in Managing Disease Activity and Guidance Therapy

Controversial results have been published on the utility of ANCA for monitoring disease activity and guidance of treatment decisions in AAV. A meta-analysis of nine studies concluded that the value of serial measurements of ANCA in patients in remission is limited. Neither the increase nor the persistence of ANCA in patients who achieved remission is highly predictive of relapse [10]. Anyway, Fussner and Specks summarized the studies on the relationship between ANCA levels and disease activity. They concluded that these various studies are difficult to compare because of many factors such as disease pattern, antigen specificity, assay used for testing, interval between taking samples, and treatment regimens [28]. Kemna et al. tested a cohort of 166 patients with PR3-ANCA or MPO-ANCA-associated vasculitis for predictive value of a rise in ANCA levels for relapsing diseases [12]. Rises of the ANCA titer were correlated with relapses in patients with renal involvement (hazard ratio 11.09; 95% CI, 5.01–24.55), whereas relapses in patients with nonrenal disease were less well associated with rise in ANCA values (hazard ratios 2.79; 95% CI, 1.30–5.98). Recently, Fussner and colleagues describe a comprehensive analysis of serial ANCA measurements in patients with AAV who were prospectively followed up after treatment with rituximab or cyclophosphamide and azathioprine within the Rituximab in ANCA-associated Vasculitis (RAVE) trial. They confirm the findings of early publications that an increase in PR3-ANCA levels is not a very sensitive and specific predictor of a subsequent relapse in general. However, an increase in PR3-ANCA titers detected by ELISA was associated with severe relapses (hazard ratio 4.57), particularly in patients with renal involvement (hazard ratio 7.94) and alveolar hemorrhage (hazard ratio 24.19) [11]. Thus, rises in ANCA titers during follow-up of AAV patients in the absence of signs of relapse should prompt intensification of monitoring measures such as more frequent urinalysis. However, the recent EULAR recommendations for the management of AAV state that treatment decisions during patient follow-up should rather be based on clinical evaluation and not on changes of the ANCA serology alone [29].

4.5 Proteinase 3-ANCA and Myeloperoxidase-ANCA Subtype: Useful Tool for Disease Classification in Small-Vessel Vasculitis

Several clinical and pathological classification systems exist that aim to define homogeneous groups among patients with AAV; however, considerable debate surrounds this classification. Existing classification systems have relied on combinations of different clinical, radiographic, and histological findings, but have not included ANCA specificity. Accumulating evidence suggests that ANCA specificity could be better than clinical diagnosis for defining groups of patients, as PR3-ANCA and MPO-ANCA are associated with different genetic backgrounds, epidemiology, and pathogenesis. The new classification approach of AAV is to use ANCA serotypes to classify disease and provide immediate diagnosis based on the presence of PR3-ANCA and/or MPO-ANCA. It was demonstrated that serotyping distinguishes distinct classes of ANCA disease: PR3-ANCA-associated vasculitides (PR3-AAV), MPO-ANCA-associated vasculitides (MPO-AAV), and ANCA-negative vasculitides (for review, see [30]).

4.5.1 Epidemiological and Genetic/Epigenetic Features vs. ANCA Specificity

Today, epidemiological evidence indicates that AAVs develop as a result of complex gene–environment interactions. The nature of these risks factors and pathogenic mechanisms involved, however, are only just beginning to be understood.

The incidence of PR3-AAV and MPO-AAV is different over the world. There is substantial heterogeneity between different geographic regions: PR3-AAV has a higher prevalence in north-western Europe and North-America, whereas MPO-AAV is more common in southern Europe and Asia [31–33]. In PR3-AAV, it has been shown that lower vitamin D levels play a role in the disease and that PR3-ANCA-positive patients but not MPO-ANCA-positive patients who carry nasal *S.*

aureus chronically are at higher risk for disease relapse. Furthermore, in MPO-AAV, silica exposure is thought to contribute to disease [32].

The genetic data from genome-wide studies (GWAS) and African-American population point to genetic differences between PR3-ANCA and MPO-ANCA patients. These studies have shown that the autoantigen specificities PR3 and MPO correlate better with different HLA risk genes (PR3-ANCA with HLA-DP, MPO-ANCA with HLA-DQ) than with the clinical and pathological phenotypes of GPA and MPA [34]. Moreover, the association with the genes encoding PR3 (PTN3) and its inhibitor α-1-antitrypsin (SERPINA1) with PR3-ANCA disease and/or GPA supports additionally a central pathogenetic role of autoantigens and their neutralizing counterparts [34].

There are also biological differences in epigenetic expression of MPO and PR3, and in glycosylation of PR3-ANCA vs. MPO-ANCA. Recently, a further epigenetic silencing defect involving DNA methylation was identified: DNA was unmethylated at CpG island in *PR3*, in both patients and controls, whereas in healthy controls, DNA was methylated at CpG island of *MPO* [35]. Altogether, these results suggest that epigenetic deregulation underlines further distinction between PR3-ANCA and MPO-ANCA-positive patients.

4.5.2 ANCA Specificity and Clinical/Histological Features

Clinical features differ both in the type and in frequency between PR3-AAV and MPO-AAV. PR3-AAV is associated with granulomatous inflammation, respiratory tract involvement, more extensive extra-renal organ manifestation, and a higher relapse rate [36, 37]. In contrast, MPO-AAV is more frequent in kidney-limited disease, displays more severe renal scarring, and is a worse renal prognosis. Furthermore, patients with MPO-ANCAs are more likely than patients with PR3-ANCAs to have renal pathology classified as mixed or sclerotic and to have a strong association with lung fibrosis [38, 39].

Among patients receiving a clinical diagnosis of GPA, those positive for MPO-ANCAs more frequently have limited disease without severe organ involvement, a higher prevalence of subglottic stenosis, a less frequent need for cyclophosphamide or rituximab therapy, and fewer relapses than patients who are positive for PR3-ANCA [40–42]. A study of more than 700 patients with GPA or MPA from five different randomized controlled trials found that the addition of ANCA specificity to a clinical-only clustering strategy improved the classification of patients into distinct categories with different outcomes (for review, see [30]). These data indicate again that ANCA specificity is a major determinant of the clinical presentation in AAV.

In summary, the classification of patients by ANCA specificity (PR3-ANCAs versus MPO-ANCAs) provides practical diagnostic criteria better aligned to patient phenotype, outcomes, and treatment responses than does their classification by clinical diagnosis (GPA vs. MPA and EGPA).

4.6 Conclusion

ANCA serology and the associated clinical manifestation of AAV continue to attract the attention of clinicians and investigators alike. In addition to be providing a useful diagnostic tool for small-vessel vasculitis, ANCA testing may be useful in predicting relapses and in guiding therapy. The revised consensus recommendations on ANCA testing state that high-quality antigen-specific immunoassays are the preferred screening methodology for the diagnosis of ANCA-associated vasculitis. When the pretest probability of the disease is high (appropriate request), performing IFT adds little to antigen-specific assays in the diagnosis of ANCA-associated vasculitis.

Notwithstanding, any testing strategy applicable to vasculitis should be able to identify relevant ANCA target antigens (PR3 and MPO) since these correlate best with the clinicopathological aspects, disease activity, propensity for relapse, and response to therapy.

References

1. Davies DJ, Moran JE, Niall JF, et al. Segmental necrotizing glomerulonephritis with antineutrophil antibody: possible arbovirus aetiology? Br Med J. 1982;285:606.
2. Van der Woude FJ, Rasmussen N, Lobatto S. Autoantibodies against neutrophils and monocytes: tool for diagnosis and marker of disease activity in Wegener's granulomatosis. Lancet. 1985;1:425–9.
3. Csernok E, Lamprecht P, Gross WL. Diagnostic significance of ANCA in vasculitis. Nat Clin Pract Rheumatol. 2006;2(4):174–5.
4. Kallenberg CGM. Usefulness of antineutrophil cytoplasmic autoantibodies in diagnosing and managing systemic vasculitis. Rheumatology. 2015;28(1):1–14.
5. Sinico RA, Radice A. Antineutrophil cytoplasmic antibodies (ANCA) testing: detection methods and clinical application. Clin Exp Rheumatol. 2014;32:S112.
6. Savige J, Gillis D, Benson E, et al. International consensus statement on testing and reporting of antineutrophil cytoplasmic antibodies (ANCA). Am J Clin Pathol. 1999;111:507–13.
7. Savige J, Dimech W, Fritzler M, et al. Addendum to the International Consensus Statement on testing and reporting of antineutrophil cytoplasmic antibodies. Quality control guidelines, comments, and recommendations for testing in other autoimmune diseases. Am J Clin Pathol. 2003;120:312–8.
8. Csernok E, Moosig F. Current and emerging techniques for ANCA detection in vasculitis. Nat Rev Rheumatol. 2014;10:494–501.
9. Cohen Tervaert JW, Damoiseaux J. Antineutrophil cytoplasmic autoantibodies: how are they detected and what is their use for diagnosis, classification and follow-up? Clin Rev Allergy Immunol. 2012;43:211–9.
10. Tomasson G, Grayson PC, Mahr AD, Lavalley M, Merkel PA. Value of ANCA measurements during remission to predict a relapse of ANCA-associated vasculitis - a meta-analysis. Rheumatology (Oxford). 2012;51:100–9.
11. Fussner LA, Hummel AM, Schroeder DR, et al. Factors determining the clinical utility of serial measurements of ANCA targeting proteinase 3. Arthritis Rheumatol. 2016;68:1700–10.
12. Kemna MJ, Damoiseaux J, Austen J, et al. ANCA as predictor of relapse: useful in patients with renal involvement but not i9n patients with nonrenal disease. J Am Soc Nephrol. 2015;26:537–42.
13. Boomsma MM, Damoiseaux FGMC, Stegeman CA, et al. Image analysis: a novel approach for the quantification of ANCA levels in patients with Wegener's granulomatosis. J Immunol Methods. 2003;274:27–35.

14. Knütter I, Hiemann R, Brumma T, et al. Automated interpretation of ANCA patterns - a new approach in the serology of ANCA-associated vasculitis. Arthritis Res Ther. 2012;14(6):R271.
15. Choi HK, Liu S, Merkel PA, et al. Diagnostic performance of antineutrophil cytoplasmic antibody tests for idiopathic vasculitides: metaanalysis with a focus on antimyeloperoxidase antibodies. J Rheumatol. 2001;28:1584–90.
16. Radice A, Bianchi L, Sinico RA. Anti-neutrophil cytoplasmic autoantibodies: methodological aspects and clinical significance in systemic vasculitis. Autoimmun Rev. 2013;12:487–95.
17. Damoiseaux J, Steller U, Buschtez M, et al. EUROPLUS ANCA BIOCHIP mosaic: PR3 and MPO antigen microdots improve the laboratory diagnostics of ANCA-associated vasculitis. J Immunol Methods. 2009;348(1-2):67–73.
18. Csernok E, Damoiseaux J, Rasmussen N, et al. Evaluation of automated multi-parametric indirect immunofluorescence assays to detect anti-neutrophil cytoplasmic antibodies (ANCA) in granulomatosis with polyangiitis (GPA) and microscopic polyangiitis (MPA). Autoimmun Rev. 2016;15:736–41.
19. Damoiseaux J, Csernok E, Rasmussen N, et al. Detection of antineutrophil cytoplasmic antibodies (ANCAs): a multicentre European Vasculitis Study Group (EUVAS) evaluation of the value of indirect immunofluorescence (IIF) versus antigen-specific immunoassays. Ann Rheum Dis. 2017;76:647–53.
20. Bossuyt X, Rasmussen N, van Paassen P, et al. A multicentre study to improve clinical interpretation of proteinase-3 and myeloperoxidase anti-neutrophil cytoplasmic antibodies. Rheumatology. 2017a;56:1533. https://doi.org/10.1093/rheumatology/kex170.
21. Bossuyt X, Cohen Tervaert JW, Arimura Y, et al. Revised 2017 international consensus on testing of ANCAs in granulomatosis with polyangiitis and microscopic polyangiitis. Nat Rev Rheumatol. 2017b;13:683. https://doi.org/10.1038/nrrheum.2017.140.
22. Wiik A, Rasmussen N, Wieslander J. Methods to detect autoantibodies to neutrophilic granulocytes. Man Biol Markers Dis. 1993;A9:1–14.
23. Holle JU, Gross WL, Holl-Ulrich K, et al. Prospective long-term follow-up of patients with localised Wegener's granulomatosis: does it occur as persistent disease stage? Ann Rheum Dis. 2010;69:1934–9.
24. Sinico RA, Di Toma L, Maggiore U, et al. Prevalence and clinical significance of antineutrophil cytoplasmic antibodies in Churg-Strauss syndrome. Arthritis Rheum. 2005;52:2926.
25. Mandl LA, Solomon DH, Smith EL, Lew RA, Katz JN, Shmerling RH. Using antineutrophil cytoplasmic antibody testing to diagnose vasculitis: can test-ordering guidelines improve diagnostic accuracy? Arch Intern Med. 2002;162:1509–14.
26. Sinclair D, Saas M, Stevens JM. The effect of a symptom related "gating policy" on ANCA requests in routine clinical practice. J Clin Pathol. 2004;57:131–4.
27. Arnold DF, Timms A, Luqmani R, Misbah SA. Does a gating policy for ANCA overlook patients with ANCA associated vasculitis? An audit of 263 patients. J Clin Pathol. 2010;63:678–80.
28. Fussner LA, Specks U. Can antineutrophil cytoplasmic antibody levels be used to inform treatment of pauci-immune vasculitis? Curr Opin Rheum. 2015;27:231–40.
29. Mukhtyar C, Guillevin L, Cid MC, et al. EULAR recommendations for the management of primary small and medium vessel vasculitis. Ann Rheum Dis. 2016;68:310–7.
30. Cornec D, Cornec-Le Gall E, Fervenza FC, Specks U. ANCA-associated vasculitis – clinical utility of using ANCA specificity to classify patients. Nat Rev Rheumatol. 2016;12:570–9.
31. Watts R, Lane S, Hanslik T, et al. Development and validation of a consensus methodology for the classification of the ANCA-associated vasculitides and polyarteritis nodosa for epidemiological studies. Ann Rheum Dis. 2007;66:222–7.
32. Ntatsaki E, Watts RA, Scott DG. Epidemiology of ANCA-associated vasculitis. Rheum Dis Clin North Am. 2010;36:447–61.
33. Scott DG, Watts RA. Epidemiology and clinical features of systemic vasculitis. Clin Exp Nephrol. 2013;17:607–10.
34. Lyons PA, Rayner TF, Trivedi S, et al. Genetically distinct subsets within ANCA-associated vasculitis. N Engl J Med. 2012;367:214–23.

35. Ciavatta DJ, Yang J, Preston G, et al. Epigenetic basis for aberrant up regulation of autoantigen genes in humans with ANCA vasculitis. J Clin Investig. 2010;120:3209–19.
36. Franssen CF, Stegeman CA, Kallenberg CG, et al. Antiproteinase 3- and antimyeloperoxidase-associated vasculitis. Kidney Int. 2000;57:2195–206.
37. Schönermarck U, Lamprecht P, Csernok E, Gross WL. Prevalence and spectrum of rheumatic diseases associated with proteinase 3-antineutrophil cytoplasmic antibodies (ANCA) and myeloperoxidase-ANCA. Rheumatology. 2001;40:178–84.
38. Hauer HA, Bajema IM, van Houwelingen HC, et al. Renal histology in ANCA-associated vasculitis: differences between diagnostic and serologic subgroups. Kidney Int. 2002;61:80–9.
39. Quintana LF, Peréz NS, De Sousa E, et al. ANCA serotype and histopathological classification for the prediction of renal outcome in ANCA-associated glomerulonephritis. Nephrol Dial Transplant. 2014;29:1764.
40. Lionaki S, Blyth ER, Hogan SL, et al. Classification of antineutrophil cytoplasmic autoantibody vasculitides: the role of antineutrophil cytoplasmic autoantibody specificity for myeloperoxidase or proteinase 3 in disease recognition and prognosis. Arthritis Rheum. 2012;64:3452–62.
41. Mahr A, Katsahian S, Varet H, et al. Revisiting the classification of clinical phenotypes of anti-neutrophil cytoplasmic antibody-associated vasculitis: a cluster analysis. Ann Rheum Dis. 2013;72:1003–10.
42. Hagen EC, Daha MR, Hermans J, et al. Diagnostic value of standardized assays for anti-neutrophil cytoplasmic antibodies in idiopathic systemic vasculitis. EC/BCR Project for ANCA Assay Standardization. Kidney Int. 1998;53:743–53.

Activity and Damage

5

Raashid A. Luqmani

5.1 Introduction

The underlying pathogenesis of the vasculitides is complex and varies between conditions, but the clinical manifestations can be similar. The pattern of disease involvement tends to vary, with a greater likelihood of significant nephritis and lung hemorrhage in MPA, while in GPA, upper airways disease is a dominant feature; by contrast, nephritis is less common in EGPA. However, in all three main forms of AAV, there is potential for overlapping clinical features; furthermore, the treatments used are similar at present, resulting in similar drug toxicity profiles for these patients. Documenting the nature of each condition and defining the severity of involvement for each patient allows the clinician to formulate a treatment plan. We will discuss how best to evaluate patients, to document their treatment needs, and to measure their response to therapy and outcome. These assessments have become a core feature of clinical trials in AAV and form the basis for sound clinical management of these complex conditions.

5.2 How Can Laboratory Measures Help?

The use of conventional inflammatory markers (C-reactive protein [CRP] and erythrocyte sedimentation [ESR]) to assess disease activity in AAV is limited by their lack of specificity, particularly in case of concomitant infections or other immune-mediated conditions. Although they are routinely used to aid clinical decisions, their

R. A. Luqmani (✉)
Nuffield Department of Orthopaedics, Rheumatology and Musculoskeletal Science, University of Oxford, Oxford, UK

Rheumatology Department, Nuffield Orthopaedic Centre, Oxford, UK
e-mail: raashid.luqmani@ndorms.ox.ac.uk

R. A. Sinico, L. Guillevin (eds.), *Anti-Neutrophil Cytoplasmic Antibody (ANCA) Associated Vasculitis*, Rare Diseases of the Immune System,
https://doi.org/10.1007/978-3-030-02239-6_5

results and changes in values should be interpreted with caution before considering any treatment modifications [1, 2].

GPA, MPA, and, to a lesser extent, EGPA are strongly associated with the presence of antineutrophil cytoplasmic antibodies (ANCAs) [3]. ANCA can be detected by indirect immunofluorescence (IIF), where a cytoplasmic pattern (C-ANCA) or a perinuclear pattern (P-ANCA) is identified, or by antigen-specific tests targeting proteinase 3 (PR3) or myeloperoxidase (MPO). PR3-ANCA, which is typically associated with a cytoplasmic pattern, is found in 80–90% of patients with the diagnosis of granulomatosis with polyangiitis (GPA); MPO-ANCA, usually associated with a perinuclear pattern, is present in 60–80% of patients with the diagnosis of microscopic polyangiitis (MPA) and 25–40% of patients with eosinophilic granulomatosis with polyangiitis (EGPA) [4]. Hence, ANCAs are an integral part of the diagnostic workup of patients with suspected AAV, even though not all cases of AAV actually have ANCA.

However, there is much less agreement over the value of measuring serial ANCA titers to assess disease activity and predict relapse. Although early studies using IIF [5, 6] advocated that serial ANCA measurements provided a sensitivity of around 100% in the prediction of relapse when a rise in the titer was observed, subsequent studies reported sensitivity below 45% [7, 8]. In 2006, a systematic review of the available literature was conducted to investigate the value of serial ANCA testing for monitoring patients with AAV [9]. However, it was unable to provide firm conclusions due to considerable methodological heterogeneity, particularly regarding the techniques used for ANCA determination, definition of ANCA increase, different frequency of sampling, and variations in the definitions of disease activity, relapse, or remission. A more recent meta-analysis [10] suggested a modest, but statistically significant, positive likelihood ratio of 2.84 (95% CI 1.65, 4.90) of a future relapse when a rise in ANCA was detected during remission. Moreover, persistently positive ANCA during remission was associated with a positive likelihood ratio of 1.97 (95% CI 1.43, 2.70) of a subsequent relapse, suggesting that serial ANCA testing might have some albeit limited value in predicting relapse.

Animal models have been used to demonstrate that ANCAs target MPO or PR3, which leads to the induction of glomerulonephritis and pulmonary capillaritis [11, 12]; by contrast, ANCAs directed against proteinase 3 fail to induce granulomatous inflammation [19]. On this basis, Kemna et al. and Fussner et al. [12, 13] investigated the role of serial ANCA measurements (PR3 or MPO) in patients with or without renal involvement and demonstrated a strong association between rise in titer and disease relapse (HR 11.09 [95% CI 5.01–24.55]) for patients with renal disease, when compared to patients without renal manifestations (HR 2.79 [95% CI 1.30–5.98]). These findings were supported by data from a clinical trial of AAV [14, 15], which showed that a rise in PR3-ANCA levels during complete remission was strongly associated with the risk of a subsequent severe relapse (HR 4.57 [95% CI 2.16–10.37]), particularly in patients with renal involvement (HR 7.94 [95% CI 2.72–29.18]) and alveolar hemorrhage (HR 24.19 [95% CI 3.05–447.2]); by contrast, there was no association between PR3-ANCA levels and disease relapse in patients with a granulomatous phenotype. Moreover, many other studies have documented that patients with PR3-ANCA have a higher risk of relapse when compared to patients with MPO-ANCA [16–22]. Therefore, although the use of serial ANCA testing remains debatable for monitoring disease activity, it may potentially aid clinical decisions by taking into account other features of the disease, such as ANCA type, specific organ involvement, and ongoing treatment.

Other laboratory markers are currently being investigated for potential use in monitoring disease activity. Urinary soluble CD163, a protein expressed by macrophages and monocytes, has been strongly associated with active renal vasculitis [23]; antibodies against lysosome-associated membrane protein 2 (LAMP-2), frequently found in patients with pauci-immune glomerulonephritis, have shown to correlate with disease activity [24]; antibodies against plasminogen [25], identified in approximately 25% of patients with AAV, have been associated with more severe glomerular involvement and a higher incidence of thrombotic events; antibodies against moesin, present in around 50% of patients with MPO-ANCA, have been reported in more severe cases of AAV [26]; and the serum proteins CXCL13, MMP-3, and TIMP-1 have been shown to discriminate active disease from remission [26]. However, further studies with larger series are required to establish the validity of these findings.

5.3 Clinical Disease Activity and Damage Measures

Given the uncertainty over use of ANCA testing or other serological measurements of disease status in AAV discussed above, the most widely used assessments to document disease status are based primarily on clinical evaluation of the patient. The Birmingham Vasculitis Activity Score (BVAS) is the most effective validated tool to document disease activity and to be used as definition for remission and response to therapy as well as flare (and is discussed in detail in the next section). The BVAS consists of typical features of active systemic vasculitis related to each body system, with each item recorded as present only if the clinician judges it to be due to active vasculitis [27, 28]. This is semisubjective because some of the active evidence is sought from the patient history and physical examination and cannot always be confirmed with more objective testing. However, the BVAS is valid, is reliable, and has been widely used in clinical trials in vasculitis to define the responsiveness to various agents, including cyclophosphamide, methotrexate, mycophenolate, intravenous immunoglobulin, and rituximab. It is a valuable tool for the clinicians and strongly recommended as a regular part of disease management in small- and medium-vessel vasculitis. Other versions of BVAS have been validated for use in individual forms of vasculitis, such as the BVAS/Wegener's granulomatosis for patients with GPA. The Disease Extent Index (DEI) is similar to the BVAS but with less items and represents a combination of activity and damage in AAV [29].

The Vasculitis Damage Index (VDI) is designed to document the damage occurring as a result of having a diagnosis of vasculitis (and is described in more detail below). VDI could be regarded as a cumulative measure to define the effectiveness of therapy (by limiting or preventing the accumulation of damage items). The VDI is strongly correlated with future mortality risk. The presence of at least five VDI items (on a scale of 0–64 items), when measured 6 months from diagnosis (and which occurs in about a third of patients) [30], is associated with a much higher future mortality (approximately sixfold higher) than patients with less than five items of damage [31]. The Combined Damage Assessment (CDA) is an expanded list of damage items, based on the VDI, with more detail, and includes weighting and reversibility of damage items. Its performance is, however, inferior to the VDI [32]. Prognosis can also be assessed using the Five-Factor Score [33] revised for use in AAV, which defines older age, the presence of renal, cardiac, or gastrointestinal involvement as adverse features, while upper airways involvement is associated with a more favorable prognosis. A score has been proposed for prognosis in MPA (Japanese Vasculitis Activity Score), based on age, creatinine, inflammatory marker levels, and the presence or absence of lung involvement [34], but not yet validated.

There is an increasing interest in the role of patient-reported outcomes as a measure of the impact of disease on patient function, and although until now the only measures in use are generic ones such as SF36 and EQ-5D, a disease-specific measure for use in AAV is being developed [35] (Table 5.1).

5.4 Disease Activity Assessment in Vasculitis

5.4.1 BVAS, BVAS WG, and PVAS

Careful assessment of disease activity in AAV is critical to guide treatment decisions, monitor progress, and ensure the appropriate use of potentially toxic therapies. We will describe the Birmingham Vasculitis Activity Score version 3 (BVAS v3) in more detail below but summarize similarities and differences with BVAS WG and PVAS in Table 5.2. BVAS v1–v3 are validated objective measures of disease activity in systemic vasculitis. BVAS is a practical, easy to use (with training) tool in standard clinical practice, recording features attributable to active vasculitis. It is based on the concept that features should be recorded if the treating clinician intends to give immunosuppressive therapy or escalate of immunosuppressive therapy due to the presence of active disease. This concept underpins the use of BVAS v3 because many of the items in BVAS v3 could result from other causes (including damage, infection, drug toxicity, or comorbidity). It is absolutely essential that the items recorded in BVAS v3 should only be recorded after consideration of the actual cause. For example, in a patient who develops a cough with purulent sputum and fever and new infiltrates on a chest X ray, it is more likely that the cause is a chest infection than a flare of vasculitis; hence, the fever and infiltrates should not be recorded in BVAS v3 if the clinician is intending to manage the problem without escalating immunosuppression (in this case, the clinician will probably treat the patient with antibiotics).

Table 5.1 Measures used to assess different aspects of disease status in AAV, it summarizes the main characteristics of these assessments

Assessment method	Status assessed				Comment
	Disease activity	Damage	Prognosis	Function	
Clinician-based evaluations					
Birmingham Vasculitis Activity Score (BVAS) Versions 1–3	x				All forms of vasculitis
Birmingham Vasculitis Activity Score (BVAS) for Wegener's granulomatosis (BVAS-WG)	x				Validated in patients with GPA, but used in other forms of vasculitis
Japanese Vasculitis Assessment Score (JVAS)			x		Predictive score for MPA for mortality risk based on renal function, lung involvement, CRP, and age
Vasculitis Damage Index (VDI)		x			Damage assessment in all forms of vasculitis
Combined Damage Assessment (CDA)		x			Not formally validated; used in some trials of patients with ANCA-associated vasculitis
Disease Extent Index (DEI)	x	x	x		Only developed for GPA
Five-Factor Score (FFS)			x		Validated and used in ANCA-associated vasculitis and PAN
Patient-reported assessments					
Short form 36				x	Generic for many conditions—has been evaluated in ANCA-associated vasculitis
EuroQOL				x	Generic for many conditions—has not been evaluated in ANCA-associated vasculitis
AAV-PRO				x	Currently being validated as a specific functional assessment in AAV

Table 5.2 Differences in items recorded in BVAS v3, BVAS WG and PVAS

System assessed	BVAS v3	BVAS WG	PVAS	Comments
General/ systemic features	Myalgia, arthralgia/arthritis, fever, weight loss	Arthritis, fever	Myalgia, arthralgia/arthritis, fever, weight loss	These are typical features in many forms of systemic vasculitis
Skin	Infarct, purpura, skin ulcer, gangrene	Purpura, skin ulcer, gangrene	Polymorphous exanthema, livedo, panniculitis, purpura, skin nodules, infarct, ulcer, gangrene, other skin vasculitis	Skin is commonly involved in most forms of small- and medium-vessel vasculitis. However, the skin manifestations in AAV are less severe compared to the effect on the kidneys, lungs, and upper airways. For skin vasculitis in children, the manifestations are more diverse
Mucous membrane/eyes	Mouth ulcers, genital ulcers, adnexal inflammation, proptosis, red eye (epi) scleritis, conjunctivitis, blepharitis, keratitis, blurred vision, visual loss, uveitis, retinal vasculitis	Mouth ulcer, conjunctivitis/ episcleritis, retro-orbital mass, uveitis, scleritis, retinal exudates	Mouth ulcers, genital ulcers, adnexal inflammation, proptosis, red eye (epi) scleritis, conjunctivitis, blepharitis, keratitis, blurred vision, visual loss, uveitis, retinal vasculitis	Eye involvement is most common in patients with GPA and less often seen in MPA or EGPA
Ear nose and throat (ENT)	Blood nasal discharge, paranasal sinus involvement, subglottic stenosis, conductive hearing loss, sensorineural hearing loss	Blood nasal discharge, paranasal sinus involvement, swollen salivary glands, subglottic inflammation, conductive hearing loss, sensorineural hearing loss	Blood nasal discharge, paranasal sinus involvement, subglottic stenosis, conductive hearing loss, sensorineural hearing loss	ENT manifestations are most common in GPA and rarely seen in MPA. EGPA is often characterized by the presence of rhinitis and nasal polyps which are inflammatory, but do not result in destructive necrotizing lesions seen in GPA

Chest	Wheeze, nodules or cavities, pleural effusion, infiltrate, endobronchial change, massive hemoptysis, respiratory failure	Nodules or cavities, pleurisy, infiltrate, endobronchial change, alveolar hemorrhage hemoptysis, respiratory failure	Wheeze, nodules or cavities, pleural effusion, infiltrate, endobronchial change, massive hemoptysis, respiratory failure	The chest is commonly affected in all three forms of AAV. Wheeze is very common in EGPA as are infiltrates. By contrast, infiltrates, nodules, and endobronchial manifestations dominate in GPA. Massive hemoptysis can occur in patients with GPA or MPA and occasionally in EGPA (of course, it is also a typical feature of patients with anti-glomerular basement membrane disease)
Cardiovascular system	Loss of pulses, ischemic cardiac pain, cardiomyopathy, congestive cardiac failure, valvular heart disease, pericarditis	Pericarditis	Loss of pulses, bruits, blood pressure discrepancy, claudication, ischemic cardiac pain, cardiomyopathy, congestive cardiac failure, valvular heart disease, pericarditis	Overt cardiovascular manifestations are probably most widely recognized in patients with EGPA and represent serious manifestations of the disease often requiring aggressive immunosuppression
Abdominal system	Ischemic abdominal pain, peritonitis, bloody diarrhea	Mesenteric ischemia	Abdominal pain, peritonitis, bloody diarrhea, bowel ischemia	Gut involvement is more typical in medium-vessel vasculitis especially polyarteritis nodosa, but is well recognized in patients with GPA especially with colitis giving rise to bloody diarrhea

(continued)

Table 5.2 (continued)

System assessed	BVAS v3	BVAS WG	PVAS	Comments
Renal system	Hypertension, proteinuria, hematuria, impaired renal function, deterioration in renal function	Hematuria, red cell casts or glomerulonephritis, deterioration in renal function	Hypertension, proteinuria, hematuria, impaired renal function, deterioration in renal function	Renal involvement is one of the major manifestations leading to organ failure and death especially in GPA and MPA (less commonly in EGPA) and should be carefully assessed
Nervous system	Headache, meningitis, organic confusion, seizures, stroke, cord involvement, cranial nerve, lesion, sensory or motor neuropathies	Meningitis, stroke, cord involvement, cranial nerve lesion, sensory or motor neuropathies	Headache, meningitis, organic confusion, seizures, stroke, cord involvement, cranial nerve, lesion, sensory or motor neuropathies	Neurological involvement is a common feature in AAV, especially EGPA; often, it does not lead to immediate loss of life. Strokes are less common features, whereas peripheral neuropathies are more common manifestations and can cause long-term residual dysfunction

BVAS v3 consists of a list of items from nine organ systems with the clinician required to document the presence or absence of each item. Each item is weighted, and a maximum score is applied to each system. When the scores from each system are added together, it gives a score from 0 to 63 (or 0–33 for persistent disease items), providing an overall measure of disease activity.

At the first assessment of vasculitis using BVAS, all features due to active vasculitis are scored irrespective of how long the features have been present. At subsequent evaluations, it is necessary to consider the duration that the features have been present before completing the form. Only those items, which are newly present or clearly worsening over the preceding 4 weeks, are scored.

The definition of persistent disease can be a difficult concept to grasp. Persistent disease for the purpose of BVAS v3 represents ongoing active vasculitis which, while it still requires immunosuppression, does not require escalation of therapy. By definition, we record items as "persistent" if they last up to 3 months, based on trials of vasculitis therapy showing that most patients no longer have any active disease features following 3 months of induction therapy. Persistent disease is not the same as damage, which should be recorded in the damage index. Persistent items should have been recorded as new or worse at a previous evaluation, but have not deteriorated since the last evaluation and which have been present for less than 3 months. If all the items to record are persistent, the "Persistent disease" box is ticked at the bottom right-hand corner of the BVAS v3 form. Persistent items have a lower weighting attached so that the overall BVAS v3 score reflects the low-grade nature of persistent disease, which usually would not require a change in treatment. However, items that have been present at a previous assessment but which have deteriorated and have been present for less than 3 months are considered as active disease and should be scored as new/worse. In general, for those items present longer than 3 months, they are often considered as due to damage and should be scored separately in the Vasculitis Damage Index (VDI) form.

In a number of patients during follow-up, there will be a mix of new/worse and persistent features present between assessments. In this case, all items are scored as representing active disease. The rationale for this is that the emergence of new features or the deterioration of existing features will likely lead to an escalation of immunosuppressive treatment, and the BVAS v3 scores should reflect this. Figure 5.1 is an algorithm to assist in completion of the BVAS v3 form.

The Paediatric Vascultis Activity Score (PVAS) is an objective measure of disease activity in childhood vasculitis. It is based on the intention to treat or escalate treatment model of BVAS and shares the same overarching principles but contains some additional items pertinent to a pediatric population [36] (Fig. 5.2).

5.5 Assessment of Damage in Vasculitis

5.5.1 VDI

The Vasculitis Damage Index (VDI) is a scoring system that records damage, irrespective of disease activity. Damage represents an irreversible state which does not

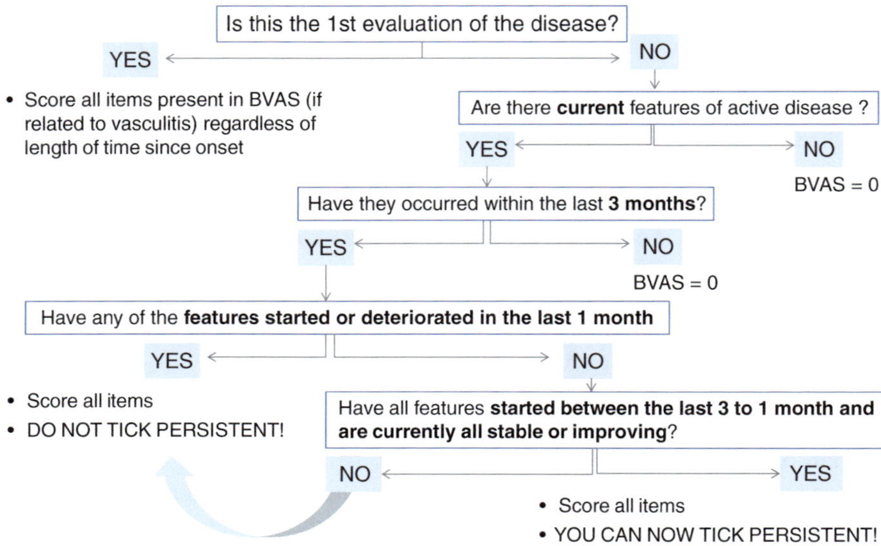

Fig. 5.1 An algorithm to indicate how to evaluate patients when using the BVAS v3 form

improve with increased immunosuppression. Regardless of whether features are attributable directly to vasculitis or not, if they occur after the onset of vasculitis and for most items, last for at least 3 months (even if they subsequently resolve), then they should be recorded in the VDI score. Some VDI items are individual events, such as a stroke or a myocardial infarction or a surgical procedure. In order to provide an equivalent way of recording these individual events, they are recorded in VDI at a time point at least 3 months after they occur. Since VDI is a cumulative measure of damage, the score never improves; it either remains stable over time or gets worse.

VDI measures the outcome of treatment in a different way from BVAS v3. It encompasses the irreversible scars of the disease as well as some of the adverse effects of treatment. If there are any items scored on VDI, we could interpret this as meaning that the instituted treatment was not enough to prevent damage, or indeed could have caused it. Although the current treatment strategies focus on controlling disease activity, in the long term, limiting the amount of damage experienced by a patient is likely to result in an improved overall outcome. High VDI values (at least five items recorded) are associated with a 6.4-fold increase in mortality risk (95% CI 2.1–19) [31] compared to patients with lower VDI values.

The VDI consists of a list of abnormalities occurring in ten systems: musculoskeletal, skin/mucous membranes, ocular, ENT, pulmonary, cardiovascular, peripheral vascular disease, gastrointestinal, renal, neuropsychiatric, and an additional 11th field for others (Fig. 5.1). The "other" section includes gonadal failure, marrow failure, diabetes, chemical cystitis, malignancy, and the opportunity to document any other unlisted feature that can be considered as damage. VDI can be performed by any health professional (see Sect. 5.8) [37].

A 62-year-old female presents for the first time with a 6 month history of nasal crusting and bloody nasal discharge. She has had a number of courses of antibiotics for extensive sinusitis confirmed on a recent CT without an improvement in her symptoms. More recently she has developed a cough associated with increasing shortness of breath. Her chest radiograph demonstrates cavitating pulmonary lesions. On systems review, arthralgia, myalgia and 10 kg of weight loss in the preceding 6 months are also noted. She is c-ANCA positive with a high titre of PR3 present. Histology from a nasal biopsy confirms a granulomatous inflammatory infiltrate, and she is commenced on appropriate therapy. Her BVAS from her initial visit is completed as follows:

Birmingham Vasculitis Activity Score (version 3)
Case Number:
Name: **Data of assessment :**

Tick an item **only** if attributable to active vasculitis. If there are no abnormalities in a section, please tick 'None' for that organ-system.

If **all** abnormalities are due to persistent disease (active vasculitis which is not new/worse in the prior 4 weeks), tick the **PERSISTENT** box at the bottom right corner

Is this the patient's first assessment? **Yes ■** **No □**

	None	Active disease
1. General	□	
Myalgia		■
Arthralgia / arthritis		■
Fever ≥38° C		□
Weight loss ≥2 kg		■
2. Cutaneous	■	
Infarct		□
Purpura		□
Ulcer		□
♦ **Gangrene**		□
Other skin vasculitis		□
3. Mucous membranes / eyes	■	
Mouth ulcers		□
Genital ulcers		□
Adnexal inflammation		□
Significant proptosis		□
Scleritis / Episcleritis		□
Conjunctivitis / Blepharitis / Keratitis		□
Blurred vision		□
Sudden visual loss		□
Uveitis		□
♦ **Retinal changes (vasculitis / thrombosis / exudate / haemorrhage)**		□
4. ENT	□	
Bloody nasal discharge / crusts / ulcers / granulomata		■
Paranasal sinus involvement		■
Subglottic stenosis		□
Conductive hearing loss		□
♦ **Sensorineural hearing loss**		□
Wheeze		□
Nodules or cavities		■
Pleural effusion / pleurisy		□
Infiltrate		□
Endobronchial involvement		□
♦ **Massive haemoptysis / alveolar haemorrhage**		□
♦ **Respiratory failure**		□

	None	Active disease
6. Cardiovascular	■	
Loss of pulses		□
Valvular heart disease		□
Pericarditis		□
♦ **Ischaemic cardiac pain**		□
♦ **Cardiomyopathy**		□
♦ **Congestive cardiac failure**		□
7. Abdominal	■	
Peritonitis		□
Bloody diarrhoea		□
♦ **Ischaemic abdominal pain**		□
8. Renal	■	
Hypertension		□
Proteinuria >1+		□
♦ **Haematuria ≥10 RBCs/hpf**		□
Creatinine 125-249μ/L(1.41-2.82mg/dl)*		□
Creatinine 250-499 μ/L(2.83-5.64mg/dl)*		□
♦ **Creatinine ≥500 μ/L (≥5.66mg/dl)***		□
♦ **Rise in serum creatinine >30% or fall in creatinine clearance >25%**		□
***Can only be scored on the first assessment**		
9. Nervous system	■	
Headache		□
Meningitis		□
Organic confusion		□
Seizures (not hypertensive)		□
♦ **Cerebrovascular accident**		□
♦ **Spinal cord lesion**		□
♦ **Cranial nerve palsy**		□
Sensory peripheral neuropathy		□
♦ **Mononeuritis multiplex**		□
10. Other	■	
a.		□
b.		□
c.		□
d.		□
PERSISTENT DISEASE ONLY: (Tick here if **all** the abnormalities are due to persistent disease)		□

♦ **Major items highlighted**

Fig. 5.2 Example of a case presentation and completed BVAS form

When completing the VDI, it is necessary to refer to previous assessments and patient records, in order to ensure that all the items previously recorded in former damage evaluations are also listed in the current record, in order to avoid underestimating the amount of damage. It is important to consider that some items of damage may develop unrelated to disease activity, such as hypertension. Although this is a common feature in patients with renal involvement, it may also develop in patients without renal involvement (due, in part, to glucocorticoid therapy).

Particular attention should be given to features that are a direct consequence of other lesions; for example, muscle wasting can be a direct consequence of peripheral neuropathy. When scoring the VDI, only the peripheral neuropathy should be recorded. Some items are always preceded by other items as is the case for the following: "Estimated/measured GFR $\leq$ 50%" prior to "end-stage renal failure"; "Subglottic stenosis (no surgery)" prior to subglottic stenosis (with surgery); "Visual impairment/diplopia" precedes "blindness"; "Blindness in one eye" precedes "Blindness in second eye" [37]. An algorithm for completing the VDI is shown in Fig. 5.3, with an example of a completed VDI in Fig. 5.4.

To limit interobserver variability, training in use of VDI is recommended (see below). A list of questions proposed for each item of the VDI score as well as other information and tips on how to complete the VDI score can be found in practical guides to using BVAS v3 and VDI [37]. The calculation for VDI is simple: each item is valued at one point and the score is cumulative. For each patient, we can calculate three possible scores—total VDI, system score, and critical damage score. Total score refers to the sum of all items and varies from 0 to 64. The system score refers to the extent of disease defined by the number of separate systems with at least one item scored. The critical damage score refers to the number of items of damage consistent with organ failure.

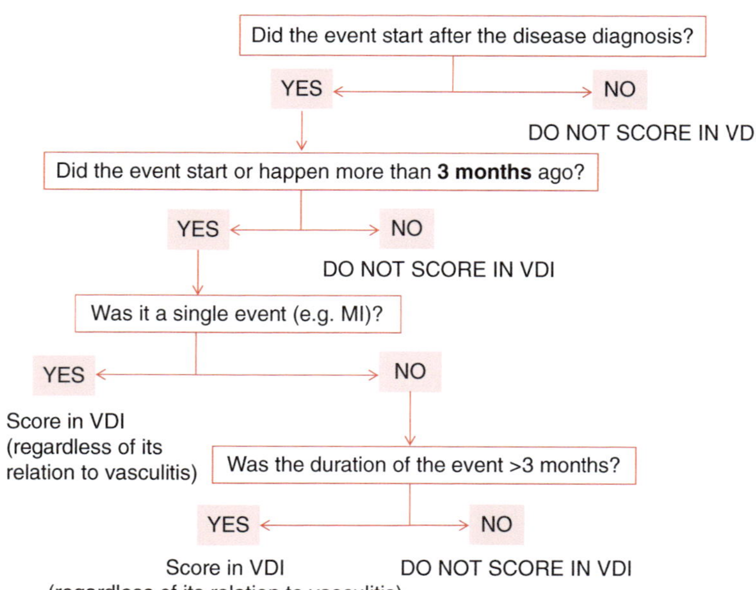

Fig. 5.3 Algorithm for completing the vasculitis damage index

An 82-year-old man presents with a 3-week history of generalised myalgia and weight loss.
On initial assessment, he is noted to have significant haematuria (+++, with 35 rbc/hpf) and proteinuria (+++) and kidney biopsy shows active glomerulonephritis. He has new onset of gangrene at the tips of the middle three fingers of the right hand and new ulcers on both legs. He is treated with glucocorticoids and cyclophosphamide. His creatinine at diagnosis is elevated at 600 μmol/L (6.78 mg/dL) and increases to >1,000 μmol/L (>11.3 mg/dL), with an estimated GFR of less than 50% of normal within 4 months of onset despite treatment.
He develops proteinuria of 3 g/24 h, which improves over the years but he has persistent proteinuria of 1.3 g/24 and reaches end-stage renal disease. He has got ulcers on his left leg, 4 months since the onset of his disease.
He sustained minor tissue loss at the pulp of the middle three fingers of the right hand, but the gangrene has otherwise healed well. He is very tired and weak with muscle wasting from atrophy (there is no neuropathy) in both legs.
He has developed a cataract in the right eye which was not previously present a month ago.
Figure adapted from Exley et al. [41].

VASCULITIS DAMAGE INDEX (VDI)
This is for recording organ damage that has occurred in patients **since the onset of vasculitis.** Patients often have co-morbidity before they develop vasculitis, **which must not be scored**. Record features of active disease using the Birmingham Vasculitis Activity Score (BVAS). A new patient should **usually have a VDI score of zero,** unless: (a) they have had vasculitis for more than three months of onset of disease and (b) the damage has developed or become worse since the onset of vasculitis.

Name
Trial Number
Date
Centre

1. Musculoskeletal	**No**	**Yes**
None	□	
Significant muscle atrophy or weakness		■
Deforming/erosive arthritis		□
Osteoporosis/vertebral collapse		□
Avascular necrosis		□
Osteomyelitis		□
Skin/Mucous membranes	**No**	**Yes**
None	□	
Alopecia		□
Cutaneous ulcers		■
Mouth ulcers		□
Ocular	**No**	**Yes**
None	■	
Cataract		□
Retinal change		□
Optic atrophy		□
Visual impairment/diplopia		□
Blindness in one eye		□
Blindness in second eye		□
Orbital wall destruction		□
ENT	**No**	**Yes**
None	■	
Hearing loss		□
Nasal blockage/chronic discharge/crusting		□
Nasal bridge collapse/septal perforation		□
Chronic sinusitis/radiological damage		□
Subglottic stenosis (no surgery)		□
Subglottic stenosis (with surgery)		□
Pulmonary	**No**	**Yes**
None	■	
Pulmonary hypertension		□
Pulmonary fibrosis		□
Pulmonary infarction		□
Pleural fibrosis		□
Chronic asthma		□
Chronic breathlessness		□
Impaired lung function		□
Cardiovascular	**No**	**Yes**
None	■	
Angina/angioplasty		□
Myocardial infarction		□
Subsequent myocardial infarction		□
Cardiomyopathy		□
Valvular disease		□
Pericarditis ≥ 3 mths or pericardectomy		□
Diastolic BP ≥ 95 or requiring antihypertensives		□

7. Peripheral vascular disease	**No**	**Yes**
None	□	
Absent pulses in one limb		□
2nd episode of absent pulses in one limb		□
Major vessel stenosis		□
Claudication >3 mths		□
Minor tissue loss		■
Major tissue loss		□
Subsequent major tissue loss		□
Complicated venous thrombosis		□
Gastrointestinal	**No**	**Yes**
None	■	
Gut infarction/resection		□
Mesenteric insufficiency/pancreatitis		□
Chronic peritonitis		□
Oesophageal stricture/surgery		□
Renal	**No**	**Yes**
None	□	
Estimated/measured GFR ≤ 50%		■
Proteinuria ≥ 0.5g/24hr		■
End stage renal disease		■
Neuropsychiatric	**No**	**Yes**
None	■	
Cognitive impairment		□
Major psychosis		□
Seizures		□
Cerebrovascular accident		□
2nd cerebrovascular accident		□
Cranial nerve lesion		□
Peripheral neuropathy		□
Transverse myelitis		□
Other	**No**	**Yes**
None	■	
Gonadal failure		□
Marrow failure		□
Diabetes		□
Chemical cystitis		□
Malignancy		□
Other		□

Total VDI Score. Record the number of positive Items (1 point for each). The VDI score can either increase or remain the same over time. **4**

Remember to carry forward any previous items of damage.

Fig. 5.4 Example of a completed VDI score

5.5.2 Main Differences When Scoring VDI Versus BVAS v3

Unlike BVAS v3, VDI records features which may not be directly caused by vasculitis as long as they occurred since the onset of vasculitis and lasted for more than 3 months.

Scoring items on VDI can be confusing, especially when a feature could apparently be scored on BVAS v3 as well. For example, a stroke is recorded in BVAS v3, if attributed to vasculitis, but it will also be scored as a damage item; however, it should not be scored on VDI until 3 months have passed since the event.

5.5.3 Key Points About VDI

1. VDI records damage and is a cumulative score, so it never improves.
2. VDI records any items that occurred and lasted for more than 3 months since the onset of vasculitis, even they subsequently resolve.
3. The same lesion should not be scored twice.
4. Some items are always preceded by other items when scoring.
5. A cumulative VDI score of ≥5 is associated with a significantly increased risk of mortality.
6. Most damage occurs early, but relapses usually result in a subsequent further increase in VDI.

5.6 Role of Assessment of Disease Status in AAV

Disease activity and damage are important concepts in vasculitis. Disease activity relates to the degree of inflammation and reflects a need for more aggressive treatment, namely immunosuppression, whereas damage represents the consequence of disease activity or its therapy and does not respond to additional immunosuppressive treatment. In order to rationalize clinical decisions in patients with AAV, it is necessary to accurately measure disease activity and monitor damage; however, there are no perfect biomarkers to help us. The elevation and decrease of CRP and ESR rate give us evidence of inflammation, but they are not specific, and given the difficulty in finding a perfect biomarker or set of biomarkers, the best way to currently measure disease activity and monitor damage is to use comprehensive clinical tools that reflect the multisystem nature of vasculitis [27]. BVAS v3 and VDI are the most widely used tools for this.

BVAS (BVAS v1–v3 and BVAS WG) and VDI have been approved by the Outcome Measures in Rheumatology (OMERACT) group and the European league against Rheumatism (EULAR), as key outcome measures to record disease activity and damage, respectively, in AAV clinical trials [38–40]. Using BVAS, we can create more robust definitions of disease status; BVAS has been employed for this purpose in a number of clinical trials. BVAS can be used to set a minimal level of disease activity to be eligible for a study (typically a minimum score on BVAS, or the presence of a minimum number of items, or the presence of at least one major item). In terms of response, this can be defined as the absence of any active BVAS items or no new or worse items appearing after a period of treatment; or a fall in BVAS from baseline of least 50%. Flares or relapses can be defined as a rise in BVAS or the appearance or worsening of at least one major item. We propose that BVAS and its variants represent the most reliable and comprehensive outcome measures available and should be evaluated in any clinical trial targeting disease activity.

All forms of BVAS (including BVAS v1, BVAS v3, and BVAS/WG) are sensitive to change in disease activity and can differentiate between disease states—remission vs. activity [39]. There are alternatives to BVAS, but these are not commonly used in clinical trials.

Like BVAS, VDI is also sensitive to change over time and is superior to other instruments in discriminating between levels of damage [41]. Damage is an important concept in vasculitis and refers to irreversible aspects of the disease that are not responsive to immunosuppression. VDI as a total score is a good predictor of mortality, as are some of its subscores, such as the critical damage score [42]. Individual items of VDI can be used as outcomes measures; for example, in the renal section, altered renal function is one of the most common and severe manifestations of AAV and is an important predictor of mortality [39].

Having reliable tools to measure activity and damage in AAV is crucial not only to monitor an individual patient's progress but also from a health economic point of view. Most of the healthcare systems are funded by public taxation, and there is a need to demonstrate value for money in terms of health gain. In the United Kingdom, the National Health Service (NHS), for example, has a commissioning system with clinically based patient pathways, requiring continuous quality assessment (https://www.england.nhs.uk/commissioning/). The ultimate goal is to provide the best possible care without compromising financial stability. Rituximab treatment in AAV is approved by NHS England but prerequisites must be met including the following: the disease has remained active or progressed, or relapsed, despite standard therapy [43]. The definitions of these disease states rely on assessment of BVAS.

5.7 Patient-Reported Outcomes

Patients with AAV, as is often the case in any chronic disease, perceive the burden of their illness differently from clinicians [44]. Constitutional features, such as fatigue, low energy level, and musculoskeletal manifestations, are considered by patients as the most important aspects of their disease, as opposed to the physicians who give greater relevance to organ damage. This highlights the need to incorporate patient-reported outcomes (PROs) in clinical management.

Patients with AAV have an impaired health-related quality of life (HRQoL) based on studies using generic PROs [39, 45–49]. The Short Form 36 (SF-36) is currently included in the AAV core set measures endorsed by the OMERACT [39]. It contains 36 questions that assess HRQoL in eight domains, with a physical and a mental component summary [50]. Both components can be of value in discriminating disease states, that is, activity vs. remission, and correlate with disease activity as measured by the BVAS WG [49, 51]. However, SF-36 is extensive and still not able to capture specific disease characteristics. More recently, the Routine Assessment of Patient Index Data 3 (RAPID3), a component of the multidimensional health assessment questionnaire (MDHAQ) which includes measures for physical function, pain, and patient global assessment, has shown to discriminate between disease states in AAV and significantly correlate with the BVAS scores with the additional advantage of taking less time to complete (<5 min) when compared to SF-36 [52]; however, larger studies are still needed to establish its role in clinical practice.

In response to the lack of a disease-specific PRO for patients with AAV, the OMERACT Vasculitis Working Group has recently developed the AAV-PRO. It consists of 29 items representing six domains: organ-specific symptoms, systemic symptoms, treatment side effects, social and emotional effect, concerns about the future, and physical function [53]. In addition, three generic Patient-Reported Outcomes Measurement Information System (PROMIS) instruments (fatigue, physical functioning, and pain interference) have been explored for use in AAV. The disease-specific AAV-PRO and the generic PROMIS are complementary instruments to each other and have both been recently endorsed by the OMERACT for use in clinical trials [35]. Future studies in prospective cohorts are needed to further assess their value and performance characteristics.

5.8 Training

For clinician-based assessments, training is recommended in order to accurately record disease status and to ensure standardization of assessments between assessors. A web-based program has been developed (bvasvdi.org) for BVAS and VDI training and certification. It comprises educational multimedia material and an interactive training module, with a collection of training and certification cases based on cohorts of patients with vasculitis. We have developed and implemented this system to provide a certification of competency in evaluating patients with vasculitis. Training in vasculitis assessment is becoming a mandatory element for a number of clinical trials in vasculitis as well as being recommended by regulatory authorities to ensure appropriate use of high-cost drugs such as rituximab or mepolizumab in clinical practice. We are currently extending the training package for use of assessment tools in pediatric patients, that is, the Paediatric Vasculitis Activity Score (PVAS) and the Paediatric Vasculitis Damage Index.

5.9 Future

Patients with AAV usually survive their initial presentation, but subsequently develop chronic problems of recurring episodes of disease and/or complicating co-morbidity, drug toxicity, and damage. Recognizing and adequately characterizing these different aspects is essential to ensure that each patient is managed appropriately, avoiding excess immunosuppression but instituting it when required. As our therapies become more targeted, we should reduce the comorbidity associated with treatment and we also anticipate that this should lead to less scarring from the disease process. It is always going to be necessary to assess the clinical status of patients with vasculitis before determining the optimal choice of therapy, but we anticipate that we will be able to make better use of existing or future biomarkers to provide further delineation of disease characteristics that would guide immunosuppressive strategies.

5.10 Conclusions

The systemic vasculitides have a significant risk of organ failure and death. The introduction of immunosuppression, particularly cyclophosphamide and more recently rituximab, has transformed the outcome, but survivors are liable to experience episodes of ongoing disease activity or relapse, as well as suffering consequences of damage from their disease and toxicity from drug therapy. This complicated set of problems is very common among the patients with AAV. Discriminating between active disease, damage, and drug toxicity can be problematic. Unfortunately, no serological markers can reliably help to inform clinical management, although in some types of disease (especially patients with GPA who are PR3-ANCA positive), there does appear to be a relationship between disease activity and levels of ANCA; however, this does not apply to other forms of AAV or indeed for patients with GPA who do not have a renal involvement. CRP is a reflection of inflammation, but also infection and has poor discriminatory value in differentiating relapse from infection. For this reason, clinical evaluation of patient status remains the current gold standard, and Birmingham Vasculitis Score is a good example of a structured protocol to allow documentation of features representing disease activity, as well as a quantification of the level of disease activity using a weighted score. In this way, we can precisely define terms such as active disease, relapse, response to treatment, and remission. BVAS has been used to define response in several clinical trials of therapies of systemic vasculitis, as well as being used as part of the eligibility criteria for studies. BVAS provides an item list of abnormities which are likely to occur in AAV, so that each patient's clinical status can be accurately assessed, providing a rational basis for treatment. Indeed for some funding authorities, there is a requirement to evaluate patient's status to ensure that there is active disease prior to use of expensive biologic therapies. Disease assessment tools can offer prognostic value, as well as being used in determining treatment response. The Vasculitis Damage Index (VDI) provides a description of features representing the cumulative burden of having had a diagnosis of vasculitis, combining not only the effects of disease but also any comorbidity occurring since the onset of disease or effects of long-term drug therapy. The association between damage and subsequent mortality is well established, and this should be regarded as an effective measurement to determine the long-term success of different therapeutic regimens.

References

1. Kalsch AI, Csernok E, Munch D, et al. Use of highly sensitive C-reactive protein for follow up of Wegener's granulomatosis. J Rheumatol. 2010;37(11):2319–25.
2. Monach PA. Biomarkers in vasculitis. Curr Opin Rheumatol. 2014;26(1):24–30.
3. Bossuyt X, Cohen Tervaert JW, Arimura Y, et al. Position paper: revised 2017 international consensus on testing of ANCAs in granulomatosis with polyangiitis and microscopic polyangiitis. Nat Rev Rheumatol. 2017;13(11):683–92.
4. Luqmani RA. ANCA-associated vasculitides and polyarteritis nodosa. In: Bijlsma JWJ, Hachulla E, editors. EULAR textbook on rheumatic diseases. 2nd ed. Zurich: EULAR; 2015. p. 717–53.
5. Tervaert JW, van der Woude FJ, Fauci AS, et al. Association between active Wegener's granulomatosis and anticytoplasmic antibodies. Arch Intern Med. 1989;149(11):2461–5.
6. Specks U, Wheatley C, McDonald TJ, et al. Anticytoplasmic autoantibodies in the diagnosis and follow-up of Wegener's granulomatosis. Mayo Clin Proc. 1989;64(1):28–36.
7. Kerr GS, Fleisher TA, Hallahan CW, Leavitt RY, Fauci AS, Hoffman GS. Limited prognostic value of changes in antineutrophil cytoplasmic antibody titer in patients with Wegener's granulomatosis. Arthritis Rheum. 1993;36(3):365–71.
8. Davenport A, Lock RJ, Wallington T. Clinical significance of the serial measurement of autoantibodies to neutrophil cytoplasm using a standard indirect immunofluorescence test. Am J Nephrol. 1995;15(3):201–7.
9. Tomasson G, Grayson PC, Mahr AD, Lavalley M, Merkel PA. Value of ANCA measurements during remission to predict a relapse of ANCA-associated vasculitis--a meta-analysis. Rheumatology (Oxford). 2012;51(1):100–9.
10. Xiao H, Heeringa P, Hu P, et al. Antineutrophil cytoplasmic autoantibodies specific for myeloperoxidase cause glomerulonephritis and vasculitis in mice. J Clin Invest. 2002;110(7):955–63.
11. Little MA, Al-Ani B, Ren S, et al. Anti-proteinase 3 anti-neutrophil cytoplasm autoantibodies recapitulate systemic vasculitis in mice with a humanized immune system. PLoS One. 2012;7(1):e28626.
12. Kemna MJ, Damoiseaux J, Austen J, et al. ANCA as a predictor of relapse: useful in patients with renal involvement but not in patients with nonrenal disease. J Am Soc Nephrol. 2015;26(3):537–42.
13. Fussner LA, Hummel A, Schroeder DR, et al. Specks factors determining the clinical utility of serial measurements of antineutrophil cytoplasmic antibodies targeting proteinase 3. Arthritis Rheum. 2016;68(7):1700–10.
14. Stone JH, Merkel PA, Spiera R, et al. Rituximab versus cyclophosphamide for ANCA-associated vasculitis. N Engl J Med. 2010;363(3):221–32.
15. Franssen C, Gans R, Kallenberg C, et al. Disease spectrum of patients with antineutrophil cytoplasmic autoantibodies of defined specificity: distinct differences between patients with antiproteinase 3 and antimyeloperoxidase autoantibodies. J Intern Med. 1998;244:209–16.
16. Hogan SL, Falk RJ, Chin H, et al. Predictors of relapse and treatment resistance in anti-neutrophil cytoplasmic antibody-associated small-vessel vasculitis. Ann Intern Med. 2005;143(9):621–31.
17. Pagnoux C, Hogan SL, Chin H, et al. Predictors of treatment resistance and relapse in antineutrophil cytoplasmic antibody-associated small-vessel vasculitis: comparison of two independent cohorts. Arthritis Rheum. 2008;58(9):2908–18.
18. Lionaki S, Blyth ER, Hogan SL, et al. Classification of antineutrophil cytoplasmic autoantibody vasculitides: the role of antineutrophil cytoplasmic autoantibody specificity for myeloperoxidase or proteinase 3 in disease recognition and prognosis. Arthritis Rheum. 2012;64(10):3452–62.
19. Specks U, Merkel PA, Seo P, et al. Efficacy of remission-induction regimens for ANCA-associated vasculitis. N Engl J Med. 2013;369(5):417–27.

20. Cao Y, Tian Z, Li W, Ma L, Yu Y, Ren W. Predictors of treatment resistance and relapse in Chinese patients with antineutrophil cytoplasmic antibody-associated disease. J Rheumatol. 2014;41(5):916–22.
21. Alberici F, Smith RM, Jones RB, et al. Long-term follow-up of patients who received repeat-dose rituximab as maintenance therapy for ANCA-associated vasculitis. Rheumatology (Oxford). 2015;54(7):1153–60.
22. O'Reilly VP, Wong L, Kennedy C, et al. Urinary soluble CD163 in active renal vasculitis. J Am Soc Nephrol. 2016;27(9):2906–16.
23. Kain R, Tadema H, McKinney EF, et al. High prevalence of autoantibodies to hLAMP-2 in anti-neutrophil cytoplasmic antibody-associated vasculitis. J Am Soc Nephrol. 2012;23(3):556–66.
24. Berden AE, Nolan SL, Morris HL, et al. Anti-plasminogen antibodies compromise fibrinolysis and associate with renal histology in ANCA-associated vasculitis. J Am Soc Nephrol. 2010;21(12):2169–79.
25. Suzuki K, Nagao T, Itabashi M, et al. A novel autoantibody against moesin in the serum of patients with MPO-ANCA-associated vasculitis. Nephrol Dial Transplant. 2014;29(6):1168–77.
26. Monach PA, Warner RL, Tomasson G, et al. Serum proteins reflecting inflammation, injury and repair as biomarkers of disease activity in ANCA-associated vasculitis. Ann Rheum Dis. 2013;72(8):1342–50.
27. Luqmani RA, Bacon PA, Moots RJ, et al. Birmingham vasculitis activity score (BVAS) in systemic necrotizing vasculitis. QJM. 1994;87(11):671–8.
28. Mukhtyar C, Lee R, Brown D, et al. Modification and validation of the Birmingham vasculitis activity score (version 3). Ann Rheum Dis. 2009;68(12):1827–32.
29. de Groot K, Gross W, Herlyn K, Reinhold-Keller E. Development and validation of a disease extent index for Wegener's granulomatosis. Clin Nephrol. 2001;55(1):31–8.
30. Robson JDH, Suppiah R, Flossmann O, et al. Damage in the anca-associated vasculitides: long-term data from the European vasculitis study group (EUVAS) therapeutic trials. Ann Rheum Dis. 2015;74(1):177–84.
31. Exley AR, Carruthers DM, Luqmani RA, et al. Damage occurs early in systemic vasculitis and is an index of outcome. QJM. 1997;90(6):391–9.
32. Suppiah R, Flossman O, Mukhtyar C, et al. Measurement of damage in systemic vasculitis: a comparison of the vasculitis damage index with the combined damage assessment index. Ann Rheum Dis. 2011;70(1):80–5.
33. Guillevin L, Pagnoux C, Seror R, et al. The five-factor score revisited: assessment of prognoses of systemic necrotizing vasculitides based on the French vasculitis study group (FVSG) cohort. Medicine (Baltimore). 2011;90(1):19–27.
34. Koike K, Fukami K, Yonemoto K, et al. A new vasculitis activity score for predicting death in myeloperoxidase-antineutrophil cytoplasmic antibody-associated vasculitis patients. Am J Nephrol. 2012;35(1):1–6.
35. Robson JC, Tomasson G, Milman N, et al. OMERACT endorsement of patient-reported outcome instruments in antineutrophil cytoplasmic antibody-associated vasculitis. J Rheumatol. 2017;44(10):1529–35.
36. Dolezalova P, Price-Kuehne F, Özen S, et al. Disease activity assessment in childhood vasculitis: development and primary validation of the Paediatric Vasculitis activity score (PVAS). Ann Rheum Dis. 2013;72(10):1628–33.
37. Luqmani R, Brown D, Hall C, O'Donoghue J, Robson J, Singh S. Clinical evaluation of systemic vasculitis. A practical guide to using BVAS and VDI. Oxford: University of Oxford; 2014. p. 32.
38. Robson J, Doll H, Suppiah R, et al. Damage in the anca-associated vasculitides: long-term data from the European vasculitis study group (EUVAS) therapeutic trials. Ann Rheum Dis. 2015;74(1):177–84.
39. Merkel PA, Aydin SZ, Boers M, et al. The OMERACT core set of outcome measures for use in clinical trials of ANCA-associated vasculitis. J Rheumatol. 2011;38(7):1480–6.
40. Hellmich B, Flossmann O, Gross WL, et al. EULAR recommendations for conducting clinical studies and/or clinical trials in systemic vasculitis: focus on anti-neutrophil cytoplasm antibody-associated vasculitis. Ann Rheum Dis. 2007;66(5):605–17.

41. Exley AR, Bacon PA, Luqmani RA, et al. Development and initial validation of the vasculitis damage index for the standardized clinical assessment of damage in the systemic vasculitides. Arthritis Rheum. 1997;40(2):371–80.
42. Exley AR, Bacon P, Luqmani RA, Kitas GD, Carruthers DM, Moots R. Examination of disease severity in systemic vasculitis from the novel perspective of damage using the vasculitis damage index (VDI). Br J Rheumatol. 1998;37(1):57–63.
43. Rheumatology NESSCRGfS. Clinical commissioning policy: rituximab for the treatment of ANCA-associated vasculitis in adults. London: NHS England; 2015.
44. Herlyn K, Hellmich B, Seo P, Merkel PA. Patient-reported outcome assessment in vasculitis may provide important data and a unique perspective. Arthritis Care Res. 2010;62(11):1639–45.
45. Koutantji M, Harrold E, Lane SE, Pearce S, Watts RA, Scott DG. Investigation of quality of life, mood, pain, disability, and disease status in primary systemic vasculitis. Arthritis Rheum. 2003;49(6):826–37.
46. Faurschou M, Sigaard L, Bjorner JB, Baslund B. Impaired health-related quality of life in patients treated for Wegener's granulomatosis. J Rheumatol. 2010;37(10):2081–5.
47. Walsh M, Mukhtyar C, Mahr A, et al. Health related quality of life in patients with newly diagnosed anti-neutrophil cytoplasm antibody associated vasculitis. Arthritis Care Res. 2011;63(7):1055.
48. Grayson PC, Amudala NA, McAlear CA, et al. Illness perceptions and fatigue in systemic vasculitis. Arthritis Care Res. 2013;65(11):1835–43.
49. Basu N, McClean A, Harper L, et al. The characterisation and determinants of quality of life in ANCA associated vasculitis. Ann Rheum Dis. 2014;73(1):207–11.
50. Ware JE Jr, Sherbourne CD. The MOS 36-item short-form health survey (SF-36). I. Conceptual framework and item selection. Med Care. 1992;30(6):473–83.
51. Tomasson G, Boers M, Walsh M, et al. Assessment of health-related quality of life as an outcome measure in granulomatosis with polyangiitis (Wegener's). Arthritis Care Res. 2012;64(2):273–9.
52. Annapureddy N, Elsallabi O, Baker J, Sreih AG. Patient-reported outcomes in ANCA-associated vasculitis. A comparison between Birmingham vasculitis activity score and routine assessment of patient index data 3. Clin Rheumatol. 2016;35(2):395–400.
53. Robson JC, Milman N, Tomasson G, et al. Exploration, development, and validation of patient-reported outcomes in antineutrophil cytoplasmic antibody-associated vasculitis using the OMERACT process. J Rheumatol. 2015;42(11):2204–9.

Eosinophilic Granulomatosis with Polyangiitis (EGPA, Churg–Strauss)

6

Yann Nguyen and Loïc Guillevin

6.1 Introduction

Eosinophilic granulomatosis with polyangiitis (EGPA), formerly called Churg–Strauss syndrome, is a systemic necrotizing vasculitis (SNV) of small- and medium-sized vessels that is characterized by asthma and blood eosinophilia [1, 2]. Jacob Churg and Lotte Strauss were the first to describe it in 1951, calling it allergic angiitis and granulomatosis. Although the presence of antineutrophil cytoplasm antibody (ANCA) is not constant, EGPA is classified as a small-sized vessel, ANCA-associated vasculitis (AAV) [3]. Clinical phenotypes and pathogenic mechanisms of this rare disease have now been partly described, but gaps in our knowledge persist. Recent advances in EGPA management include several novel immunomodulatory drugs and biotherapies, the efficacies of which are currently being evaluated. In this review, EGPA epidemiology, pathophysiology, clinical manifestations, outcomes, and the different therapeutic options, including therapeutic perspectives, are addressed.

6.2 Epidemiology

EGPA is a rare disease and its prevalence in inhabitants ranges between 7.3 and 17.8/million [4, 5] and annual incidence ranges between 0.9 and 2.4/million [6]. Some authors found higher EGPA incidences in urban than rural regions [7], but provided no clear explanation for the cause. Its prevalence seems to be similar in Europe, Japan, and the USA [5]. Patients' mean age of ~50 years at diagnosis [8] is lower than those for microscopic polyangiitis (MPA), granulomatosis with polyangiitis

Y. Nguyen · L. Guillevin (✉)
Department of Internal Medicine, Referral Center for Rare Systemic and Autoimmune Diseases, Hôpital Cochin, AP-HP, Université Paris Descartes, Paris, France

R. A. Sinico, L. Guillevin (eds.), *Anti-Neutrophil Cytoplasmic Antibody (ANCA) Associated Vasculitis*, Rare Diseases of the Immune System,
https://doi.org/10.1007/978-3-030-02239-6_6

(GPA), and polyarteritis nodosa (PAN). Childhood-onset EGPA is extremely rare [9]. No male/female sexual predominance has been reported.

According to a French EGPA study [10], most patients have asthma for a mean of 9.3 years before the first vasculitis manifestations appear. The EGPA incidence among asthma patients was 34.6 (range: 21.4–53)/million person-years. Because of their asthma, most patients are nonsmokers, so smoking is not a factor associated with EGPA.

6.3 Triggering Factors

Although no common EGPA-triggering event or cause has yet been identified, many environmental factors implicated in its pathogenesis have been described, for example, inhalation of antigens (dark diesel fumes, grain dust, cereal dust, and dust), desensitization, or vaccination [11, 12]. However, those exposures may merely be disease accelerators in patients, with already present but undiagnosed EGPA, rather than its true cause.

Because of EGPA's asthmatic phase, allergens are thought to be its triggers. But less than one-third of EGPA patients had documented allergies, when frequent allergens were systematically tested. That finding suggests that the potentially responsible molecules have not yet been identified or their mechanism to induce EGPA manifestations is not the only one [13].

Certain medications, mainly leukotriene-receptor antagonists (e.g., montelukast) or, more recently, anti-IgE antibodies (e.g., omalizumab), are still possible suspects because they are often prescribed during corticosteroid tapering but their role remains unclear [14–18].

6.4 Pathophysiology

EGPA pathogenesis is still incompletely understood, but genetic background, environmental factors, and immune dysregulation seem to be implicated.

Genetic studies revealed associations between EGPA patients and specific human leukocyte antigen (HLA) alleles. Indeed, genetically distinct subsets within AAVs, with major-histocompatibility-complex (MHC) and non-MHC associations, were identified in a genome-wide association study (GWAS) on GPA and MPA, but not EGPA [19], with the strongest associations being with the ANCA-antigen specificities but not the clinical phenotype. Anti-myeloperoxidase (MPO) and anti-proteinase 3 (PRS) ANCA, respectively, were associated with *HLA–DQ* and *HLA–DP*. An earlier study had found an association with the *HLA–DRB4* gene, for EGPA patients harboring an *HLA–DRB1∗04*, *HLA–DRB1∗07,* or *HLA–DRB1∗09* allele (odds ratio (OR) 2.49; 95% confidence interval (CI) 1.58–3.09), but *HLA–DRB3*-gene frequency was lower in EGPA patients than controls (OR 0.54, 95% CI 0.35–0.84) [20].

Although allergy–EGPA associations have been described for many years, allergy does not represent a constant predisposing factor because the quasi-totality of patients have asthma as their first EGPA sign and their total serum IgE levels are elevated but less than a third of them have documented allergies [13].

Because blood and tissue eosinophilia are among the major EGPA characteristics, eosinophils are thought to be key players in EGPA pathogenesis. That immune dysfunction results in massive eosinophilic proliferation, impaired apoptosis, and elevated tissue toxicity attributed to eosinophil products. Defective CD95 (Apo-1/Fas)-mediated apoptosis seems to be involved in eosinophil proliferation [21]. Blood eosinophils from patients with active EGPA have less expression of primarily pro-apoptotic genes (e.g., *BLC2L13* (mitochondrially localized protein with conserved B-cell lymphoma 2 homology motifs), *CASP2* (*Caspase* 2), and *CARD4* (caspase recruitment domain family member 4)) involved in NF-κB (nuclear factor-kappa B) regulation [22]. EGPA patients also have elevated concentrations of eosinophil-synthesized interleukin (IL)-25, which maintains eosinophil proliferation via T-helper cell type 2 (Th2)-predominant stimulation by cytokines synthesized by CD4+ T-lymphocytes [23]. Eosinophilic cytotoxic proteins (e.g., eosinophil cationic protein, eosinophil peroxidase) directly involved in damaging tissues, are also found at high levels in EGPA patients' sera, urine, and tissues [24].

As seen in asthma, EGPA patients' CD4+ T lymphocytes, mostly Th2 phenotype, are activated. EGPA patients' sera and bronchoalveolar lavage (BAL) fluid also contain elevated concentrations of Th2 ILs (e.g., IL-4, IL-5, and IL-13) [25]. IL-5 plays major roles in eosinophil maturation and survival, and strong associations have been established between IL-5 expression and clinical parameters of EGPA activity (Birmingham Vasculitis Activity Score, eosinophilia). Moreover, EGPA pathogenesis also seems to implicate Th1 and Th17 responses [26].

Although the precise role of B lymphocytes has not yet been fully elucidated, their involvement in EGPA pathogenesis is being more thoroughly examined, in light of the efficacy of anti-CD20 monoclonal antibodies against GPA and MPA [27, 28]. Higher percentages of CD80+, CD27+, or CD95+ B cells and lower rates CD19+ B cells were described in patients with frequently relapsing EGPA [29]. Furthermore, IgG4 levels, indirect surrogate signs of B-lymphocyte activation, were elevated during EGPA flares [30].

Pertinently, ANCA-positivity, albeit in only one-third of EGPA patients, is also indicative of B-lymphocyte activation. Direct EGPA pathogenesis via anti-MPO ANCA was demonstrated in vitro and in mouse models [31, 32].

6.5 Clinical Manifestations

EGPA generally evolves in three stages, with asthma or sometimes symptoms attributed to allergy appearing first, then eosinophilia and lung infiltrates, and later systemic vasculitis manifestations. The time between the first asthma manifestations and EGPA is usually around 9 years, but the onset of all manifestations can be simultaneous in some patients (Table 6.1).

Table 6.1 EGPA patients' clinical features according to the main published series

Feature	Chumbley et al. [81]	Lanham et al. [48]	Guillevin et al. [12]	Gaskin et al. [82]	Guillevin et al. [39]	Solans et al. [83]	Comarmond et al. [8]	Durel et al. [84]
Patient demographics								
Number included	30	16	43	21	96	32	383	101
Male/Female sex ratio, *n*	21/9	12/4	24/19	14/7	45/51	9/23	199/184	43/58
Mean age (year)	47	38	43.2	46.5	48.2	42	50.3	49.2
[Range]	[15–69]		[7–66]	[23–69]	[17–74]	[17–85]	[35–66]	
Clinical features								
General symptoms			72		70	69		
Arthritis, arthralgias	20	51	28	43	41		29.8	68.3
Myalgias		68			54		38.9	82.2
Allergic rhinitis and/or ENT involvement	70	70	21		47		48	96
Asthma	100	100	100	100	100	100	91.1	53.4
Pulmonary infiltrates	27	72	77	43	38	53	38.6	53.5
Pleural effusion		29				19	8.9	3
Skin involvement	67			50	51	69	39.7	46.5
Purpura		48	28		31	41	22.5	24.7
Nodules	27	30	21		19	6	9.7	8.9
Mononeuritis multiplex	63	66	67	70	78	44	46	54.5
GI involvement	17	59	37	58	33	38	23.2	25
CV involvement	16	47	49	15	30	28	27.4	20.8
Renal involvement	20	49	16	80	16	13	21.7	26

Values are expressed as percentages, unless stated otherwise
ENT ear, nose and throat, *GI* gastrointestinal, *CV* cardiovascular

6.5.1 General Symptoms

Fever, asthenia, and weight loss commonly occur before systemic manifestations, as for our EGPA series at diagnosis: 38.9% had fever and myalgias, 29.8% had arthralgias, and almost 50% had lost weight, with mean loss at 7.8 ± 4.7 kg [8].

6.5.2 Pulmonary and Ear, Nose, and Throat (ENT) Manifestations

Asthma is the major EGPA characteristic, affecting 91–100% of the patients, most often before systemic vasculitis (mean interval: 9.3 ± 10.8 years). It is often late-onset asthma, starting around 30–40 years of age, but can start during childhood. Asthma is generally severe and corticosteroid-dependent. During the weeks preceding the onset of systemic EGPA manifestations, asthma often worsens, despite inhaled and oral corticosteroids. In a retrospective study on 157 EGPA patients, at diagnosis, 3 years and the final visit, respectively, 57%, 48%, and 56% of them had severe asthma, and 38%, 30%, and 46% had persistent airflow obstruction [33].

Asthma can be associated with ENT symptoms. Maxillary sinusitis is common in EGPA and is one of the American College of Rheumatology (ACR) classification criteria defining this vasculitis. Allergic rhinitis and nasal polyposis, found in 17% and 41% of EGPA patients, must be distinguished from the ENT manifestations of GPA, which are often destructive and severe.

Alveolar hemorrhage, resulting from pulmonary vasculitis, is rare (4%) but can sometimes be severe with massive hemoptysis (often associated with renal involvement); however, it is usually mild in most patients, with only bloody sputum or diagnosed by BAL. Pulmonary infiltrates can be seen on computed-tomography (CT) scans and the most severely affected patients can be anemic. Pleural involvement, with eosinophilic exudative pleural effusions, has been described. Pleural biopsy, rarely obtained, can show signs of vasculitis, with eosinophilic infiltrates [34]. Lung infiltrates are common (38.6%), and can be uni- or bilateral, transitory and often disappear after a few days of corticosteroids [35]. Phrenic paralysis has been described, but is extremely rare [36].

6.5.3 Neurological Manifestations

Peripheral neuropathies are frequent (affecting 46–75%), mainly mononeuritis multiplex (46% in our series) [8]. These result from vasculitis of the *vasa nervorum* of peripheral nerves, most frequently involving common peroneal nerves, sometimes internal popliteal nerves and less frequently, radial, cubital, and median nerves. Patients may complain of paresthesia or sometimes painful hyperesthesia before the onset of sensory and motor deficiencies. When mild, only superficial sensitivity is affected. Recovery is long and unpredictable. Cranial nerve involvement occurs rarely (3.1%) [8]. As for PAN and MPA, EGPA peripheral neuropathy is not a poor-prognosis factor and does not influence mortality, as evaluated by the Five-Factor Score (FFS) [37], but motor or sensitive deficiency sequelae can worsen the functional prognosis.

Central nervous system involvement is uncommon (5.2%), with nonspecific clinical manifestations of cerebral vasculitis: hemiplegia, brain hemorrhage, sub-arachnoid hemorrhages, and seizures. Although CT scans visualize ischemic or hemorrhagic events, magnetic resonance imaging (MRI) can detect T2-weighted cortical and subcortical signals, more specific to cerebral vasculitis. Since the FFS was revised in 2011, central nervous system involvement is no longer considered as a poor-prognosis factor.

6.5.4 Skin Manifestations

Skin involvement is frequent (affecting 40–70%), due to small-vessel vasculitis or extravascular granuloma, with vascular purpura, preferentially affecting the lower limbs, being the most common (22–50%). Subcutaneous nodules, often bilateral, symmetrical, red, and predominantly affecting the fingers, elbows and upper limbs, are found in 10–30% of EGPA patients. Nodules can also develop on the fore-head. Nodule biopsies contain extravascular granuloma(s), but they are not specific to EGPA, as they can also be seen in other vasculitides or inflammatory bowel diseases. Other skin manifestations are known: Raynaud's phenomenon, urticaria, livedo reticularis (3.9%), and gangrenous necrotic lesions.

6.5.5 Gastrointestinal Involvement

Gastrointestinal involvement is often severe and is an FFS poor-prognosis factor [37, 38]. Clinical manifestations are often nonspecific, with abdominal pain (30–60%), nausea, vomiting, diarrhea, and/or intestinal hemorrhage. Bowel perforation, the most severe digestive manifestation, is associated with high mortality. In a French study on 96 EGPA patients, four required surgical interventions for ischemic colitis or mesenteric ischemia [39].

Histological findings can include vasculitis, extravascular granulomas, and sometimes mimicking pseudopolypoid lesions and eosinophilic infiltrates.

Vascular stenosis and microaneurysms can be seen on angiograms, although much less frequently than in PAN.

6.5.6 Cardiac Manifestations

Heart involvement, one of the most severe EGPA manifestations and its primary cause of death, is also a FFS prognostic item. In our series, 16.4% and 15.1% of the patients, respectively, had cardiomyopathy and pericarditis [8]. The prev-alence of EGPA cardiac manifestations may be underestimated. Based on 32 ambulatory patients in EGPA remission, detailed cardiac work-ups revealed that 62% had cardiac involvement, 26% were clinically symptomatic, but 66% had electrocardiogram abnormalities, 60% had echocardiographic defects, and 62% had MRI abnormalities [40]. Cardiac involvement is more frequent in ANCA-negative patients [39]. Cardiac manifestations derive pathophysiologically from coronary vasculitis, extravascular granuloma(s), and eosinophilic interstitial infiltrate.

The clinical manifestations can include eosinophilic myocarditis, pericarditis, hypertension, valvulopathy, and/or congestive heart failure, which were implicated in 14 (31%) of the 45 deaths that occurred in our series [8]. Despite coronary vasculitis, myocardial infarcts remain rare. Moreover, the absence of symptoms or electrocardiogram abnormalities does not exclude cardiac involvement; notably, echocardiography or cardiac MRI still detected abnormalities in 38% of those patients [40].

Although T1-weighted cardiac MRI sequences can reveal centromyocardial, subepicardial, and/or subendocardial myocardial late gadolinium enhancement, its/their meaning in EGPA patients remains unelucidated, especially for asymptomatic patients with cardiac abnormalities. In a retrospective study on 42 EGPA patients who had systematically undergone cardiac MRI, 82.4% with cardiomyopathy (diagnosed independently of MRI findings) had myocardial late gadolinium enhancement and 56% has no cardiomyopathy. Noncardiomyopathic patients with or without MRI abnormalities had comparable EGPA outcomes and cardiac manifestations. MRI findings should not be the only criteria used to diagnose cardiomyopathy [41, 42]. For patients with symptomatic cardiomyopathy, cardiac MRI can help detect those with less favorable cardiac outcomes. Coronary arteriography may be necessary to differentiate EGPA cardiomyopathy from underlying ischemic cardiopathy.

6.5.7 Renal Manifestations

Renal involvement is relatively uncommon in EGPA (affecting 16–22%), compared with other AAVs. In our series, mean creatininemia at diagnosis was 89.1 ± 38.6 μmol/L (1.01 ± 0.44 mg/dL), and 12.8% of the patients had proteinuria above 0.4 g/24 h [8]. Renal biopsies mainly show crescentic glomerulonephritis, which can be focal or diffuse, and less frequent renal vasculitis, eosinophilic infiltrates, or granuloma(s) [43]. Dialysis may be required temporarily or definitively. Glomerulonephritis in EGPA is usually associated with anti-MPO ANCA-positivity. Ureteral stenosis has been described but rarely [44].

6.5.8 Other Manifestations

Ophthalmological disease, with uveitis, episcleritis, ischemic vasculitis, and/or orbital inflammatory pseudotumor with conjunctival involvement, has been described [45].

6.6 Complementary Investigations

Blood eosinophilia is a constant EGPA symptom, with counts exceeding 1,500/ mm^3 or 10% of total leukocytes as diagnostic criteria. In the French series, the mean eosinophil count was 7569 ± 6428/mm^3 [8], but eosinophil counts exceeding 50,000/mm^3 have been reported [46]. Eosinophilia may decline rapidly, within a few days, under corticosteroids. Although eosinophilia can be a marker of EGPA evolution, when isolated, it may not be sufficient to diagnose a relapse. During follow-up, eosinophil counts rise frequently without clinical manifestations, usually when corticosteroids are being tapered, making close surveillance necessary.

Approximately, 80% of EGPA patients have signs of an inflammatory syndrome, with elevated C-reactive protein (66.9 ± 61.8 mg/L) or erythrocyte sedimentation rate [8].

BAL is indicated when alveolar hemorrhage is suspected; it contains red blood cells and has an elevated Golde score (Prussian blue-stained macrophages). When BAL was performed for other indications, inflammatory fluid contained a mean total of 296 leukocytes/mm^3, with a mean (± standard deviation; SD) 33 ± 29% eosinophils [33].

Antinuclear antibodies are not present, but rheumatoid factor can be detected [47]. About a third of EGPA patients are ANCA-positive, with mostly perinuclear immunofluorescence-staining P-ANCA and approximately 70% with myeloperoxidase (MPO) specificity, as determined by enzyme-linked immunosorbent assay.

Skin, nerve, and/or muscle biopsy can confirm EGPA diagnosis, with good sensitivity (48–67%) [39, 48]. Biopsies may contain three types of lesions: (1) necrotizing small- to medium-sized vessel vasculitis, which is typified by fibrinoid necrosis of the media and pleomorphic cellular infiltrate(s), predominantly composed of eosinophils; (2) extravascular granuloma(s), with central necrosis and epithelioid cells, are quite typical, but nonspecific, of EGPA and can be seen in other vasculitides (e.g., GPA) or autoimmune diseases; and (3) eosinophil infiltration(s) of arterial walls and adjacent tissues that can be seen in any organ [49]. Finding all three lesion types in the same specimen is very rare (<20% of EGPA patients).

Among imaging techniques, chest radiographs can be useful. In a study on 91 patients, chest X-ray abnormalities, for example, ground-glass attenuation (29%), nodules or mass (9%), consolidation (29%), and/or pleural effusion (10%), were seen in 58% of the patients at diagnosis, and they were frequently bilateral (58%) [33]. Chest CT scans can further evaluate lung abnormalities, being able to visualize ground-glass opacities (39%), bronchial wall thickening (32%), and/or micronodules less than 3 mm (24%).

Angiography, if done, may reveal typical stenosis consistent with vasculitis; it can be particularly useful to detect mesenteric vasculitis. Microaneurysms are rarely seen in EGPA.

6.7 Diagnosis

6.7.1 Diagnostic Criteria

Initially, the three EGPA-defining pathological lesions mentioned above served as the basis of the diagnosis. Because finding all three lesions in one biopsy is very rare, less stringent diagnostic criteria were devised.

Today, EGPA diagnosis remains clinical: vasculitis and systemic manifestations in a previously asthmatic patient with eosinophilia and sometimes, anti-MPO ANCA-positivity. In 1984, to help clinicians diagnose EGPA with good specificity and sensitivity, Lanham et al. formulated a clinical redefinition of EGPA [48] combining the following criteria: asthma, blood eosinophilia >1500/mm^3 and at least two organs with manifestations suggestive of vasculitis. However, those criteria have been considered insufficient because asthma onset can follow the vasculitic phase, eosinophilia sometimes varies, and vasculitis documentation is difficult to confirm without biopsy.

Other criteria have been devised for classification: ACR (Table 6.2) and more recently, the Chapel Hill Consensus Conference criteria [2, 3], which define EGPA as an eosinophil-rich and necrotizing granulomatous inflammation, frequently involving the respiratory tract, and necrotizing vasculitis predominantly affecting small- to medium-sized vessels, and associated with asthma and eosinophilia. However, those criteria are not diagnostic; they are intended for classification of patients with probable EGPA, once vasculitis has already been diagnosed. They are more useful in clinical studies.

Table 6.2 1990 American College of Rheumatology criteria for the classification of Churg–Strauss syndrome (Reproduced with permission from [2])

Criterion		Definition
1.	Asthma	History of wheezing or diffuse high-pitched rales on expiration
2.	Eosinophilia	Eosinophilia >10% of white blood cell differential count
3.	Mononeuropathy or polyneuropathy	Development of mononeuropathy, multiple mononeuropathies, or polyneuropathy (i.e., glove/stocking distribution) attributable to vasculitis
4.	Pulmonary infiltrates, nonfixed	Migratory or transitory pulmonary infiltrates on radiographs (not including fixed infiltrates), attributable to systemic vasculitis
5.	Paranasal sinus abnormality	History of acute or chronic paranasal sinus pain or tenderness or radiographic opacification of the paranasal sinuses
6.	Extravascular eosinophils	Biopsy including artery, arteriole or venule, showing accumulations of eosinophils in extravascular areas

For classification purposes, a patient with vasculitis shall be said to have EGPA, when at least four of these six criteria are present. The presence of any four or more criteria yields 85% sensitivity of and 99.7% specificity

6.7.2 Differential Diagnosis

Clinical manifestations dictate the entities included in the differential diagnosis of EGPA. Prior to the onset of vasculitic manifestations, it may be difficult to differentiate EGPA among eosinophilic asthma, parasitic infections, or allergic bronchopulmonary aspergillosis.

Once vasculitis symptoms have become overt, the main differential diagnoses are other systemic vasculitides, especially GPA and PAN. Although eosinophilia is also seen in GPA, EGPA can usually be differentiated by concomitant asthma or previous atopic allergies, nondestructive sinus manifestations, and anti-MPO specificity, if ANCA are detected (as opposed to anti-PR3 in GPA).

Another potentially difficult differential diagnostic entity to consider is hypereosinophilic syndrome (HES), which can also be associated with cardiopathy, pulmonary manifestations, and/or nerve involvement. The main differences between the two are the vasculitis symptoms and/or biopsy confirmation of EGPA but not HES [50]. Because HES myeloid variants have specifically elevated tryptase and vitamin B_{12} levels, those biological determinations can be useful to exclude HES, the diagnosis of which can be confirmed by genetic testing for *FIP1L1–PDGFRA* fusion and *JAK2* mutations [51]. HES lymphocytic variant typically has a predominance of skin-and-soft tissue involvements, resulting from abnormal $CD3^{-}CD4^{+}$ T-cell subsets that are responsible for IL-5 synthesis [52]. To exclude at least differential diagnoses, the EGPA Consensus Task Force experts recommended [53] toxocariasis and human immunodeficiency virus serology, specific IgE and IgG dosages for *Aspergillus* spp., the search for *Aspergillus* spp. in sputum and/or BAL specimens, tryptase and vitamin B_{12} dosages, peripheral blood smears to look for dysplastic eosinophils or blasts, and thoracic CT scan.

6.8 Prognosis

Corticosteroids and immunosuppressants have revolutionized EGPA prognoses. In the 1950s, the five-year survival rate for PAN (still grouped together with EGPA) patients was 10%, whereas overall EGPA survival at 7 years now reaches 90%.

However, prognosis is not the same for all EGPA patients and varies according to the presence or not of several identified prognostic factors. The original 1996 prognostic FFS, based on multivariate analyses of the characteristics of 260 PAN and 82 EGPA patients, retained five items significantly associated with outcome and accorded each presence with one point: proteinuria >1 g/day; gastrointestinal bleeding, perforation, infarction and/or pancreatitis; renal insufficiency (with creatininemia >1.58 mg/dL or 140 μmol/L); central nervous system involvement; and cardiomyopathy. Adding the accorded points, an FFS of 0, 1, or 2 led to five-year mortality rates of 12%, 26%, or 46%, respectively. In 2011, a new analysis of 1108 vasculitis patients (230 with EGPA as well as those with GPA or MPA), generated the revised FFS [37], which retained five factors associated with a higher mortality-risk rate: serum creatinine >150 μmol/L; severe gastrointestinal involvement;

myocardial involvement; age >65 years; and the absence of ENT manifestations. Again, each factor was accorded one point and the sum of those points is strong prognostic indicator of death, with FFS = 0, 1, or 2 associated with respective five-year mortality rates of 9%, 21%, or 40%. Hence, simple determination of the revised FFS can contribute to identifying vasculitis patients at high risk of death, who require aggressive therapy with immunosuppressants.

In our series, 11.7% of the patients died with a mean ± SD of 50.4 ± 60.1 (median: 21.4) months postdiagnosis. The leading cause of death (31%) was heart-related (i.e., myocardial infarction, cardiac insufficiency, or arrhythmia), followed by infections or malignancies (11% each), active vasculitis, and respiratory failure (severe asthma attacks and/or end-stage chronic pulmonary obstructive disease, 9% each) [8].

EGPA relapses were defined as the new appearance, recurrence or worsening of clinical EGPA manifestations (excluding asthma and/or ENT) that required adjunction, change, or intensification of the corticosteroid and/or other immunosuppressant dose(s). They represent another major concern [53]. Although almost 90% of EGPA patients achieve remission, 25.3% of our series relapsed, and 18% experienced asthma flares, sinusitis, and/or enhanced eosinophilia levels, justifying prolonged use of corticosteroids for about 85% of the series. The relapse-free survival rate was 78.6% (95% CI: 64.3–84.3) for all patients, and most relapses occurred during the first year postdiagnosis.

6.9 Phenotypes According to ANCA Status

EGPA clinical findings and prognosis differ depending on the patient's ANCA status, which defined two phenotypes [54, 55].

Sinico et al.'s analysis of 93 patients showed that ANCA-positivity was associated with more frequent renal involvement (51.4% vs. 12.1%, $P < 0.001$), pulmonary hemorrhages (20% vs. 0%, $P = 0.001$), purpura, and mononeuritis multiplex, but less frequent lung infiltrates (34.2% vs. 60.3%) and cardiac involvement (5.7% vs. 22.4%, $P = 0.042$) [54]. Those findings suggested that ANCA-positivity might be associated with more frequent vasculitis-associated symptoms, whereas ANCA-negativity would be associated with eosinophilic infiltrates. In our series, prognoses differed according to the ANCA phenotype: positivity was associated with more frequent relapses (35.2% vs. 22.5%, $P = 0.01$) but fewer deaths (5.6% vs. 12.5%, $P < 0.5$) [8].

Recent genetic findings (Lyons et al., unpublished personal data) indicated that different genes were involved in EGPA and corresponded to biological and clinical parameters, establishing EGPA clusters/phenotypes able to differentiate genetically and clinically two subentities, based on ANCA-positivity with distinct genetic features. ANCA-positive EGPA was associated with *HLA-DQ*, whereas ANCA-negative EGPA had no HLA association. Those observations indicate that, in future clinical trials, EGPA patients should be stratified based on their ANCA profile.

6.10 Treatment

Corticosteroids, immunosuppressants, and now targeted therapies can be prescribed for EGPA patients. In our opinion, each patient should receive a tailored regimen adapted to different parameters, for example, disease severity, organ involvement, age, and predictable outcomes, with the aim of inducing, as rapidly as possible, clinical remission, defined as the absence of clinical manifestations of vasculitis. As for most SNVs, EGPA's treatment comprises induction and maintenance phases, as recommended by the EGPA Consensus Task Force in its 2015 recommendations for evaluation and management of these patients [53].

6.10.1 Remission Induction

Corticosteroids are the foundation of induction therapy. When life-threatening symptoms are present, methylprednisolone pulses (usually 7.5–15 mg/kg/day, administered intravenously (IV) over 1 h on days 1–3) should be given, because of that drug's rapid action and relative safety. As induction or relay therapy, prednisone (or its equivalent of methylprednisolone), starting at 1 mg/kg/day, should be taken for 2–3 weeks, followed by gradual tapering. A therapeutic response is usually achieved very rapidly, with rapid attenuation of asthma and vasculitis symptoms and reduction of eosinophilia levels. No standard regimen has been accorded consensus for corticosteroid tapering, but the maintenance corticosteroid dose should be slowly reduced to the lowest effective dose, or when possible, until withdrawal. A daily dose less than 7.5 mg could be the goal to avoid corticosteroid-related adverse events (AEs). However, the chronic steroid-dependent asthma often accompanying EGPA frequently makes long-term prednisone intake essential. AEs may occur even when corticosteroid doses are low and it should be kept in mind that corticosteroid toxicity is cumulative.

For patients without poor-prognosis factors (1996 FFS = 0), induction and maintenance regimens of corticosteroids alone were shown to be safe and effective in the CHUSPAN trial [56, 57]. Indeed, 92% of the patients enrolled in that prospective study were still alive at 5 years, which also further validated the FFS. However, the complete remission rate was only 56% and 35% eventually required recourse to immunosuppressant use. Good-prognosis patients were prescribed different immunosuppressants to limit relapses but their efficacies remain controversial. The recently reported results of the prospective, randomized CHUSPAN2 trial demonstrated that adding azathioprine to corticosteroid neither improved the remission rate nor limited the relapse rate, that is, azathioprine is not an effective steroid-sparing agent [58].

For high-risk patients, defined as having FFS ≥ 1, adjunction of cytotoxic agents is recommended [59]. Although not FFS items, other life- and/or organ-threatening disease manifestations (i.e., alveolar hemorrhage, eye involvement and fulminant mononeuritis multiplex) should encourage physicians to also prescribe an immunosuppressant.

Cyclophosphamide was evaluated prospectively in a study on 48 EGPA patients with FFS-defined poor-prognosis factors, comparing 12 vs. 6 cyclophosphamide pulses, both combined with corticosteroids, but no maintenance therapy [59]. Among them, 42 (78.5%) entered complete remission, with the two regimens being comparably effective. However, the 12-pulse arm had fewer mild relapses (6/21 (28.6%) vs. 14/21 (66.7%), $P < 0.02$). Since then, maintenance therapy has become the standard of care, by analogy with other AAVs: a 6-pulse induction regimen (three infusions at 0.6 g/m^2 or 15 mg/kg every 2 weeks, followed by 3–6 additional pulses at 15 mg/kg or 0.7 g/m^2 every 3 weeks) is now followed by maintenance therapy. To induce remission, IV pulses or continuous oral cyclophosphamide (2 mg/kg/day) are equally effective, in analogy to GPA and MPA induction therapy in the CYCLOPS trial [60], but oral administration has been associated with a higher leukopenia rate and a higher cumulative cyclophosphamide dose. However, long-term follow-up of that study found that the IV-pulse regimen was associated with a higher risk of relapse (39.5% vs. 29.8%, hazard ratio = 0.50 [95% CI: 0.26–0.93]; $P = 0.029$), but not with increased mortality [61], and might favor compliance and, hence, less long-term morbidity and mortality. The results of the prospective randomized CORTAGE trial on 108 SNV patients (including 14 with EGPA) ≥65 year-old given fixed low-dose IV cyclophosphamide pulses (500 mg/m^2 every 2–3 weeks until remission) and limiting corticosteroid exposure [62] showed no difference, compared to the standard regimen for achieving remission, but fewer severe AEs with the "lighter" regimen.

Physicians should strive to prevent cyclophosphamide-associated severe AEs (e.g., hemorrhagic cystitis and gonadal toxicity, for which cryopreservation and GnRH-analog treatment for women is recommended). Prophylaxis against *Pneumocystis jiroveci* pneumonia with co-trimoxazole (or pentamidine aerosols in the case of intolerance to sulfa drugs) should be prescribed and screening for cyclophosphamide-related neutropenia may be useful.

6.10.2 Maintenance Therapy

Once remission has been achieved, poor-prognosis EGPA patients (FFS ≥ 1) should be prescribed maintenance therapy, because of their high risk of relapse. Without maintenance therapy, relapse rates are high, ranging from 73.8% to 85.7% depending on how many cyclophosphamide pulses were administered [59]. Unlike other AAVs, no randomized trial for EGPA has compared immunosuppressants as optimal maintenance agents or determined the best duration of their administration.

Maintenance therapy with an immunosuppressant should be started 2 weeks after the last cyclophosphamide pulse, or a few days after stopping oral cyclophosphamide, when the leukocyte count is acceptable.

Azathioprine, at an initial maintenance dose of 2 mg/kg/day, can be used, in analogy to that prescribed for GPA and MPA. Its dose can be adjusted to the clinical response, being upped to 3 mg/kg/day, or tapered if toxicity occurs.

Methotrexate, at a dose 0.25 mg/kg/week, seems to be a comparable maintenance alternative, based on findings of a prospective trial comparing azathioprine to methotrexate for GPA and MPA remission-maintenance therapy [63].

Mycophenolate mofetil is prescribed less frequently for maintenance because of its poorer efficacy in this context for patients with GPA and MPA [64].

How long maintenance therapy should last to be optimal remains unknown. It does not seem untoward to recommend 18–24 months after remission has been obtained. However, to date, no consensus criteria exist for completely stopping treatment.

6.10.3 Other Treatments

Although therapeutic plasma exchanges are usually ineffective against EGPA [65], they can be used for selected ANCA-positive patients with rapidly progressive glomerulonephritis or severe pulmonary–renal syndrome [66]. Whether they have long-term benefits for these patients is unknown [67].

The efficacy of rituximab, a chimeric monoclonal antibody directed against CD20-expressing B lymphocytes, to induce GPA and MPA remissions and maintain them was demonstrated [27, 28], but EGPA patients were not enrolled in those studies, and data on rituximab treatment of EGPA are limited to case reports and case series [68–70]. Rituximab EGPA-remission induction seems to be effective and safe, mainly for ANCA-positive patients. However, bronchospasms after the first infusion were reported [71]. The French Vasculitis Study Group is currently conducting the prospective, randomized REOVAS trial. Until its results become available, rituximab use seems reasonable for patients with severe refractory EGPA despite conventional therapy or when it is contraindicated.

According to case reports and case series [72, 73], IV immunoglobulins (IVIg) can be a second-line therapy option for patients with EGPA flares, especially those with myocardial or neural involvement, that fail to respond to other therapeutics.

Interferon-alpha has successfully induced EGPA remission but seems to have limited efficacy in preventing major relapses, and because of its numerous AEs, its use should be avoided [74, 75]. It could be considered a second- or third-line therapy for selected patients.

Omalizumab, an anti-IgE monoclonal antibody, has successfully treated allergic asthma and allergic rhinitis. Available information on its use to treat EGPA is scarce and contradictory, with some case reports suggesting that it was beneficial against active disease, but others claiming an association between omalizumab intake and EGPA onset [17, 18, 76, 77]. A more recent French retrospective study [78] on 17 patients indicated that omalizumab might have a corticosteroid-sparing effect, allowing lowering of the median prednisone dose of 16 mg/day at baseline to 9 mg/day at 12 month; however, eight patients stopped taking it because of refractory disease (25%), relapse (50%), or severe asthma flare for two, raising the question of its safety.

Mepolizumab, an anti-IL-5 monoclonal antibody, was assessed in a multicenter, double-blind, phase 3 trial that enrolled 136 relapsing/refractory EGPA patients, who had received a stable prednisone dose for at least 4 weeks. Mepolizumab, compared to placebo, achieved significantly more weeks in remission, a higher percentage of patients in remission (respectively: 32% vs. 3%; OR: 16.7 [95% CI: 3.61–77.56]; $P < 0.001$), and the corticosteroid dose could also be diminished.

Lastly, other therapeutic supportive care is important. The improved EGPA prognosis means it has become a chronic relapsing disease for most patients, despite the need for long-term steroids. Thus, other supplemental agents, for example, as calcium, vitamin D, and bisphosphonates, should be added to the therapeutic regimen to prevent corticosteroid-related complications. Patients must also be warned to avoid tobacco smoke and other respiratory irritants.

Immunization with inactivated vaccines against influenza and pneumococcal pneumonia should be strongly encouraged. In a large prospective study on patients with autoimmune diseases, vaccines against pandemic A/H1N1 influenza strains seemed safe and well tolerated in EGPA patients [79]. Optimized vaccination regimens against pneumococcal pneumonia are currently being tested in GPA and MPA patients, who received corticosteroids and rituximab remission-induction therapy in the prospective French PNEUMOVAS trial.

Finally, implementation of patient-education programs is strongly encouraged to help patients' improve their knowledge of the disease [80].

6.11 Conclusion

The notable progress made over the past three decades, in our understanding of EGPA pathophysiology and the management of affected patients, has substantially improved their prognoses.

Two subsets of EGPA patients, defined by their ANCA status but also different clinical findings, prognoses, and genetic backgrounds are now distinguished, and can contribute to better individually tailoring each patient's therapeutic regimen. Nonetheless, the EGPA-relapse rate remains high and long-term damage is consequential. Further investigations are needed to improve overall care of EGPA patient.

References

1. Churg J, Strauss L. Allergic granulomatosis, allergic angiitis, and periarteritis nodosa. Am J Pathol. 1951;27(2):277–301.
2. Masi AT, Hunder GG, Lie JT, et al. The American College of Rheumatology 1990 criteria for the classification of Churg–Strauss syndrome (allergic granulomatosis and angiitis). Arthritis Rheum. 1990;33(8):1094–100.
3. Jennette JC, Falk RJ, Bacon PA, et al. 2012 Revised International Chapel Hill Consensus Conference Nomenclature of Vasculitides. Arthritis Rheum. 2013;65:1):1–11.
4. Mahr A, Guillevin L, Poissonnet M, Aymé S. Prevalences of polyarteritis nodosa, microscopic polyangiitis, Wegener's granulomatosis, and Churg–Strauss syndrome in a French urban multiethnic population in 2000: a capture–recapture estimate. Arthritis Rheum. 2004;51(1):92–9.

5. Sada K-E, Amano K, Uehara R, et al. A nationwide survey on the epidemiology and clinical features of eosinophilic granulomatosis with polyangiitis (Churg–Strauss) in Japan. Mod Rheumatol. 2014;24(4):640–4.
6. Watts RA, Lane SE, Scott DG, et al. Epidemiology of vasculitis in Europe. Ann Rheum Dis. 2001;60(12):1156–7.
7. Gonzalez-Gay MA, Garcia-Porrua C, Guerrero J, Rodriguez-Ledo P, Llorca J. The epidemiology of the primary systemic vasculitides in northwest Spain: implications of the Chapel Hill Consensus Conference definitions. Arthritis Rheum. 2003;49(3):388–93.
8. Comarmond C, Pagnoux C, Khellaf M, et al. Eosinophilic granulomatosis with polyangiitis (Churg–Strauss): clinical characteristics and long-term followup of the 383 patients enrolled in the French Vasculitis Study Group cohort. Arthritis Rheum. 2013;65(1):270–81.
9. Iudici M, Puéchal X, Pagnoux C, et al. Brief report: childhood-onset systemic necrotizing vasculitides: long-term data from the French Vasculitis Study Group Registry. Arthritis Rheumatol. 2015;67(7):1959–65.
10. Harrold LR, Andrade SE, Go AS, Buist AS, Eisner M, Vollmer WM, et al. Incidence of Churg–Strauss syndrome in asthma drug users: a population-based perspective. J Rheumatol. 2005;32(6):1076–80.
11. Mouthon L, Khaled M, Cohen P, Guillevin L, Subra J. Systemic small sized vessel vasculitis after massive antigen inhalation. Ann Rheum Dis. 2001;60(9):903–4.
12. Guillevin L, Guittard T, Bletry O, Godeau P, Rosenthal P. Systemic necrotizing angiitis with asthma: causes and precipitating factors in 43 cases. Lung. 1987;165(1):165–72.
13. Bottero P, Bonini M, Vecchio F, et al. The common allergens in the Churg–Strauss syndrome. Allergy. 2007;62(11):1288–94.
14. Franco J, Artés MJ. Pulmonary eosinophilia associated with montelukast. Thorax. 1999;54(6):558–60.
15. Hauser T, Mahr A, Metzler C, et al. The leucotriene receptor antagonist montelukast and the risk of Churg–Strauss syndrome: a case–crossover study. Thorax. 2008;63(8):677–82.
16. Wechsler ME, Finn D, Gunawardena D, et al. Churg–Strauss syndrome in patients receiving montelukast as treatment for asthma. Chest. 2000;117(3):708–13.
17. Puéchal X, Rivereau P, Vinchon F. Churg–Strauss syndrome associated with omalizumab. Eur J Intern Med. 2008;19(5):364–6.
18. Wechsler ME, Wong DA, Miller MK, Lawrence-Miyasaki L. Churg-Strauss syndrome in patients treated with omalizumab. Chest. 2009;136(2):507–18.
19. Lyons PA, Rayner TF, Trivedi S, et al. Genetically distinct subsets within ANCA-associated vasculitis. N Engl J Med. 2012;367(3):214–23.
20. Vaglio A, Martorana D, Maggiore U, et al. *HLA-DRB4* as a genetic risk factor for Churg–Strauss syndrome. Arthritis Rheum. 2007;56(9):3159–66.
21. Müschen M, Warskulat U, Perniok A, et al. Involvement of soluble CD95 in Churg–Strauss syndrome. Am J Pathol. 1999;155(3):915–25.
22. Jakiela B, Szczeklik W, Sokolowska B, et al. Intrinsic pathway of apoptosis in peripheral blood eosinophils of Churg–Strauss syndrome. Rheumatology. 2009;48(10):1202–7.
23. Terrier B, Bièche I, Maisonobe T, et al. Interleukin-25: a cytokine linking eosinophils and adaptive immunity in Churg–Strauss syndrome. Blood. 2010;116(22):4523–31.
24. Tai PC, Holt ME, Denny P, Gibbs AR, Williams BD, Spry CJ. Deposition of eosinophil cationic protein in granulomas in allergic granulomatosis and vasculitis: the Churg–Strauss syndrome. Br Med J (Clin Res Ed). 1984;289(6442):400–2.
25. Jakiela B, Szczeklik W, Plutecka H, et al. Increased production of IL-5 and dominant Th2-type response in airways of Churg–Strauss syndrome patients. Rheumatology. 2012;51(10):1887–93.
26. Jakiela B, Sanak M, Szczeklik W, et al. Both Th2 and Th17 responses are involved in the pathogenesis of Churg–Strauss syndrome. Clin Exp Rheumatol. 2011;29(1 Suppl 64):S23–34.
27. Stone JH, Merkel PA, Spiera R, et al. RAVE: rituximab versus cyclophosphamide for ANCA-associated vasculitis. N Engl J Med. 2010;363(3):221–32.
28. Guillevin L, Pagnoux C, Karras A, et al. MAINRITSAN: rituximab versus azathioprine for maintenance in ANCA-associated vasculitis. N Engl J Med. 2014;371(19):1771–80.

29. Tsurikisawa N, Saito H, Oshikata C, Tsuburai T, Akiyama K. Decreases in the numbers of peripheral blood regulatory T cells, and increases in the levels of memory and activated B cells, in patients with active eosinophilic granulomatosis and polyangiitis. J Clin Immunol. 2013;33(5):965–76.
30. Vaglio A, Strehl JD, Manger B, et al. IgG4 immune response in Churg–Strauss syndrome. Ann Rheum Dis. 2012;71(3):390–3.
31. Falk RJ, Terrell RS, Charles LA, Jennette JC. Anti-neutrophil cytoplasmic autoantibodies induce neutrophils to degranulate and produce oxygen radicals in vitro. Proc Natl Acad Sci U S A. 1990;87(11):4115–9.
32. Xiao H, Heeringa P, Hu P, et al. Antineutrophil cytoplasmic autoantibodies specific for myeloperoxidase cause glomerulonephritis and vasculitis in mice. J Clin Invest. 2002;110(7):955–63.
33. Cottin V, Bel E, Bottero P, et al. Respiratory manifestations of eosinophilic granulomatosis with polyangiitis (Churg–Strauss). Eur Respir J. 2016;48(5):1429–41.
34. Erzurum SC, Underwood GA, Hamilos DL, Waldron JA. Pleural effusion in Churg–Strauss syndrome. Chest. 1989;95(6):1357–9.
35. Choi YH, Im JG, Han BK, Kim JH, Lee KY, Myoung NH. Thoracic manifestation of Churg–Strauss syndrome: radiologic and clinical findings. Chest. 2000;117(1):117–24.
36. Herreman G, Ferme I, Puech H, Caubarrère I. Churg and Strauss' allergic granulomatous angiitis with phrenic paralysis. 2 cases. Nouv Presse Med. 1980;9(47):3631.
37. Guillevin L, Pagnoux C, Seror R, et al. The Five-Factor Score revisited: assessment of prognoses of systemic necrotizing vasculitides based on the French Vasculitis Study Group (FVSG) cohort. Medicine (Baltimore). 2011;90(1):19–27.
38. Guillevin L, Lhote F, Gayraud M, et al. Prognostic factors in polyarteritis nodosa and Churg–Strauss syndrome. A prospective study in 342 patients. Medicine (Baltimore). 1996;75(1):17–28.
39. Guillevin L, Cohen P, Gayraud M, Lhote F, Jarrousse B, Casassus P. Churg–Strauss syndrome. Clinical study and long-term follow-up of 96 patients. Medicine (Baltimore). 1999;78(1):26–37.
40. Dennert RM, van Paassen P, Schalla S, et al. Cardiac involvement in Churg–Strauss syndrome. Arthritis Rheum. 2010;62(2):627–34.
41. Dunogué B, Terrier B, Cohen P, et al. Impact of cardiac magnetic resonance imaging on eosinophilic granulomatosis with polyangiitis outcomes: a long-term retrospective study on 42 patients. Autoimmun Rev. 2015;14(9):774–80.
42. Pugnet G, Gouya H, Puéchal X, et al. Cardiac involvement in granulomatosis with polyangiitis: a magnetic resonance imaging study of 31 consecutive patients. Rheumatolgy (Oxford). 2017;56(6):947–56.
43. Sinico RA, Di Toma L, Maggiore U, et al. Renal involvement in Churg–Strauss syndrome. Am J Kidney Dis. 2006;47(5):770–9.
44. Azar N, Guillevin L, Lê Thi Huong D, Herreman G, Meyrier A, Godeau P. Symptomatic urogenital manifestations of polyarteritis nodosa and Churg–Strauss angiitis: analysis of 8 of 165 patients. J Urol. 1989;142(1):136–8.
45. Takanashi T, Uchida S, Arita M, Okada M, Kashii S. Orbital inflammatory pseudotumor and ischemic vasculitis in Churg–Strauss syndrome: report of two cases and review of the literature. Ophthalmology. 2001;108(6):1129–33.
46. Dietz A, Hübner C, Andrassy K. Makrolid-Antibiotika induzierte Vaskulitis (Churg–Strauss-Syndrom). Laryngol-Rhinol-Otologie (Stuttg). 1998;77(02):111–4.
47. Yokoyama A, Kohno N, Fujino S, Inoue Y, Hiwada K. IgG and IgM rheumatoid factor levels parallel interleukin-6 during the vasculitic phase in a patient with Churg–Strauss syndrome. Intern Med Tokyo Jpn. 1995;34(7):646–8.
48. Lanham JG, Elkon KB, Pusey CD, Hughes GR. Systemic vasculitis with asthma and eosinophilia: a clinical approach to the Churg–Strauss syndrome. Medicine (Baltimore). 1984;63(2):65–81.
49. Churg A. Recent advances in the diagnosis of Churg–Strauss syndrome. Mod Pathol. 2001;14(12):1284–93.

50. Kahn J-E, Grandpeix-Guyodo C, Ackermann F, Charles P, Legrand F, Blétry O. Syndromes hyperéosinophiliques: actualités physiopathologiques et thérapeutiques. Rev Méd Intern. 2010;31(4):268–76.
51. Ogbogu PU, Bochner BS, Butterfield JH, et al. Hypereosinophilic syndromes: a multicenter, retrospective analysis of clinical characteristics and response to therapy. J Allergy Clin Immunol. 2009;124(6):1319–25.
52. Roufosse F, Cogan E, Goldman M. Lymphocytic variant hypereosinophilic syndromes. Immunol Allergy Clin North Am. 2007;27(3):389–413.
53. Groh M, Pagnoux C, Baldini C, et al. Eosinophilic granulomatosis with polyangiitis (Churg–Strauss) (EGPA) Consensus Task Force recommendations for evaluation and management. Eur J Intern Med. 2015;26(7):545–53.
54. Sinico RA, Di Toma L, Maggiore U, et al. Prevalence and clinical significance of antineutrophil cytoplasmic antibodies in Churg–Strauss syndrome. Arthritis Rheum. 2005;52(9):2926–35.
55. Sablé-Fourtassou R, Cohen P, Mahr A, et al. Antineutrophil cytoplasmic antibodies and the Churg–Strauss syndrome. Ann Intern Med. 2005;143(9):632–8.
56. Ribi C, Cohen P, Pagnoux C, et al. Treatment of Churg–Strauss syndrome without poor-prognosis factors: a multicenter, prospective, randomized, open-label study of seventy-two patients. Arthritis Rheum. 2008;58(2):586–94.
57. Samson M, Puéchal X, Devilliers H, et al. Long-term outcomes of 118 patients with eosinophilic granulomatosis with polyangiitis (Churg–Strauss syndrome) enrolled in two prospective trials. J Autoimmun. 2013;43(Suppl C):60–9.
58. Puéchal X, Pagnoux C, Baron G, et al. CHUSPAN2: adding azathioprine to remission-induction glucocorticoids for eosinophilic granulomatosis with polyangiitis (Churg–Strauss), microscopic polyangiitis, or polyarteritis nodosa without poor prognosis factors: a randomized, controlled trial. Arthritis Rheumatol. 2017;69(11):2175–86.
59. Cohen P, Pagnoux C, Mahr A, et al. Churg–Strauss syndrome with poor-prognosis factors: a prospective multicenter trial comparing glucocorticoids and six or twelve cyclophosphamide pulses in forty-eight patients. Arthritis Rheum. 2007;57(4):686–93.
60. de Groot K, Harper L, Jayne DRW, et al. Pulse versus daily oral cyclophosphamide for induction of remission in antineutrophil cytoplasmic antibody-associated vasculitis: a randomized trial. Ann Intern Med. 2009;150(10):670–80.
61. Harper L, Morgan MD, Walsh M, et al. Pulse versus daily oral cyclophosphamide for induction of remission in ANCA-associated vasculitis: long-term follow-up. Ann Rheum Dis. 2012;71(6):955–60.
62. Pagnoux C, Quéméneur T, Ninet J, et al. CORTAGE: treatment of systemic necrotizing vasculitides in patients aged sixty-five years or older: results of a multicenter, open-label, randomized controlled trial of corticosteroid and cyclophosphamide-based induction therapy. Arthritis Rheumatol. 2015;67(4):1117–27.
63. Pagnoux C, Mahr A, Hamidou MA, et al. Azathioprine or methotrexate maintenance for ANCA-associated vasculitis. N Engl J Med. 2008;359(26):2790–803.
64. Hiemstra TF, Walsh M, Mahr A, et al. Mycophenolate mofetil vs azathioprine for remission maintenance in antineutrophil cytoplasmic antibody-associated vasculitis: a randomized controlled trial. JAMA. 2010;304(21):2381–8.
65. Guillevin L, Lhote F, Cohen P, et al. Corticosteroids plus pulse cyclophosphamide and plasma exchanges versus corticosteroids plus pulse cyclophosphamide alone in the treatment of polyarteritis nodosa and Churg–Strauss syndrome patients with factors predicting poor prognosis. Arthritis Rheum. 1995;38(11):1638–45.
66. Klemmer PJ, Chalermskulrat W, Reif MS, Hogan SL, Henke DC, Falk RJ. Plasmapheresis therapy for diffuse alveolar hemorrhage in patients with small-vessel vasculitis. Am J Kidney Dis. 2003;42(6):1149–53.
67. Walsh M, Casian A, Flossmann O, et al. Long-term follow-up of patients with severe ANCA-associated vasculitis comparing plasma exchange to intravenous methylprednisolone treatment is unclear. Kidney Int. 2013;84(2):397–402.

68. Pepper RJ, Fabre MA, Pavesio C, et al. Rituximab is effective in the treatment of refractory Churg–Strauss syndrome and is associated with diminished T-cell interleukin-5 production. Rheumatology. 2008;47(7):1104–5.
69. Thiel J, Hässler F, Salzer U, Voll RE, Venhoff N. Rituximab in the treatment of refractory or relapsing eosinophilic granulomatosis with polyangiitis (Churg–Strauss syndrome). Arthritis Res Ther. 2013;15(5):R133.
70. Mohammad AJ, Hot A, Arndt F, et al. Rituximab for the treatment of eosinophilic granulomatosis with polyangiitis (Churg–Strauss). Ann Rheum Dis. 2016;75(2):396–401.
71. Bouldouyre M-A, Cohen P, Guillevin L. Severe bronchospasm associated with rituximab for refractory Churg–Strauss syndrome. Ann Rheum Dis. 2009;68(4):606.
72. Danieli M, Cappelli M, Malcangi G, Logullo F, Salvi A, Danieli G. Long term effectiveness of intravenous immunoglobulin in Churg–Strauss syndrome. Ann Rheum Dis. 2004;63(12):1649–54.
73. Tsurikisawa N, Taniguchi M, Saito H, et al. Treatment of Churg–Strauss syndrome with high-dose intravenous immunoglobulin. Ann Allergy Asthma Immunol. 2004;92(1):80–7.
74. Metzler C, Csernok E, Gross WL, Hellmich B. Interferon-alpha for maintenance of remission in Churg–Strauss syndrome: a long-term observational study. Clin Exp Rheumatol. 2010;28(1) Suppl 57):24–30.
75. Metzler C, Schnabel A, Gross WL, Hellmich B. A phase II study of interferon-alpha for the treatment of refractory Churg–Strauss syndrome. Clin Exp Rheumatol. 2008;26(3) Suppl 49):S35–40.
76. Bargagli E, Rottoli P. Omalizumab treatment associated with Churg–Strauss vasculitis. Int Arch Allergy Immunol. 2008;145(3):268.
77. Detoraki A, Di Capua L, Varricchi G, Genovese A, Marone G, Spadaro G. Omalizumab in patients with eosinophilic granulomatosis with polyangiitis: a 36-month follow-up study. J Asthma. 2016;53(2):201–6.
78. Jachiet M, Samson M, Cottin V, et al. Anti-IgE monoclonal antibody (omalizumab) in refractory and relapsing eosinophilic granulomatosis with polyangiitis (Churg–Strauss): data from 17 patients. Arthritis Rheumatol. 2016;68(9):2274–82.
79. Kostianovsky A, Charles P, Alves J-F, et al. Immunogenicity and safety of seasonal and 2009 pandemic A/H1N1 influenza vaccines for patients with autoimmune diseases: a prospective, monocentre trial on 199 patients. Clin Exp Rheumatol. 2012;30(1 Suppl 70):S83–9.
80. Herlyn K, Gross WL, Reinhold-Keller E. Longitudinale Effekte des strukturierten Patientenschulungsprogramms für Vaskulitispatienten. Z Für Rheumatol. 2008;67(3):206.
81. Chumbley LC, Harrison EG, DeRemee RA. Allergic granulomatosis and angiitis (Churg–Strauss syndrome). Report and analysis of 30 cases. Mayo Clin Proc. 1977;52(8):477–84.
82. Gaskin G, Clutterbuck EJ, Pusey CD. Renal disease in the Churg–Strauss syndrome. Diagnosis, management and outcome. Contrib Nephrol. 1991;94:58–65.
83. Solans R, Bosch JA, Pérez-Bocanegra C, et al. Churg–Strauss syndrome: outcome and long-term follow-up of 32 patients. Rheumatology (Oxford). 2001;40(7):763–71.
84. Durel C-A, Berthiller J, Caboni S, Jayne D, Ninet J, Hot A. Long-term followup of a multicenter cohort of 101 patients with eosinophilic granulomatosis with polyangiitis (Churg–Strauss). Arthritis Care Res. 2016;68(3):374–87.

Granulomatosis with Polyangiitis

7

Christian Pagnoux

7.1 Introduction

Granulomatosis with polyangiitis (GPA; previously called Wegener's granulomatosis) is a necrotizing systemic vasculitis characterized by granulomatous inflammation of small-vessel walls [1, 2]. Although GPA is rare, its incidence seems to have increased over the past decades, at least in some Nordic countries [3, 4]. It mainly affects adults between 45 and 60 years old. The ear, nose, and throat (ENT), pulmonary, and/or renal manifestations represent the cardinal signs of the disease [5, 6]. The origin of GPA remains unknown, although knowledge of the main pathogenic mechanisms has greatly improved, particularly since the discovery of antineutrophil cytoplasmic antibodies (ANCA) in 1985 and their possible pathogenic role, and in recent years [7]. GPA is typically associated with the presence in serum of these autoantibodies directed against cytoplasmic granules of neutrophils, as detected by indirect immunofluorescence (mainly cANCA) or ELISA (mainly antiproteinase 3 [PR3]-ANCA).

In the mid-1950s, the median survival of GPA patients was only 5 months [8], with 82% of deaths occurring within 1 year of the first symptoms. With current treatments, when respected, remission can be achieved in most cases, with limited side effects [9, 10]. However, the risk of relapse is still an issue and requires prolonged prescription of immunosuppressive treatments for maintenance, the optimal duration still unclear [11, 12]. Some patients also carry GPA forms that are refractory to "classical" treatments or experience multiple relapses, the treatment of which can be challenging.

C. Pagnoux (✉)
Division of Rheumatology, Vasculitis Clinic, Mount Sinai Hospital, Toronto, ON, Canada
e-mail: cpagnoux@mtsinai.on.ca

R. A. Sinico, L. Guillevin (eds.), *Anti-Neutrophil Cytoplasmic Antibody (ANCA) Associated Vasculitis*, Rare Diseases of the Immune System,
https://doi.org/10.1007/978-3-030-02239-6_7

7.2 Epidemiology

The global incidence of GPA is estimated at 2–12 cases per year per million population and its prevalence 23–160 cases per million inhabitants [3, 13, 14]. GPA affects both sexes with equal frequency, although a few studies suggested a relatively higher frequency among women. The median age of patients at diagnosis is in the fifth decade, but children and older people can be affected. White Caucasian individuals represent 93–98% of the GPA population [5, 15].

The incidence of GPA appears to show a North–South gradient, at least in Europe: indeed, the reported incidence of GPA is twice as high in Norway as in Spain (10.6 vs. 4.9 new cases per year per million inhabitants) [4, 16]. The incidence seems to have increased in recent years, as suggested by several Scandinavian studies [16, 17], but remained stable between 1990 and 2005 in an English study, at around 8.4 new cases of GPA per year per million inhabitants (8.8 for men and 8.1 for women), although the prevalence had increased (from 28.8 per million inhabitants in 1990 to 64.8 in 2005) [18]. These changes in incidence and prevalence rates could be related, at least in part, to better knowledge of the disease, especially since the discovery of the ANCA and the reduced mortality under treatment. Seasonal variations in the incidence of GPA have also been reported but remain uncertain [19]. The existence of these geographical differences and temporal variations of incidence suggest possible pathogenic environmental factors, including occupational exposures, allergens, toxic and/or infectious agents, and/or genetic predisposing factors (see Chaps. 2 and 3) [20].

7.3 Pathogeny

The pathophysiological mechanisms of GPA are more extensively detailed in Chaps. 3 and 4. They are not all known and, above all, the *primum movens* of the disease remains to be identified [21, 22].

GPA remains considered an inflammatory autoimmune disease, and 80% of patients with systemic GPA are positive for PR3-ANCA. The current theory remains that the disease could be triggered by one or more antigenic stimuli (such as infections or exposure to environmental and/or toxic agents) in patients with some genetic predispositions. The hypothesis of an infectious agent, especially *Staphylococcus aureus*, responsible for the activation or the persistent activation of the immune system has been suggested by a few studies [23, 24]. Family forms are exceptional, which supports GPA as not an inherited or genetic disease, although the relative risk of GPA in first-degree relatives of GPA patients compared to the general population is 1.56 times higher (95% confidence interval 0.35–6.90) [25]. A few genetic predisposing factors or associations have been demonstrated with certain alleles, such as those encoding PR3 (*PRTN3* (rs62132295)), intracellular tyrosine phosphatase *PTPN22* (620W allele) or alpha-1 antitrypsin (*serpine A1*), the natural inhibitor of PR3 [26, 27]. Various associations with molecules of the major histocompatibility complex, in particular, with *HLA-DPB1∗0401*, have also been described [26–29].

Following this initial triggering signal(s), the synthesis and subsequent secretion of pro-inflammatory cytokines (tumor necrosis factor α [TNF-α], interleukin 8 [IL-8], and IL-1, in particular) would lead to the activation of neutrophils, then the translocation of cytoplasmic PR3 to the neutrophil membrane, the increased expression of membrane adhesion molecules, and the migration and fixation of neutrophils to endothelial cells. Once attached to the endothelium, neutrophils secrete oxygenated radicals and externalize proteolytic enzymes (including PR3), which are toxic to endothelial cells, and eventually release neutrophil extracellular traps (NETs), loaded in PR3, which may perpetuate PR3 presentation and therefore the production of PR3-ANCA [30–32]. The release and binding of ANCA also lead to the activation of the alternative complement pathway, which amplifies the local inflammatory response and thus increases endothelial lesions.

However, the mechanistic pathogenic role of PR3-ANCA remains uncertain or at least less well demonstrated than that of anti-myeloperoxidase ANCA (MPO-ANCA), which is more characteristic of microscopic polyangiitis and can induce vasculitis in relatively simple animal models [33]. In addition, 10–20% of patients with GPA are negative for ANCA or MPO-ANCA positive. Numerous other dysregulations of the immunological systems have been reported in GPA, including functional abnormalities of T lymphocytes CD4+ CD25+ FoxP3+ regulators [34, 35], whose pathogenic role and frequency are variable. Functional abnormalities of endothelial cells have also been described, and serum endothelial cell autoantibodies have been found in some patients [36, 37].

The formation of granuloma, another histological feature of GPA, involves various cell subpopulations, whose role and action are still poorly elucidated. This granulomatous reaction is thought to be related to a preferential cytokine secretion pattern of T helper 1 (TH1)-type T cells, whereas the predominant TH2-type reactions (IL-4 and IL-10) rather lead to "vasculitic" systemic manifestations (alveolar hemorrhage or glomerulonephritis) [38]. Cytokine imbalances during GPA are probably much more complex, and other types of lymphocytes and cytokines are involved, such as TH17 lymphocytes, the source of IL-17 [39].

7.4 Clinical Manifestations

The main clinical manifestations of GPA and their frequencies are summarized in Table 7.1 [5, 6, 40–42]. The three main target organs or systems are the upper (ENT) and lower (lung) respiratory airways and the kidneys (necrotizing extracapillary, pauci-immune glomerulonephritis).

Table 7.1 Main characteristics of granulomatosis with polyangiitis

Clinical manifestations	
Constitutional symptoms (fever, arthralgia, myalgia)	70–100%
Skin	Purpura (10–50%)
Ear, nose, and throat (ENT) manifestations	Frequent (50–95%): crusting rhinitis, destructive sinusitis, saddle-nose deformity, nasal septum deformity, otitis media
Lung involvement	Frequent (60–80%): lung solid and/or excavated nodules, alveolar hemorrhage, bronchial and/or subglottic stenosis
Kidney involvement	Frequent (60–80%): glomerulonephritis (pauci-immune, necrotizing extracapillary)
Peripheral neuropathy (mononeuritis multiplex)	Possible (25%)
Other "classical" manifestations	Eye manifestations (scleritis, orbital tumor); pachymeningitis; venous thrombosis (7–8%)
Biology	
Standard	Nonspecific inflammatory syndrome; check creatinine and urine analysis (red blood cell casts?)
ANCA	Yes (90% if systemic disease): mainly PR3-ANCA (cytoplasmic ANCA in immunofluorescence)
Radiology	
	Check chest X-ray and/or CT scan for lung nodules, cavitary or not, alveolar hemorrhage (ground-glass opacities), subglottic and/or bronchial stenosis; sinus X-ray and/or CT scan for erosive sinusitis, pseudotumor; other imaging according to clinical presentation
Histology	
	Granuloma (frequent but not always); necrotizing vasculitis of small-sized vessels

ANCA antineutrophil cytoplasmic antibodies, *PR3-ANCA* antiproteinase 3-ANCA

7.4.1 ENT Manifestations

Noted in 70% of patients, ENT manifestations often reveal the disease and include persistent nasal obstruction, nasal pain, sinusitis, rhinitis, possibly hemorrhagic and/or crusting, repeated epistaxis, serous otitis media and/or hypoacousia, conductive, neurosensorial or mixed and sometimes definitive [43]. Hyposmia and/or hypogeusia are not exceptional [44]. Sinus CT may reveal unilateral or bilateral sinusitis, bone destruction, and/or lysis of the cartilage of the nose, which may result in perforation of the nasal septum (Figs. 7.1 and 7.2) and clinically manifest as a "saddle nose" (Fig. 7.3), observed in 4% of patients at diagnosis but up to 23% afterward [15, 45]. The cartilage of the ears can also be affected (chondritis). Erosion of sinus bone and cartilage can be accompanied by the development of granulomatous inflammatory pseudotumors, which can infiltrate the sinuses, the base of the skull, and/or the orbits (Figs. 7.1, 7.2, and 7.4) and be responsible for pain, exophthalmia, pachymeningitis by contiguity, and/or compress surrounding structures, such as cranial nerves (ophthalmoplegia) or optic nerves.

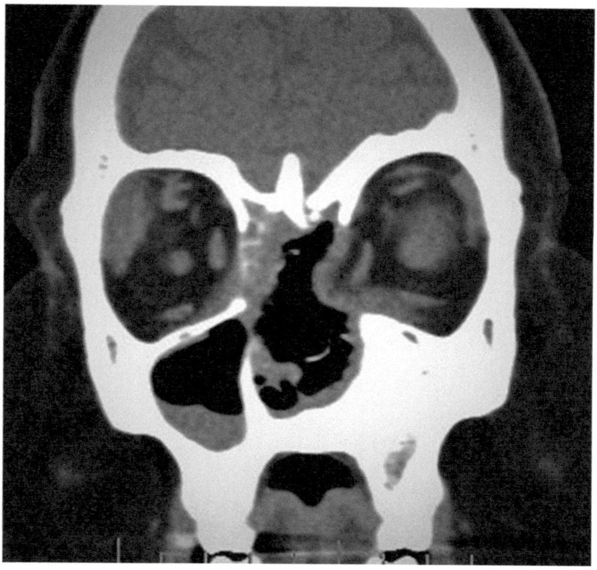

Fig. 7.1 Head CT (coronal view). Erosive destruction of the midline sinonasal cartilaginous structures, atrophy of left maxillary sinus, mild right maxillary sinusitis, erosion of lamina papyracea, and right supero-orbital pseudotumor in a patient with granulomatosis with polyangiitis (GPA)

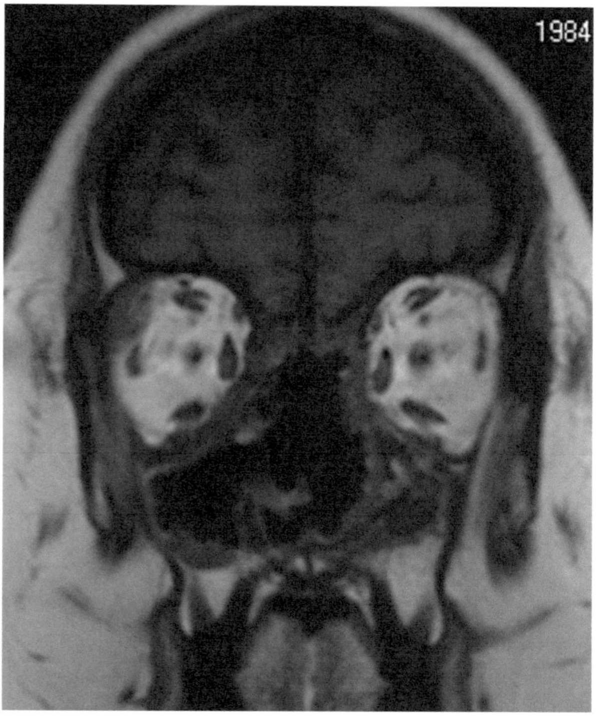

Fig. 7.2 Head MRI (coronal view) (same patient as in Fig. 7.7). Erosive destruction of the midline sinonasal cartilaginous structures, atrophy of left maxillary sinus, mild right maxillary sinusitis, erosion of lamina papyracea, and right supero-orbital pseudotumor in a patient with GPA

Subglottic stenosis (7–15% of patients) can be responsible for dysphonia and dyspnea, with or without stridor, and may occasionally require local urgent procedures (dilation with local injections of glucocorticoids or surgery with tracheostomy) and are sometimes associated with endobronchial lesions [46, 47] (Figs. 7.5, 7.6, and 7.7).

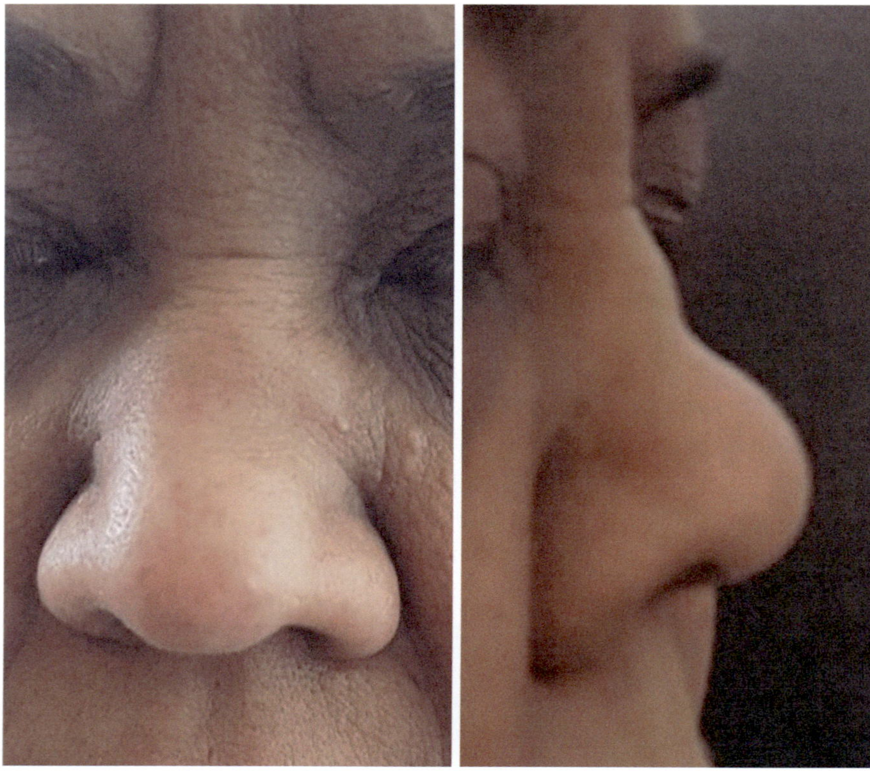

Fig. 7.3 Saddle nose deformity in a patient with GPA

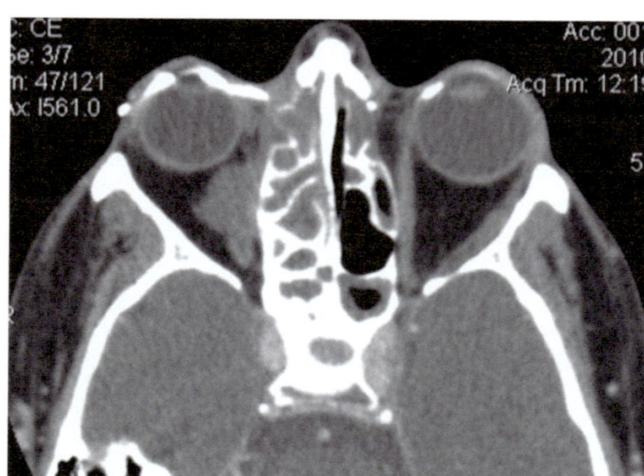

Fig. 7.4 Head CT (axial view). Right orbital, retro-ocular pseudotumor in a patient with GPA

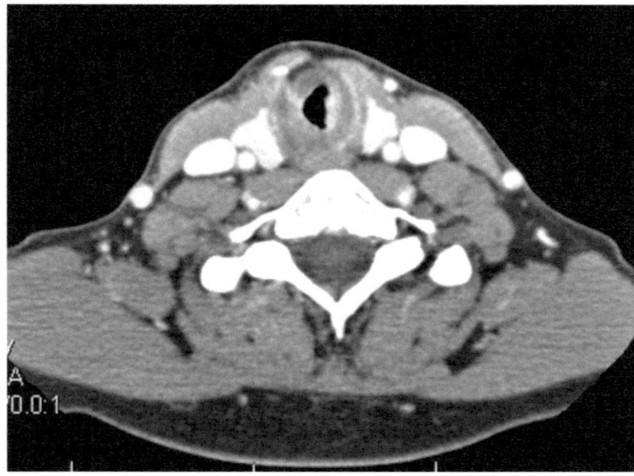

Fig. 7.5 Chest/neck CT (axial view). Subglottic narrowing, with submucosal infiltration

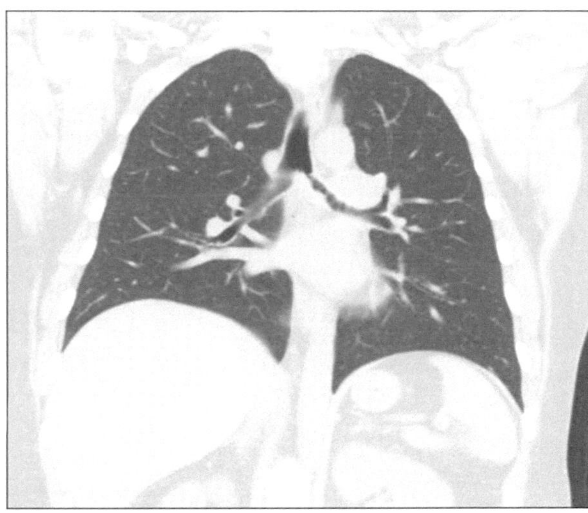

Fig. 7.6 Chest CT (coronal view). Main bronchial stenosis in a patient with GPA (especially the main left bronchus, with compensatory dilation of the end portion of the trachea)

7.4.2 Pulmonary Manifestations

Pulmonary manifestations, present in 70% of patients, can be asymptomatic or present clinically as simple cough, moderate dyspnea, chest pain, or acute respiratory distress with hemoptysis due massive alveolar hemorrhage. Pulmonary nodules are characteristic signs of GPA, observed on X-rays and CT scan of the thorax in 40–66% of patients [5, 48], unilateral or bilateral, single or multiple (generally <10), and excavated in half of the cases (Figs. 7.8, 7.9, and 7.10). Alveolar hemorrhage (8–30% of patients)

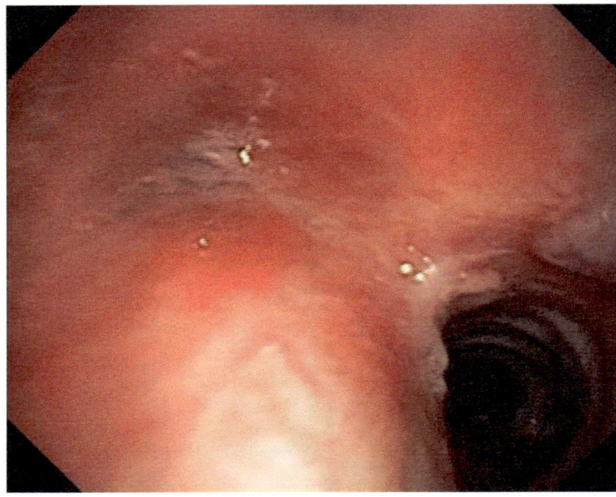

Fig. 7.7 Bronchoscopic appearance of the left main bronchus stenosis (almost completely occluded) in a patient with GPA (same patient as Fig. 7.5)

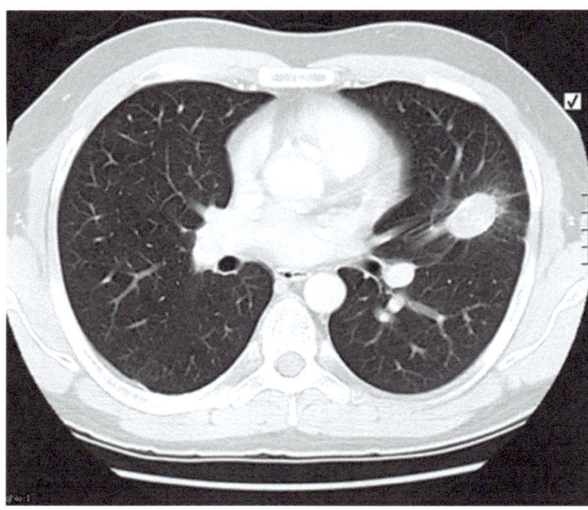

Fig. 7.8 Chest CT (axial view). Plain nodule in the left lung of a patient with GPA

may be limited to a few hemoptoic expectorations or be more massive, responsible for acute respiratory failure and anemia (Fig. 7.11). Unilateral or bilateral pulmonary infiltrates are observed in 30–50% of patients and pleural effusion in 9–28%. Bronchial stenoses are not uncommon, often combined with subglottic stenosis [49] (Figs. 7.5, 7.6, and 7.7). Pneumothorax or hemopneumothorax has also been reported.

7.4.3 Renal Involvement

The most typical and earliest sign of renal involvement during GPA is microscopic hematuria, before the development of proteinuria and renal function impairment.

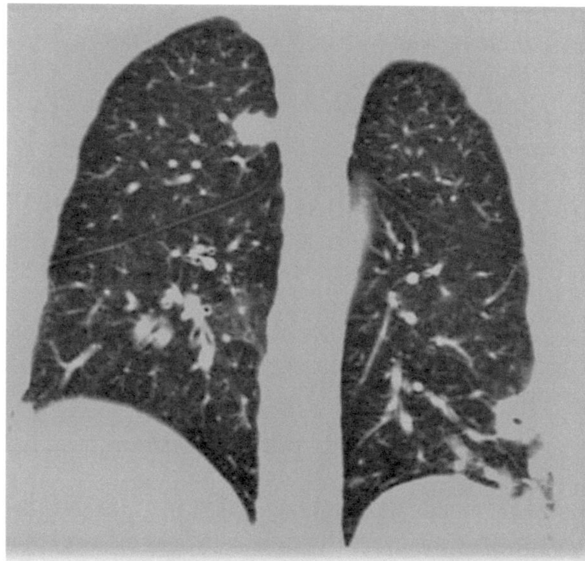

Fig. 7.9 Chest CT (coronal view). Multiple, bilateral lung nodules in a patient with GPA

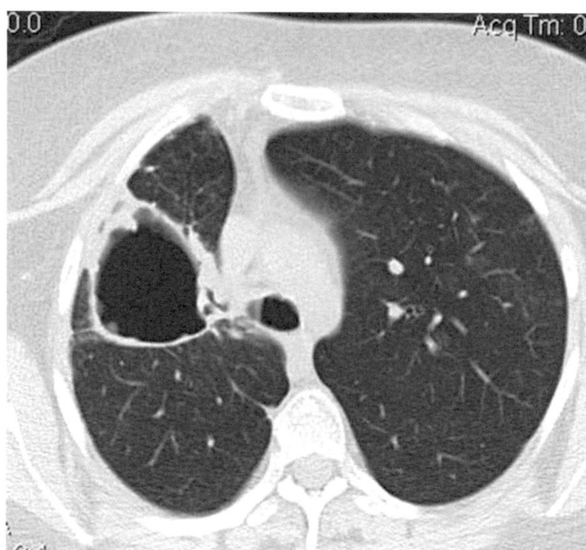

Fig. 7.10 Chest CT (axial view). Large cavitary lesion in the left lung of a patient with GPA

Segmental and focal necrotizing glomerulonephritis, associated with extracapillary proliferation with crescents, with no (or very little) detectable deposits in immunofluorescence (pauci-immune glomerulonephritis) are the classical histological findings on renal biopsy. The combination of alveolar hemorrhage and renal involvement defines the pneumorenal syndrome, the occurrence of which evokes a number of vasculitides, including GPA and microscopic polyangiitis but also anti-glomerular

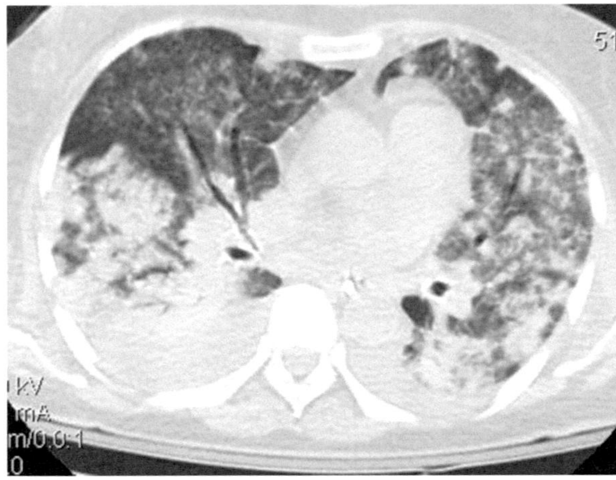

Fig. 7.11 Chest CT (axial view). Diffuse ground glass opacities and posterior consolidation areas in a patient with GPA and alveolar hemorrhage

basement membrane antibody (antiGBM) disease (overlaps exist between renal ANCA-associated vasculitis and antiGBM disease). Rarer renal manifestations during GPA include interstitial granulomatous nephritis, granulomatous renal masses, or renal artery branch aneurysms, especially parenchymal [50].

7.4.4 Other Manifestations

General signs are common during GPA, especially asthenia, fever, myalgia, arthralgia, and/or weight loss but are nonspecific.

Peripheral neuropathy, related to ischemic axonal vasculitis of *vasa nervorum*, is noted in 11–68% of the patients [51, 52], at the time of diagnosis in more than half of the cases [53], and most typically mononeuritis multiplex. Sensorimotor polyneuropathy is less common. Central neurological system involvement is rarer (6–13% of the patients, on average) and occurs often later than peripheral involvement, 8 months on average, after GPA diagnosis [52, 54]. Central nervous system involvement can result from the contiguous extension of sinus or orbital granulomatous lesions or the development of authentic granulomatous lesions of the meninges (pachymeningitis) and/or intracranial vasculitis. These lesions can clinically manifest with headaches, meningeal syndrome, cranial nerve palsies, hypoacousia, ischemic or rarely hemorrhagic stroke, or comitiality [55]. Pituitary involvement is a rare but well-known manifestation and may result in optic chiasma compression or diabetes insipidus [56]. Medullary involvement is rare, related to compression by a granulomatous meningeal infiltrate or to ischemic medullary vasculitis [52]. Cranial nerve palsies, mainly of the optic nerves (II), VI, and/or VII, unilateral or bilaterally, is found in 4–14% of patients [53].

Skin lesions, observed 10–50% of patients, are mainly vascular purpura, declive, petechial, infiltrated, and palpable (Figs. 7.12 and 7.13) but sometimes ulcerative, necrotic, and extensive and, more rarely, subcutaneous nodules [57]. Lesions on the elbows and hands, including the pulp of the fingertips, are not uncommon. Pyoderma gangrenosum or hidradenitis suppurativa (Fig. 7.14) has also been reported [58].

Oral mucosal lesions such as ulcerations have been reported in 10–50% of patients. "Raspberry" gingival hypertrophy is rarer but very suggestive of GPA. Genital ulcerations are less common.

Ocular and/or orbital involvement is reported in 14–60% of patients [59], sometimes inaugural and/or isolated (Fig. 7.4). Exophthalmia, possibly associated

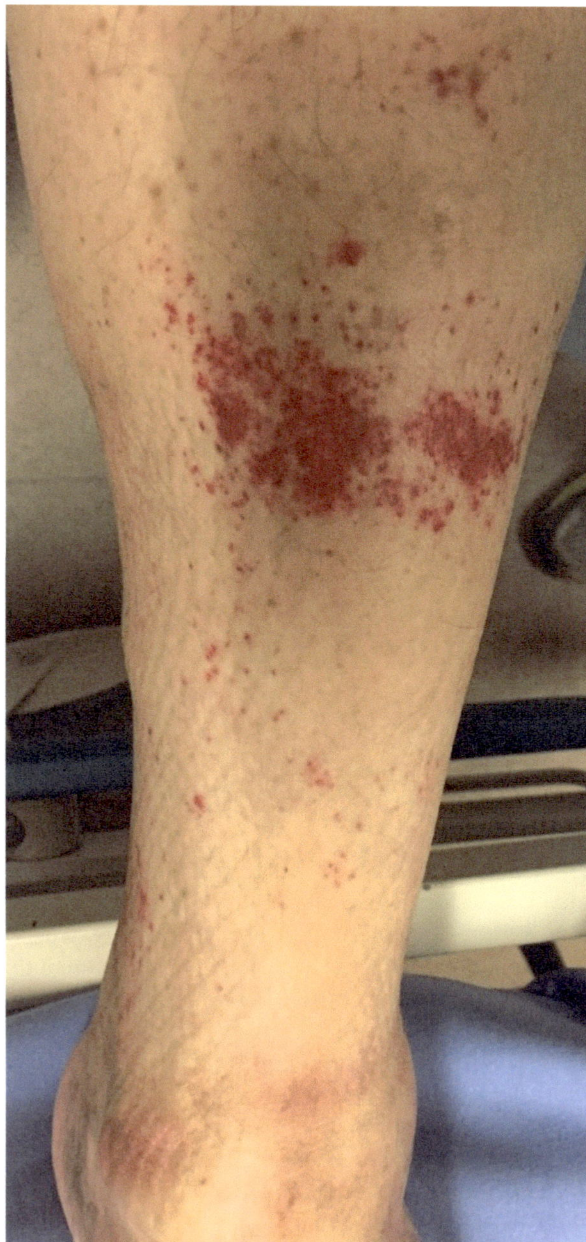

Fig. 7.12 Purpuric-ecchymotic lesions of the legs (left leg on the picture) in a patient with GPA

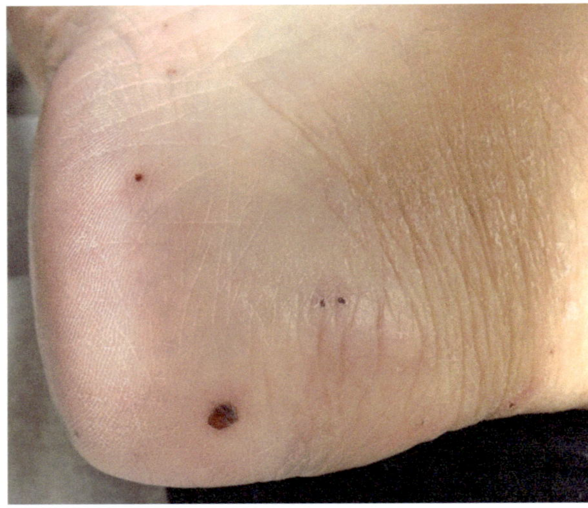

Fig. 7.13 Small necrotic purpuric lesion of the talus in a patient with GPA

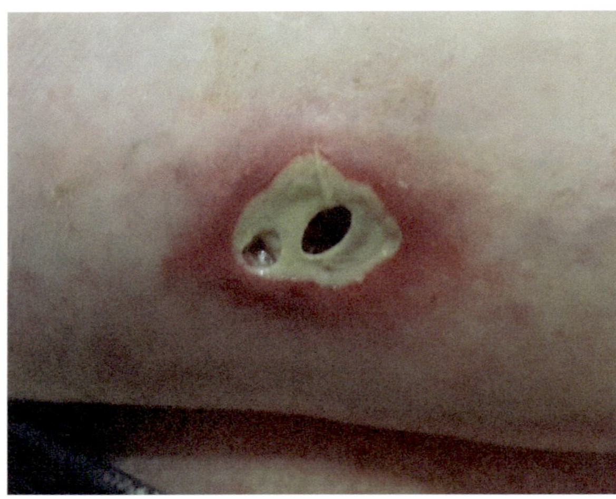

Fig. 7.14 Hidradenitis suppurativa lesion of the abdominal pannus in a patient with GPA

with ophthalmoplegia, can result from the local extension of a contiguous granulomatous lesion within the orbital frame. Conjunctivitis and/or episcleritis are relatively frequent and of no particular gravity, whereas corneal ulcerations, necrotizing nodular scleritis (with risk of perforation of the eye and endophthalmitis), and/or, more rarely, retinal vasculitis represent more serious manifestations that may lead to vision loss. Dacryocystitis can be responsible for obstruction of the lacrimal ducts and require surgical debridement and stenting of lacrimal canals. Xanthelasma may develop, spontaneously or after regression of an ipsilateral orbital pseudotumor [57].

Clinically manifested cardiac manifestations are rare during GPA (0–12%) [8, 60]. Pericardial effusion, tamponade and/or constrictive pericarditis, and coronary artery disease, mostly clinically silent, account for half of these cases. Valvular lesions, mainly aortic, are reported with a frequency of 21% in some ultrasonography studies [61]. Sinus tachycardia is common, as is atrial fibrillation; granulomatous involvement of conduction tissues (sinus node: 13%, atrioventricular node: 13%) can lead to atrioventricular blocks or bundle branch blocks, generally regressing rapidly after initiation of medical treatment for GPA. Cardiac abnormalities may be more frequent on MRI imaging, yet of undetermined clinical significance [62, 63].

Gastrointestinal (GI) manifestations concern 5–11% of patients, ranging from simple, nonspecific abdominal pain to more severe ischemic digestive perforations, especially of the small bowel [64, 65]. Granulomatous ileocolitis, anorectitis, or gastritis have also been reported, sometimes mimicking Crohn's disease or ulcerative colitis [66]. Granulomatous, vasculitic appendicitis or pancreatic lesions (sometimes with a pseudotumoral appearance), and/or cholecystitis have been reported. Hepatic involvement is rare and usually remains biological and subclinical, as are splenic lesions [67], although they may be responsible for infarction or nontraumatic rupture of the spleen [68]. Aneurysms of GI arteries, which may rupture, have rarely been reported in GPA [69].

Various other and rarer manifestations described during GPA include thyroid granulomatous lesions; ureteral stenosis related to ischemic fibrosing lesions, ureteral or periureteral arteriolitis, granulomatous infiltrates, or retroperitoneal fibrosis; granulomatous prostatitis, cystitis, orchitis, urethritis, and penile ulcerations; mastitis, vulvar, ovarian, or uterine localizations; periostitis or prevertebral dorsal lesions; and aortitis [70, 71].

Finally, increased risk of thromboembolic venous accidents (7.6% of patients with GPA in a French cohort) was demonstrated in several studies, 20 times more than in the general population, particularly within 2–3 months after the initial diagnosis or a relapse [72–75].

7.4.5 Limited/Localized Forms Versus Diffuse/Systemic/Severe Forms

Systemic/diffuse/severe forms of GPA are characterized by the involvement of one or more major organs, particularly progressive renal disease and/or extensive and progressive alveolar hemorrhage. Limited/localized forms are mainly ENT (rhinitis, sinusitis) and/or respiratory (lung nodules), sometimes also cutaneous [40, 76], and do not involve the life prognosis. These localized/limited forms would represent up to 29% of GPA patients at diagnosis, particularly women, slightly younger than those with diffuse forms (41 years vs. 50 years, on average, at diagnosis) [42, 77]. From a biological point of view, ANCAs are found in more than 90% of patients with systemic/diffuse/severe forms but only 50–78% of those with the limited/localized forms [78, 79].

Although limited/localized, these forms of GPA are no less difficult to treat, and the transition to a systemic/diffuse/severe form is possible, and vice versa, during the course of the disease. GPA strictly localized to an organ or system and remaining as such is indeed rather exceptional in practice. In the German and French cohorts, patients with GPA remaining with localized disease after 3 years of follow-up (with treatments adapted to these forms) represented less than 5% of all GPA patients [78, 79].

7.4.6 Pediatric Patients

GPA is exceptional in children. The disease presentations remain very similar to that in adults, although girls appear to be more often affected than boys. As well, nasal deformities and subglottic stenosis are more common, thereby being integrated in the criteria for classification of GPA of the European research groups EULAR/PReS [80]. Renal damage is also common, and venous thrombosis may occur more often than in adults (up to 16% of children with GPA) as well as ischemic abdominal pain (20% vs. 6% in adults). However, neurological disorders appear to be slightly less frequent (18% of cases) [81, 82]. The short-term overall prognosis seems quite comparable, but with significant morbidity related to the disease and the side effects of treatments [83, 84].

7.5 Diagnosis

The diagnosis of GPA can be straightforward in patients with a combination of classical features such as crusting rhinitis, pulmonary nodules, renal involvement with microscopic hematuria and proteinuria, necrotic purpura of the lower limbs, and mononeuritis multiplex. PR3-ANCA positivity then makes the diagnosis certain. However, especially in those less obvious situations, histological confirmation of the diagnosis can be preferable. Renal biopsy, in case of renal impairment, may also provide prognostic information about the chance of renal function recovery [50].

A nonspecific inflammatory syndrome with neutrophilia is usual (about 9500–12,500/mm^3), with anemia in 50–73% of patients, more pronounced with alveolar hemorrhage [5]. The erythrocyte sedimentation rate is increased, as is C-reactive protein level [85]. Transient and moderate eosinophilia is possible (<12% of cases), which, however, should prompt discussion of an alternative diagnosis of eosinophilic granulomatosis with polyangiitis or immunoglobulin G4 (IgG4)-related disease [86].

The presence of cANCA (diffuse cytoplasmic type in immunofluorescence) directed against PR3 on ELISA is a major argument for the diagnosis of GPA. The ANCA search by two techniques combined (immunofluorescence and ELISA) has excellent specificity (95%) and sensitivity (80–90%) for the diffuse forms of the disease, less so in the "limited" forms (sensitivity 50–60% and specificity 95%). Recent recommendation is to prioritize ELISA as the primary screening method [87]. Some cases of GPA are called ANCA negative, especially in patients with "limited" disease forms, and some patients are positive for pANCA (perinuclear type in immunofluorescence) directed against MPO on ELISA (less than 5% of patients but more in Asian GPA patients). Patients with both types, PR3-ANCA and

MPO-ANCA, are exceptional, and this double positivity should raise suspicion for cocaine-levamisole–induced vasculopathy, during which anti-elastase antibodies, cross-reacting with PR3-ANCA tests, can be detected. Importantly, the detection of ANCA is possible under other conditions or pathologies, some of which may mimic or be accompanied by genuine vasculitis, such as infectious endocarditis or ulcerative colitis (see Chap. 6) [66, 87, 88].

Imaging of the chest should always be performed. CT imaging will be ordered in case of abnormal chest X-ray findings or systematically. Other radiological examinations, such as brain MRI or angio-MRI, cerebral arteriography, abdominopelvic ultrasonography, or CT, are prescribed according to the clinical findings. The presence of micro-aneurysms of the renal, splenic, and/or hepatic arteries is characteristic of polyarteritis nodosa, although a few cases of microaneurysms have been reported in GPA [69]. Endoscopic examinations should also be considered in case of ENT, bronchial, and/or lung involvement, with caution in case of subglottic or bronchial stenosis (risk of spasm or subacute edematous inflammatory reaction). Bronchoalveolar lavage can confirm alveolar hemorrhage and rule out infection (or neoplasia). Bronchial biopsy can be performed, with sensitivity lower than that of surgical lung biopsy [5, 89]. In cases of GI manifestations, endoscopy can be used to detect ulcerations, especially ileocolic or anorectal, sometimes resembling those found in Crohn's disease, but also gastric and/or esophageal. GI tract biopsy is not without risk (perforations), and the sensitivity is low in practice [64–66].

Electromyography exploration (nerve conduction studies) may confirm or rule out axonal peripheral neuropathy, most typically manifesting as asymmetric mononeuritis multiplex or, less commonly, polyneuropathy [52].

Histological confirmation of the diagnosis can be obtained by biopsy of an organ affected by the disease. Naso-sinus biopsy is simple to perform but requires a large number of samples (only half of sinus biopsies and only 20% of nasal biopsies are contributory) [43]. Tracheal biopsy, in case of subglottic stenosis, can be hazardous, and therefore, findings often remain superficial; as a result, less than 18% are contributive [90]. Biopsy of pulmonary nodules is more difficult and can sometimes be performed only surgically. However, they can show necrotizing arteriolar vasculitis in more than 60% of cases, sometimes associated with palisade granulomas and/or giant cells [89]. Renal biopsy (in case of renal involvement) typically shows pauci-immune glomerulonephritis (little or no Ig and complement deposits), also known as extracapillary necrotizing glomerulonephritis. Granulomas can be observed in less than 20% of cases. The amount of damage observed is associated with the probability of kidney recovery [50]. Focal glomerular involvement and/or numerous glomerular crescents (>50% of glomeruli) carry better prognosis than highly sclerotic (>50% glomeruli) or mixed cases (<50% sclerotic or crescent glomeruli). Muscle or neuromuscular biopsies have a sensitivity of about 60% in patients with peripheral neuropathy [91]. Biopsy of cutaneous lesions often reveals leucocytoclastic vasculitis, which remains nonspecific. A few patients with GPA-related temporal arteritis and granulomatous findings on biopsy, similar to giant cell arteritis, have been reported [92].

7.6 Treatment

Untreated, GPA is almost always fatal, at least in its diffuse form [8]. With current treatments, remission is achieved in more than 80% of cases, with an overall mortality rate of 10–15% at 5 years [10]. This mortality rate remains higher than that of the general population of the same age, with a standardized mortality ratio (SMR) of 1.58 (95% confidence interval 1.14–2.13), particularly for males (SMR 1.8 vs. 1.23 for women) [6]. The main causes of early mortality include infections and poor disease control [93]. Beyond the first year after the diagnosis, the main causes of death include cardiovascular complications (from treatments and/or disease), infections, and late cancers [94, 95].

The risk of relapse, sometimes multiple in the same patient, is one of the main outcome features of GPA. Relapse is almost guaranteed in the absence of prolonged treatments to maintain remission. However, even with maintenance treatments, relapse remains frequent. The relapse-free survival rate does not exceed 42–57% at 5 years with conventional treatments, although it has improved over the last decades [6, 96]. Moreover, only 11–14% of patients do not show damage or definitive adverse effects from the treatments received [15].

7.6.1 Induction Treatment of Diffuse/Systemic/Severe Forms

The treatment of GPA has two phases: first the induction treatment, based on the combination of corticosteroids and an immunosuppressant, then, once remission has been achieved, maintenance treatment (to maintain remission); however, optimal regimens and durations are not fully established.

Since the late 1970s, the combination of corticosteroids and cyclophosphamide has been considered the standard induction treatment for severe forms of GPA [97, 98], allowing for remission in more than 80% of cases. The initial corticosteroid dose is 1 mg/kg/day prednisone equivalent, sometimes preceded by one to three methylprednisolone boluses (15 mg/kg/day) [11, 12, 99]. After the first 2–4 weeks of treatment, the dose of corticosteroids should be reduced rapidly, by approximately 10% every 1–2 weeks, to reach a half-dose after 1–3 months. The optimal duration and tapering pace of treatment with corticosteroids remain debated [100]. In the United States, some centers consider that treatment beyond 6 months is useless and even dangerous [101, 102].

Cyclophosphamide can be administered in two modalities: intravenous “pulsed” (bolus at regular intervals) or continuous oral, usually for a total of 3–6 months. Pulsed oral administration at regular intervals is another possibility, unusually chosen in practice. The intravenous boluses of cyclophosphamide are administered every 15 days for 1 month at 0.6 g/m^2 or 15 mg/kg (on days 1, 15, and 30), then at 0.7 g/m^2 or 15 mg/kg every 3 weeks [97, 103]. Oral cyclophosphamide is prescribed at 2 mg/kg/day [11, 12, 104, 105]. Doses must be adjusted to renal function and the patient’s age, then according to the therapeutic response and side effects, regardless of the route used [12, 106]. Good hydration should be ensured when intravenous boluses of cyclophosphamide are used, when the bolus dose exceeds 600 mg, in combination with mesna to reduce the bladder toxicity of the cyclophosphamide [107]. In France and most European countries, the most often used regimen is intravenous boluses of cyclophosphamide [108]. The continuous oral route is then a possible "rescue" option for patients who do not achieve remission with intravenous cyclophosphamide boluses. Several studies have established that the two routes of administration of cyclophosphamide (intravenous boluses or oral continuous) are comparable in terms of achieving remission [103, 104, 109]. However, cumulative doses of cyclophosphamide are higher with the continuous oral route, which is associated in some studies with greater risk of neutropenia and infections [103, 104] but also, in the long term, with a lower rate of subsequent relapse [110]. The risk of infertility and/or long-term delayed complications (cancer) are also directly associated with the cumulative dose of cyclophosphamide received.

Rituximab was approved in 2012 by the US Food and Drug Administration for adults with severe forms of GPA as an alternative to cyclophosphamide for induction therapy, combined with corticosteroids. Indeed, two randomized prospective studies showed that rituximab was not inferior in efficacy to cyclophosphamide as induction therapy for remission [101, 111, 112]. At 6 and 18 months, the rates of adverse events, particularly infectious, were also quite comparable in patients with rituximab or cyclophosphamide induction [101]. The primary reason for choosing rituximab over cyclophosphamide is to limit exposure to the latter in patients with contraindication to cyclophosphamide, those with GPA relapse, and/or those who previously received significant cumulative doses of cyclophosphamide (>20 or 30 g, despite no consensual threshold dose to date). Another preferential indication for rituximab is for women of childbearing age (the risk of infertility in a 20-year-old woman receiving a cumulative dose of 6–9 g of cyclophosphamide is probably minimal but not null). The use of rituximab in children with GPA remains limited to date [82, 113]. Other factors may influence the preference for rituximab over cyclophosphamide. The response to rituximab seems better in patients positive for PR3-ANCA and/or with relapsing GPA but less and/or slower in patients with granulomatous lesions (such as ENT lesions or lung nodules), as opposed to vasculitis manifestations (such as alveolar hemorrhage) [114]. The choice between cyclophosphamide and rituximab is also based on economic parameters; of note, rare cases of progressive multifocal leukoencephalopathy have been reported in patients receiving rituximab for other pathologies (lymphoma, lupus) as well as allergic reactions, sometimes very serious, and interstitial "immunoallergic" pneumopathies. Rituximab for induction can be given as four infusions of 375 mg/m^2 at 1-week intervals each or as two infusions of 1 g at 15-day intervals, with comparable efficacy [115]. Maintenance treatment should be considered 4–6 months later.

Plasma exchange has been proposed with rapidly progressive glomerulonephritis and/or alveolar hemorrhage [99, 116, 117]. However, the exact benefit of plasma exchange in patients with ANCA-associated vasculitis has not been formally demonstrated to date. A single small randomized study suggested that in patients with severe renal impairment, plasma exchange (with the classical scheme of "seven exchanges over 15 days") could improve the chance of renal function recovery at 12 months, but the benefit was not sustained beyond this time [118, 119]. The final results of the PEXIVAS trial, expected in late 2019, should help determine the exact place of plasma exchange [120]. Preliminary data suggest no overt benefit of plasma exchange in term of overall or renal survival. The latter study will also inform on the optimal dosing of prednisone during the first months of induction, because it also compared a standard regimen, as described above, to one with faster dose tapering.

7.6.2 Maintenance Treatment of Diffuse/Systemic/Severe Forms

The simple continuation of cyclophosphamide beyond remission is associated with a relatively low rate of relapse of 13% at 5 years [98, 103], but its cumulative toxicity over the long term clearly overweighs its efficacy. Other immunosuppressants, less toxic than cyclophosphamide, should be prescribed for maintenance, after induction therapy with cyclophosphamide [97], usually started within 2 to a maximum of 4 weeks after the last dose of cyclophosphamide. The current choice of conventional maintenance therapy is primarily between oral azathioprine (2–3 mg/kg/day) and methotrexate (orally, intramuscularly, or subcutaneously, 0.3 mg/kg/week, up to 25 mg/week) [97, 121, 122]. Leflunomide (20 mg/day) and mycophenolate mofetil (2 g/day) have also been evaluated for maintenance but in smaller series and, for the latter, with inferior results at maintaining remission over time than azathioprine [123, 124]. Therefore, leflunomide and mycophenolate are usually considered only for patients intolerant to or with a history of relapse(s) with azathioprine and methotrexate.

The optimal duration of maintenance with these agents remains debated, and despite their use, the global relapse rates remain at about 16% at 18 months, 37% at 25 months, and 51–64% at 7 years [6, 97, 121, 125, 126]. Some studies showed no overt benefit in pursuing them beyond 2 years, whereas the largest randomized prospective REMAIN study showed that 4 years of combined maintenance with low-dose prednisone and azathioprine was superior to 2 years in preventing relapse (22% of relapse vs. 63% at year 4), especially in patients who are persistently ANCA-positive at the time of remission (when cyclophosphamide is discontinued) [127]. A few other studies also suggested higher risk of relapse for patients positive for PR3-ANCA than MPO-ANCA (and thus possibly candidates for longer maintenance therapy), although in these studies, MPO-ANCA–positive patients mostly had microscopic polyangiitis rather than GPA [128–130].

The same debate exists regarding the optimal duration of low-dose corticosteroids. In some centers, corticosteroids are stopped early, by months 4–6, especially to reduce the risk of steroid-related infections [131]. However, the continuation of low-dose corticosteroid therapy (prednisone 5 mg/day) beyond 6 and 12 months may also reduce the risk of relapse [100]. Several prospective studies are ongoing and/or planned to more definitely answer this question.

Meanwhile, several studies reported that routine maintenance infusions of rituximab, instead of the conventional azathioprine, could reduce the relapse rate to only

7% or 22% at 2–3 years [132–136]. In the MAINRITSAN study, rituximab was given at 500 mg every 6 months for a total of 5 infusions, after induction with corticosteroids and cyclophosphamide [137]. Rituximab was superior to azathioprine in preventing major relapse, in newly diagnosed as well as relapsing patients. In the ongoing RITAZAREM study, rituximab is given at 1 g every 4 months for 18 months (results expected late 2019), for patients with relapse, induced with rituximab [138]. If confirmed superior to the conventional azathioprine or methotrexate for maintenance, the next question will also be to determine the optimal duration of rituximab use and that of the associated low-dose corticosteroid therapy. Because of the high cost of rituximab, it would also be useful to have definitive answers as to which patient subsets would benefit the most from rituximab maintenance therapy and whether rituximab could be given with a more sparing approach (i.e., only with B-cell repopulation and/or ANCA reappearance or significant titer increase). The MAINRITSAN-2 study showed that this later sparing approach was grossly as effective as systematic infusions every 6 months (17.3% vs. 9.9% of major relapses at 28 months postremission; $P = 0.22$), although this "on-demand" strategy requires a closer biologic monitoring (CD19-B-cell count and ANCA testing every 3 months) [139].

As stated earlier, the therapeutic maintenance strategy when remission is achieved with rituximab is not well defined at this time. In the RAVE trial, no maintenance treatment was given after induction [101]. Hence, a simple monitoring of patients is one option, with repeat treatment only with disease relapse. A few groups suggested that repeat treatments could be given with B-cell repopulation and/or ANCA reappearance or titer increase, as was done in the MAINRITSAN-2 trial mentioned above, although relapse can also occur in patients persistently B-cell depleted and ANCA negative [132, 140]. Conventional maintenance treatments can be considered but with conflicting results on their efficacy in two separate retrospective studies [111, 141]. Finally, systematic maintenance infusions of rituximab, as in the previously mentioned MAINRITSAN (in which cyclophosphamide was used for induction) and (ongoing) RITAZAREM trials, can be considered, especially in patients in remission after a GPA relapse [137, 138].

Cotrimoxazole (trimethoprim-sulfamethoxazole) is not a substitute for maintenance immunosuppressants and is clearly not as effective in this indication [142]. However, its prescription at high dose (trimethoprim 320 mg/day, sulfamethoxazole 1600 mg/day), combined with or after the usual maintenance treatments for GPA, allowed for a further reduction of the relapse rate of 40% at 1 year in a small study, regardless of the presence or absence of *S. aureus* in nasal swabs [143]. Therefore, it can be prescribed in combination (although not with methotrexate, because the renal toxicity of these two drugs could be increased) and/or continued after stopping the other maintenance agent for several months or years [144, 145].

The prevention of relapses and adjustments of the maintenance strategy should also take into account some of the patient's and disease's characteristics. Patients with GPA and PR3-ANCA experience relapse more often than do those with MPO-ANCA microscopic polyangiitis in published studies of ANCA-associated vasculitis [128, 130, 140, 146]. However, in GPA patients only, this distinction between PR3-ANCA and MPO-ANCA is not as obvious. The persistence or reappearance of ANCA under treatment, particularly when switching to maintenance treatment, is associated with a higher subsequent relapse rate. However, relapses are not systematic in case of persistent ANCA, and even patients who become ANCA-negative can relapse [147, 148]. Hence, the consensus is that the treatment should not be adjusted based solely on the ANCA titer, at least when using conventional immunosuppressants, but patients should be monitored closely [11, 12]. In patients receiving rituximab for maintenance, the follow-up of ANCA and CD19 B-cell count may be more reliable [132, 148, 149]. As mentioned earlier, few studies suggested that repeat rituximab infusions for maintenance could be given cost effectively based on ANCA and CD19 B-cell count monitoring every 3 months [132, 139]. Several other clinical predictors of relapse have been identified in several patient cohorts but not uniformly, and none has since been studied prospectively. Among them, the existence of cardiac involvement at diagnosis, a "less intense" initial treatment (cumulative dose of cyclophosphamide <10 g after the first 6 months of treatment and/or reduction of the dose of corticosteroids to <20 mg/day before the third month), previous relapses, pulmonary involvement, especially cavitary lung nodules, and/or ENT involvement have been associated with frequent relapses. Conversely, the presence of initial renal impairment (serum creatinine level >100 μmol/L) seems associated with low risk of relapse [85, 146, 150, 151].

7.6.3 Treatment of Localized/Limited Forms

Lighter treatment may be attempted for localized/limited forms of GPA, mainly granulomatous ENT manifestations. Corticosteroids alone provide improvement in more than 50% of cases but exceptionally, sustained remission [77]. For some patients, treatment has been successful with cotrimoxazole (trimethoprim 320 mg/day, sulfamethoxazole 1600 mg/day) alone or combined with corticosteroids [144], but the results with this treatment were disappointing in a few subsequent prospective studies, some of which had to be stopped early [42, 142]. Moreover, these limited forms are often recurrent, destructive, and/or eventually evolve into a diffuse form; therefore, treatment with a combination of corticosteroids and an immunosuppressant may be preferable [79, 114].

These limited forms may be treated with cyclophosphamide or another, less toxic immunosuppressant, particularly methotrexate, which can achieve remission as frequently and rapidly as cyclophosphamide in these limited forms [152, 153]. More recently, similar results were observed with mycophenolate mofetil, which achieved a similar rate of remission as cyclophosphamide in nonsevere forms [11]. However, the relapse rates were high after methotrexate or mycophenolate mofetil treatment, which should likely be continued for years when effective.

The place of rituximab for limited forms remains to be determined (at present, it is mainly considered for patients with refractory/relapsing limited forms, rather than as a first-line option).

7.6.4 Principles of Treating Relapses and Refractory Forms

When a relapse is suspected, it is first (and concomitantly) necessary to rule out an infection or another associated pathology, particularly neoplasm. Treatment of a relapse occurring under maintenance treatment or when the patient no longer takes immunosuppressants is based on the same type of induction treatment as detailed above. However, results of the RAVE study suggested that rituximab is more often effective than cyclophosphamide in achieving remission in relapsing patients [101, 112]. The cumulative dose of cyclophosphamide previously received must also be considered in the choice between these two induction immunosuppressants. The subsequent switch to maintenance treatment is again based on azathioprine or methotrexate, although maintenance with rituximab may then also be more effective [133, 134, 137, 141]. The results of the ongoing RITAZAREM study should further determine the place of rituximab for maintenance in relapsing patients [138].

For patients with the most severe, refractory, and/or multirelapsing disease, other strategies or combinations can be discussed on a case-by-case basis and in consultation with reference centers for the management of GPA, ideally as part of prospective therapeutic protocols.

7.6.5 Other Treatments and Special Situations

7.6.5.1 Polyvalent Intravenous Immunoglobulins

Intravenous Ig treatment is mainly used in patients with refractory, relapsing GPA, and/or those with ongoing infections, at 2 g/kg/month, given over 2–5 days, with good immediate results but usually only transient, nonsustained efficacy [154, 155]. The treatment has the advantage of being less toxic, particularly in terms of infection and does not cause delayed neoplastic complications, which are other reasons for its occasional use in children or pregnant women with GPA.

7.6.5.2 Treatments Under Investigation and/or Development

Ofatumumab is another fully humanized monoclonal antibody directed against B cells that targets CD20 and has slower dissociation kinetics than rituximab. Ofatumumab is a more potent activator of complement-dependent cytotoxicity in vitro. Combined with low-dose pulsed intravenous cyclophosphamide and corticosteroids, it achieved remission in small group of eight patients with GPA ($n = 3$) or other ANCA-associated vasculitis [156].

Avacopan is an orally administered, selective complement C5a receptor inhibitor tested in small randomized trials in systemic GPA, with promising results, and it is now under investigation in a larger study [157]. In this latter study, it is given orally (30 mg × 2/day) for 12 months, combined with cyclophosphamide (then azathioprine for maintenance) or rituximab (then no maintenance immunosuppressant) and no (or a very brief) corticosteroid treatment and compared with the conventional regimen with the same immunosuppressant(s) and corticosteroids for 20 weeks (and placebo of avacopan). Other complement inhibitors or blocking monoclonal antibodies are also under investigations.

Abatacept is a selective T-cell co-stimulation modulator that consists of the extracellular domain of human cytotoxic T-lymphocyte–associated antigen 4 (CTLA-4) linked to the modified Fc (hinge, CH2, and CH3 domains) portion of human IgG1. It has been tested in a small open-label study in patients with relapsing limited/nonsevere GPA, with promising results (intravenous infusions of 10 mg/kg on days 1, 15, 29 then every 4 weeks) [158]. A larger placebo-controlled randomized study of subcutaneous injections of abatacept (125 mg every week) combined with corticosteroids for relapsing nonsevere GPA is ongoing (ClinicalTrials.gov Identifier: NCT02108860).

Belimumab is a human monoclonal antibody that inhibits B-cell activating factor (BAFF), also known as B-lymphocyte stimulator (BLyS). It has been tested in combination with low-dose corticosteroids and azathioprine for maintenance (intravenous infusions of 10 mg/kg on days 1, 15, and 30, then monthly). This addition of belimumab, as compared with placebo, to the conventional maintenance regimen had no obvious benefit, although a slightly lower relapse rate was observed in the subset of patients induced with rituximab before switching to azathioprine for maintenance [159]. Thus, other studies with belimumab may be considered in GPA patients, especially those receiving rituximab for induction.

Tocilizumab, a humanized monoclonal antibody against the IL-6 receptor, has been used with some benefit in a few patients with GPA or microscopic polyangiitis [160, 161]. A small randomized trial in Japan is further determining whether tocilizumab could have a place for treatment of nonlimited, severe but not-life-threatening GPA (intravenous infusions of 8 mg/kg ever 2 weeks for 4 months, then every 2 months [162]).

New potential therapeutic targets are being identified at an increasing pace, and hence, new agents will likely be investigated in the near future, possibly directed against IL-17, IL-23, NETs, or the Janus kinase/signal transducers and activators of transcription (JAK-STAT) signaling pathway [31, 163, 164].

7.6.5.3 Other Treatments

Both infliximab and etanercept, the two anti-TNF-alpha drugs, have been investigated in ANCA-associated vasculitides but are no longer used today for GPA, despite some beneficial results with infliximab (prescribed at 5 mg/kg on days 0, 15, and 45, then every 1–2 months) in patients with refractory forms [165, 166]. The results of the WGET study, in which etanercept was studied in combination with usual induction and then maintenance treatments, showed no benefit in preventing relapses as compared with placebo. Also, solid cancers developed in several patients who received etanercept combined with corticosteroids and cyclophosphamide, including several years after the end of the study [102, 167].

Deoxyspergualin was also used in patients with relapsing or refractory GPA, and in a prospective, multicenter open-label study, it achieved at least partial remission in most patients and complete remission in almost half of them (0.5 mg/kg per day, subcutaneously, for six cycles of up to 21 days with a 7-day washout between cycles) [95]. However, relapse occurred in 43% of the patients after a median of approximately 6 months after achieving remission, and severe or life-threatening adverse events, mostly leukopenias, occurred in 53%.

Alemtuzumab (CAMPATH-1H) is a humanized monoclonal anti-CD52 antibody rarely used to treat relapsing/refractory GPA or MPA. In a single series from Cambridge, UK, 85% of the 71 patients receiving alemtuzumab (doses of 4, 10, 40, 40, and 40 mg on five consecutive days) achieved remission, but 43 showed relapse (median 9.2 months), and adverse events, mainly infections, were common [168].

7.6.5.4 Adjuvant Measures

Other therapies may be indicated according to the clinical manifestations and in combination with corticosteroids and immunosuppressive treatments, such as dialysis and then renal transplant in the absence of recovery of renal function [169], surgery for intestinal perforation or ischemic gangrene of limb(s) extremities, insertion of a pacemaker in patients with severe conduction disorders, local treatments with corticosteroids and/or anti-inflammatory agents for episcleritis, and cosmetic surgical repair of nasal deformities.

The treatment of subglottic and bronchial stenoses is complex, especially because this manifestation is often isolated and not accompanied by other signs of disease activity [46, 47, 90]. Systemic treatment is often disappointing because of the fibrotic and atrophic component of the lesions. Endoscopic dilations with bougies, balloons, and repeated local injections of corticosteroids, with or without mitomycin application, may be effective. Stents and surgery (in referral and specialized centers) can be considered in refractory patients.

The adverse effects of prolonged systemic corticosteroid therapy are numerous and require at least the preventative prescription of calcium, vitamin D, and, often, bisphosphonates, according to the current recommendations for preventing osteoporosis [11, 12]. The management of the usual factors of cardiovascular risk is essential, from the beginning of treatment (smoking, dyslipidemia, diabetes, etc.) and to limit the cardiovascular consequences of the corticosteroid therapy, which are added to those related to the vascular inflammation of GPA [170, 171].

During the induction phase, cotrimoxazole should be prescribed as prophylaxis against *Pneumocystis jiroveci* infection (sulfamethoxazole 400 mg/day and trimethoprim 80 mg/day, or 800 mg and 160 mg, respectively, 3 days per week) systematically according to most teams, at least for patients receiving both corticosteroids and cyclophosphamide or rituximab. In addition, this risk persists for several months (3–6 months) after discontinuation of cyclophosphamide or rituximab and when the prednisone dose is less than 10 mg/day [11, 12, 144]. Therefore, this treatment should be maintained 3–6 months after stopping cyclophosphamide or rituximab if possible. In case of cotrimoxazole allergy, contraindication, or intolerance, the prevention of pneumocystosis can be based on pentamidine aerosolizations (300 mg every 3–4 weeks), oral disulone (100 mg/day), which can cause hemolytic anemia even in the absence of glucose-6-dehydrogenase deficiency (or more rarely methemoglobinemia), or atovaquone (1500 mg/day). Other opportunistic infections have been reported during GPA treatment, including bacterial infections (community-acquired pneumonia, urinary sepsis, nocardiosis, etc.), disseminated histoplasmosis, oral or mucosal candidiasis, and progressive multifocal leukoencephalitis with JC virus [172]. Most cannot be prevented, but annual vaccination against influenza, pneumococcal and *Haemophilus influenzae*, and shingles is good practice, as is ensuring that the mandatory vaccines are up-to-date [173].

In addition, the risk of treatment-induced neoplasia, teratogenicity, and/or infertility must be taken into account in therapeutic decisions and follow-up of patients [174, 175].

7.7 Conclusion

GPA is a severe, chronic, and often recurrent disease. However, with appropriate and extended treatment, as detailed in this chapter, patient survival now exceeds 80–90% at 5 years and relapse rates can be lowered. Relapse-free survival at 5 years varies from 30% to 40% with more "conventional" maintenance regimens to 60–70% with newer maintenance strategies such as rituximab. Many therapeutic protocols have been and are still being investigated by international groups to further improve the management and overall prognosis of GPA patients and to limit the damage related to the disease or, very often, the treatments. Epidemiological and fundamental research is in continual progress, which will allow for better understanding the pathophysiological mechanisms of the disease, thereby enabling the identification of new therapeutic targets and more precisely adapting the treatments to each form of the disease and, eventually, each patient individually. Also, one (or a combination of several) biological marker(s), more reliable than ANCA status and titers, to monitor disease activity and predict the risk of relapse may finally be identified and further help guide treatments.

References

1. Jennette JC, Falk RJ, Bacon PA, et al. 2012 revised International Chapel Hill Consensus Conference Nomenclature of Vasculitides. Arthritis Rheum. 2013;65:1–11.
2. Jennette JC, Falk RJ, Andrassy K, et al. Nomenclature of systemic vasculitides. Proposal of an international consensus conference. Arthritis Rheum. 1994;37:187–92.
3. Mohammad AJ, Jacobsson LT, Westman KW, Sturfelt G, Segelmark M. Incidence and survival rates in Wegener's granulomatosis, microscopic polyangiitis, Churg-Strauss syndrome and polyarteritis nodosa. Rheumatology (Oxford). 2009;48:1560–5.
4. Watts RA, Mahr A, Mohammad AJ, Gatenby P, Basu N, Flores-Suarez LF. Classification, epidemiology and clinical subgrouping of antineutrophil cytoplasmic antibody (ANCA)-associated vasculitis. Nephrol Dial Transplant. 2015;30(Suppl 1):i14–22.
5. Hoffman GS, Kerr GS, Leavitt RY, et al. Wegener granulomatosis: an analysis of 158 patients. Ann Intern Med. 1992;116:488–98.
6. Holle JU, Gross WL, Latza U, et al. Improved outcome in 445 patients with Wegener's granulomatosis in a German vasculitis center over four decades. Arthritis Rheum. 2011;63:257–66.
7. Jennette JC, Falk RJ, Gasim AH. Pathogenesis of antineutrophil cytoplasmic autoantibody vasculitis. Curr Opin Nephrol Hypertens. 2011;20:263–70.

8. Walton EW. Giant-cell granuloma of the respiratory tract (Wegener's granulomatosis). Br Med J. 1958;2:265–70.
9. Wallace ZS, Lu N, Unizony S, Stone JH, Choi HK. Improved survival in granulomatosis with polyangiitis: a general population-based study. Semin Arthritis Rheum. 2016;45:483–9.
10. Flossmann O, Berden A, de Groot K, et al. Long-term patient survival in ANCA-associated vasculitis. Ann Rheum Dis. 2011;70:488–94.
11. Yates M, Watts RA, Bajema IM, et al. EULAR/ERA-EDTA recommendations for the management of ANCA-associated vasculitis. Ann Rheum Dis. 2016;75:1583–94.
12. McGeoch L, Twilt M, Famorca L, et al. CanVasc Recommendations for the Management of Antineutrophil Cytoplasm Antibody-associated Vasculitides. J Rheumatol. 2016;43:97–120.
13. Mahr AD. Epidemiological features of Wegener's granulomatosis and microscopic polyangiitis: two diseases or one 'anti-neutrophil cytoplasm antibodies-associated vasculitis' entity? APMIS Suppl. 2009;(127):41–7.
14. Mohammad AJ, Jacobsson LT, Mahr AD, Sturfelt G, Segelmark M. Prevalence of Wegener's granulomatosis, microscopic polyangiitis, polyarteritis nodosa and Churg-Strauss syndrome within a defined population in southern Sweden. Rheumatology (Oxford). 2007;46:1329–37.
15. Abdou NI, Kullman GJ, Hoffman GS, et al. Wegener's granulomatosis: survey of 701 patients in North America. Changes in outcome in the 1990s. J Rheumatol. 2002;29:309–16.
16. Koldingsnes W, Nossent H. Epidemiology of Wegener's granulomatosis in northern Norway. Arthritis Rheum. 2000;43:2481–7.
17. Takala JH, Kautiainen H, Malmberg H, Leirisalo-Repo M. Incidence of Wegener's granulomatosis in Finland 1981-2000. Clin Exp Rheumatol. 2008;26:S81–5.
18. Watts RA, Al-Taiar A, Scott DG, Macgregor AJ. Prevalence and incidence of Wegener's granulomatosis in the UK general practice research database. Arthritis Rheum. 2009;61:1412–6.
19. Watts RA, Mooney J, Skinner J, Scott DG, Macgregor AJ. The contrasting epidemiology of granulomatosis with polyangiitis (Wegener's) and microscopic polyangiitis. Rheumatology (Oxford). 2012;51:926–31.
20. Lane SE, Watts R, Scott DG. Epidemiology of systemic vasculitis. Curr Rheumatol Rep. 2005;7:270–5.
21. van Timmeren MM, Heeringa P. Pathogenesis of ANCA-associated vasculitis: recent insights from animal models. Curr Opin Rheumatol. 2012;24:8–14.
22. Jennette JC, Falk RJ. Pathogenesis of antineutrophil cytoplasmic autoantibody-mediated disease. Nat Rev Rheumatol. 2014;10:463–73.
23. Pendergraft WF III, Pressler BM, Jennette JC, Falk RJ, Preston GA. Autoantigen complementarity: a new theory implicating complementary proteins as initiators of autoimmune disease. J Mol Med (Berl). 2005;83:12–25.
24. Stegeman CA, Tervaert JW, Sluiter WJ, Manson WL, de Jong PE, Kallenberg CG. Association of chronic nasal carriage of *Staphylococcus aureus* and higher relapse rates in Wegener granulomatosis. Ann Intern Med. 1994;120:12–7.
25. Knight A, Sandin S, Askling J. Increased risk of autoimmune disease in families with Wegener's granulomatosis. J Rheumatol. 2010;37:2553–8.
26. Jagiello P, Gross WL, Epplen JT. Complex genetics of Wegener granulomatosis. Autoimmun Rev. 2005;4:42–7.
27. Wieczorek S, Holle JU, Epplen JT. Recent progress in the genetics of Wegener's granulomatosis and Churg-Strauss syndrome. Curr Opin Rheumatol. 2010;22:8–14.
28. Lyons PA, Rayner TF, Trivedi S, et al. Genetically distinct subsets within ANCA-associated vasculitis. N Engl J Med. 2012;367:214–23.
29. Rahmattulla C, Mooyaart AL, van Hooven D, et al. Genetic variants in ANCA-associated vasculitis: a meta-analysis. Ann Rheum Dis. 2016;75:1687–92.
30. Hong Y, Eleftheriou D, Hussain AA, et al. Anti-neutrophil cytoplasmic antibodies stimulate release of neutrophil microparticles. J Am Soc Nephrol. 2012;23:49–62.
31. Kessenbrock K, Krumbholz M, Schonermarck U, et al. Netting neutrophils in autoimmune small-vessel vasculitis. Nat Med. 2009;15:623–5.

32. Kraaij T, Kamerling SWA, van Dam LS, et al. Excessive neutrophil extracellular trap formation in ANCA-associated vasculitis is independent of ANCA. Kidney Int. 2018;94:139.
33. Xiao H, Heeringa P, Hu P, et al. Antineutrophil cytoplasmic autoantibodies specific for myeloperoxidase cause glomerulonephritis and vasculitis in mice. J Clin Invest. 2002;110:955–63.
34. Abdulahad WH, Stegeman CA, Limburg PC, Kallenberg CG. CD4-positive effector memory T cells participate in disease expression in ANCA-associated vasculitis. Ann N Y Acad Sci. 2007;1107:22–31.
35. Abdulahad WH, Stegeman CA, van der Geld YM, Doornbos-van der Meer B, Limburg PC, Kallenberg CG. Functional defect of circulating regulatory CD4+ T cells in patients with Wegener's granulomatosis in remission. Arthritis Rheum. 2007;56:2080–91.
36. Regent A, Lofek S, Dib H, et al. Identification of target antigens of anti-endothelial cell antibodies in patients with anti-neutrophil cytoplasmic antibody-associated vasculitides: a proteomic approach. Clin Immunol. 2014;153:123–35.
37. Holmen C, Elsheikh E, Christensson M, et al. Anti endothelial cell autoantibodies selectively activate SAPK/JNK signalling in Wegener's granulomatosis. J Am Soc Nephrol. 2007;18:2497–508.
38. Popa ER, Franssen CF, Limburg PC, Huitema MG, Kallenberg CG, Tervaert JW. In vitro cytokine production and proliferation of T cells from patients with anti-proteinase 3- and antimyeloperoxidase-associated vasculitis, in response to proteinase 3 and myeloperoxidase. Arthritis Rheum. 2002;46:1894–904.
39. Abdulahad WH, Stegeman CA, Limburg PC, Kallenberg CG. Skewed distribution of Th17 lymphocytes in patients with Wegener's granulomatosis in remission. Arthritis Rheum. 2008;58:2196–205.
40. Stone JH. Limited versus severe Wegener's granulomatosis: baseline data on patients in the Wegener's granulomatosis etanercept trial. Arthritis Rheum. 2003;48:2299–309.
41. Solans-Laque R, Fraile G, Rodriguez-Carballeira M, et al. Clinical characteristics and outcome of Spanish patients with ANCA-associated vasculitides: impact of the vasculitis type, ANCA specificity, and treatment on mortality and morbidity. Medicine (Baltimore). 2017;96:e6083.
42. Reinhold-Keller E, Beuge N, Latza U, et al. An interdisciplinary approach to the care of patients with Wegener's granulomatosis: long-term outcome in 155 patients. Arthritis Rheum. 2000;43:1021–32.
43. Pagnoux C, Wolter NE. Vasculitis of the upper airways. Swiss Med Wkly. 2012;142:w13541.
44. Fasunla JA, Hundt W, Lutz J, Forger F, Thurmel K, Steinbach S. Evaluation of smell and taste in patients with Wegener's granulomatosis. Eur Arch Otorhinolaryngol. 2012;269:179–86.
45. Martinez Del Pero M, Walsh M, Luqmani R, et al. Long-term damage to the ENT system in Wegener's granulomatosis. Eur Arch Otorhinolaryngol. 2011;268:733–9.
46. Langford CA, Sneller MC, Hallahan CW, et al. Clinical features and therapeutic management of subglottic stenosis in patients with Wegener's granulomatosis. Arthritis Rheum. 1996;39:1754–60.
47. Terrier B, Dechartres A, Girard C, et al. Granulomatosis with polyangiitis: endoscopic management of tracheobronchial stenosis: results from a multicentre experience. Rheumatology (Oxford). 2015;54:1852–7.
48. Russell BA, Mohan S, Chahal R, Carette S, Pagnoux C, Canadian Vasculitis N. Prognostic significance of cavitary lung nodules in granulomatosis with polyangiitis - a clinical and imaging study of 225 patients. Arthritis Care Res. 2018;70:1082.
49. Girard C, Charles P, Terrier B, et al. Tracheobronchial stenoses in granulomatosis with polyangiitis (Wegener's): a report on 26 cases. Medicine (Baltimore). 2015;94:e1088.
50. Berden AE, Ferrario F, Hagen EC, et al. Histopathologic classification of ANCA-associated glomerulonephritis. J Am Soc Nephrol. 2010;21:1628–36.
51. Pagnoux C, Guillevin L. Peripheral neuropathy in systemic vasculitides. Curr Opin Rheumatol. 2005;17:41–8.
52. Nishino H, Rubino FA, DeRemee RA, Swanson JW, Parisi JE. Neurological involvement in Wegener's granulomatosis: an analysis of 324 consecutive patients at the Mayo Clinic. Ann Neurol. 1993;33:4–9.

53. de Groot K, Schmidt DK, Arlt AC, Gross WL, Reinhold-Keller E. Standardized neurologic evaluations of 128 patients with Wegener granulomatosis. Arch Neurol. 2001;58: 1215–21.
54. De Luna G, Terrier B, Kaminsky P, et al. Central nervous system involvement of granulomatosis with polyangiitis: clinical-radiological presentation distinguishes different outcomes. Rheumatology (Oxford). 2015;54:424–32.
55. Younger DS. Vasculitis of the nervous system. Curr Opin Neurol. 2004;17:317–36.
56. Goyal M, Kucharczyk W, Keystone E. Granulomatous hypophysitis due to Wegener's granulomatosis. AJNR Am J Neuroradiol. 2000;21:1466–9.
57. Frances C, Du LT, Piette JC, et al. Wegener's granulomatosis. Dermatological manifestations in 75 cases with clinicopathologic correlation. Arch Dermatol. 1994;130:861–7.
58. Le Hello C, Bonte I, Mora JJ, Verneuil L, Noel LH, Guillevin L. Pyoderma gangrenosum associated with Wegener's granulomatosis: partial response to mycophenolate mofetil. Rheumatology (Oxford). 2002;41:236–7.
59. Rothschild PR, Pagnoux C, Seror R, Brezin AP, Delair E, Guillevin L. Ophthalmologic manifestations of systemic necrotizing vasculitides at diagnosis: a retrospective study of 1286 patients and review of the literature. Semin Arthritis Rheum. 2013;42:507–14.
60. McGeoch L, Carette S, Cuthbertson D, et al. Cardiac Involvement in Granulomatosis with Polyangiitis. J Rheumatol. 2015;42:1209–12.
61. Morelli S, Gurgo Di Castelmenardo AM, Conti F, et al. Cardiac involvement in patients with Wegener's granulomatosis. Rheumatol Int. 2000;19:209–12.
62. Mavrogeni S, Schwitter J, van Rossum A, et al. Cardiac magnetic resonance imaging in myocardial inflammation in autoimmune rheumatic diseases: an appraisal of the diagnostic strengths and limitations of the Lake Louise criteria. Int J Cardiol. 2018;252:216–9.
63. Pugnet G, Gouya H, Puechal X, et al. Cardiac involvement in granulomatosis with polyangiitis: a magnetic resonance imaging study of 31 consecutive patients. Rheumatology (Oxford). 2017;56:947–56.
64. Pagnoux C, Mahr A, Cohen P, Guillevin L. Presentation and outcome of gastrointestinal involvement in systemic necrotizing vasculitides: analysis of 62 patients with polyarteritis nodosa, microscopic polyangiitis, Wegener granulomatosis, Churg-Strauss syndrome, or rheumatoid arthritis-associated vasculitis. Medicine (Baltimore). 2005;84:115–28.
65. Soowamber M, Weizman AV, Pagnoux C. Gastrointestinal aspects of vasculitides. Nat Rev Gastroenterol Hepatol. 2017;14:185–94.
66. Sy A, Khalidi N, Dehghan N, et al. Vasculitis in patients with inflammatory bowel diseases: a study of 32 patients and systematic review of the literature. Semin Arthritis Rheum. 2016;45:475–82.
67. Gal AA, Masor JJ. Splenic involvement in Wegener's granulomatosis. Arch Pathol Lab Med. 1996;120:974–7.
68. McCain M, Quinet R, Davis W, et al. Splenic rupture as the presenting manifestation of vasculitis. Semin Arthritis Rheum. 2002;31:311–6.
69. Arlet JB, Le Thi Huong D, Marinho A, Cluzel P, Wechsler B, Piette JC. Arterial aneurysms in Wegener's granulomatosis: case report and literature review. Semin Arthritis Rheum. 2008;37:265–8.
70. Lie JT. Wegener's granulomatosis: histological documentation of common and uncommon manifestations in 216 patients. Vasa. 1997;26:261–70.
71. Barreto P, Pagnoux C, Luca L, et al. Dorsal prevertebral lesions in Wegener granulomatosis: report on four cases. Joint Bone Spine. 2011;78:88–91.
72. Merkel PA, Lo GH, Holbrook JT, et al. Brief communication: high incidence of venous thrombotic events among patients with Wegener granulomatosis: the Wegener's Clinical Occurrence of Thrombosis (WeCLOT) Study. Ann Intern Med. 2005;142:620–6.
73. Allenbach Y, Seror R, Pagnoux C, Teixeira L, Guilpain P, Guillevin L. High frequency of venous thromboembolic events in Churg-Strauss syndrome, Wegener's granulomatosis and microscopic polyangiitis but not polyarteritis nodosa: a systematic retrospective study on 1130 patients. Ann Rheum Dis. 2009;68:564–7.

74. Kronbichler A, Leierer J, Leierer G, et al. Clinical associations with venous thromboembolism in anti-neutrophil cytoplasm antibody-associated vasculitides. Rheumatology (Oxford). 2017;56:704–8.
75. Berti A, Matteson EL, Crowson CS, Specks U, Cornec D. Risk of Cardiovascular disease and venous thromboembolism among patients with incident ANCA-associated vasculitis: a 20-year population-based cohort study. Mayo Clin Proc. 2018;93:597.
76. Hellmich B, Flossmann O, Gross WL, et al. EULAR recommendations for conducting clinical studies and/or clinical trials in systemic vasculitis: focus on anti-neutrophil cytoplasm antibody-associated vasculitis. Ann Rheum Dis. 2007;66:605–17.
77. Hoffman GS. Immunosuppressive therapy is always required for the treatment of limited Wegener's granulomatosis. Sarcoidosis Vasc Diffuse Lung Dis. 1996;13:249–52.
78. Holle JU, Gross WL, Holl-Ulrich K, et al. Prospective long-term follow-up of patients with localised Wegener's granulomatosis: does it occur as persistent disease stage? Ann Rheum Dis. 2010;69:1934–9.
79. Pagnoux C, Stubbe M, Lifermann F, et al. Wegener's granulomatosis strictly and persistently localized to one organ is rare: assessment of 16 patients from the French Vasculitis Study Group database. J Rheumatol. 2011;38:475–8.
80. Cabral DA, Uribe AG, Benseler S, et al. Classification, presentation, and initial treatment of Wegener's granulomatosis in childhood. Arthritis Rheum. 2009;60:3413–24.
81. Akikusa JD, Schneider R, Harvey EA, et al. Clinical features and outcome of pediatric Wegener's granulomatosis. Arthritis Rheum. 2007;57:837–44.
82. Cabral DA, Canter DL, Muscal E, et al. Comparing presenting clinical features in 48 children with microscopic polyangiitis to 183 children who have granulomatosis with polyangiitis (Wegener's): an ARChiVe cohort study. Arthritis Rheumatol. 2016;68:2514–26.
83. Morishita KA, Moorthy LN, Lubieniecka JM, et al. Early outcomes in children with antineutrophil cytoplasmic antibody-associated vasculitis. Arthritis Rheumatol. 2017;69:1470–9.
84. Iudici M, Pagnoux C, Quartier P, et al. Childhood- versus adult-onset ANCA-associated vasculitides: a nested, matched case-control study from the French Vasculitis Study Group Registry. Autoimmun Rev. 2018;17:108–14.
85. Koldingsnes W, Nossent JC. Baseline features and initial treatment as predictors of remission and relapse in Wegener's granulomatosis. J Rheumatol. 2003;30:80–8.
86. Karim AF, Verdijk RM, Nagtegaal AP, et al. To distinguish IgG4-related disease from seronegative granulomatosis with polyangiitis. Rheumatology (Oxford). 2017;56:2245–7.
87. Bossuyt X, Cohen Tervaert JW, Arimura Y, et al. Position paper: revised 2017 international consensus on testing of ANCAs in granulomatosis with polyangiitis and microscopic polyangiitis. Nat Rev Rheumatol. 2017;13:683–92.
88. Mahr A, Batteux F, Tubiana S, et al. Brief report: prevalence of antineutrophil cytoplasmic antibodies in infective endocarditis. Arthritis Rheumatol. 2014;66:1672–7.
89. Duna GF, Galperin C, Hoffman GS. Wegener's granulomatosis. Rheum Dis Clin North Am. 1995;21:949–86.
90. Gluth MB, Shinners PA, Kasperbauer JL. Subglottic stenosis associated with Wegener's granulomatosis. Laryngoscope. 2003;113:1304–7.
91. Gwathmey KG, Burns TM, Collins MP, Dyck PJ. Vasculitic neuropathies. Lancet Neurol. 2014;13:67–82.
92. McGeoch L, Silecky WB, Maher J, Carette S, Pagnoux C. Temporal arteritis in the young. Joint Bone Spine. 2013;80:324–7.
93. Bourgarit A, Le Toumelin P, Pagnoux C, et al. Deaths occurring during the first year after treatment onset for polyarteritis nodosa, microscopic polyangiitis, and Churg-Strauss syndrome: a retrospective analysis of causes and factors predictive of mortality based on 595 patients. Medicine (Baltimore). 2005;84:323–30.
94. Faurschou M, Sorensen IJ, Mellemkjaer L, et al. Malignancies in Wegener's granulomatosis: incidence and relation to cyclophosphamide therapy in a cohort of 293 patients. J Rheumatol. 2008;35:100–5.

95. Flossmann O, Jayne DR. Long-term treatment of relapsing Wegener's granulomatosis with 15-deoxyspergualin. Rheumatology (Oxford). 2010;49:556–62.
96. Puechal X, Pagnoux C, Perrodeau E, et al. Long-Term Outcomes Among Participants in the WEGENT Trial of Remission-Maintenance Therapy for Granulomatosis With Polyangiitis (Wegener's) or Microscopic Polyangiitis. Arthritis Rheumatol. 2016;68:690–701.
97. Jayne D, Rasmussen N, Andrassy K, et al. A randomized trial of maintenance therapy for vasculitis associated with antineutrophil cytoplasmic autoantibodies. N Engl J Med. 2003;349:36–44.
98. Fauci AS, Haynes BF, Katz P, Wolff SM. Wegener's granulomatosis: prospective clinical and therapeutic experience with 85 patients for 21 years. Ann Intern Med. 1983;98:76–85.
99. Pagnoux C, Guillevin L. Treatment of granulomatosis with polyangiitis (Wegener's). Expert Rev Clin Immunol. 2015;11:339–48.
100. Walsh M, Merkel PA, Mahr A, Jayne D. Effects of duration of glucocorticoid therapy on relapse rate in antineutrophil cytoplasmic antibody-associated vasculitis: a meta-analysis. Arthritis Care Res. 2010;62:1166–73.
101. Stone JH, Merkel PA, Spiera R, et al. Rituximab versus cyclophosphamide for ANCA-associated vasculitis. N Engl J Med. 2010;363:221–32.
102. WGET. Etanercept plus standard therapy for Wegener's granulomatosis. N Engl J Med. 2005;352:351–61.
103. Guillevin L, Cordier JF, Lhote F, et al. A prospective, multicenter, randomized trial comparing steroids and pulse cyclophosphamide versus steroids and oral cyclophosphamide in the treatment of generalized Wegener's granulomatosis. Arthritis Rheum. 1997;40: 2187–98.
104. de Groot K, Harper L, Jayne DR, et al. Pulse versus daily oral cyclophosphamide for induction of remission in antineutrophil cytoplasmic antibody-associated vasculitis: a randomized trial. Ann Intern Med. 2009;150:670–80.
105. Lapraik C, Watts R, Bacon P, et al. BSR and BHPR guidelines for the management of adults with ANCA associated vasculitis. Rheumatology (Oxford). 2007;46:1615–6.
106. Pagnoux C, Quemeneur T, Ninet J, et al. Treatment of systemic necrotizing vasculitides in patients aged sixty-five years or older: results of a multicenter, open-label, randomized controlled trial of corticosteroid and cyclophosphamide-based induction therapy. Arthritis Rheumatol. 2015;67:1117–27.
107. Monach PA, Arnold LM, Merkel PA. Incidence and prevention of bladder toxicity from cyclophosphamide in the treatment of rheumatic diseases: a data-driven review. Arthritis Rheum. 2010;62:9–21.
108. Pagnoux C, FVSG. Vascularites nécrosantes systémiques - protocole national de diagnostic et de soins. 2009. https://www.has-sante.fr.
109. Haubitz M, Schellong S, Gobel U, et al. Intravenous pulse administration of cyclophosphamide versus daily oral treatment in patients with antineutrophil cytoplasmic antibody-associated vasculitis and renal involvement: a prospective, randomized study. Arthritis Rheum. 1998;41:1835–44.
110. Harper L, Morgan MD, Walsh M, et al. Pulse versus daily oral cyclophosphamide for induction of remission in ANCA-associated vasculitis: long-term follow-up. Ann Rheum Dis. 2012;71:955–60.
111. Jones RB, Furuta S, Tervaert JW, et al. Rituximab versus cyclophosphamide in ANCA-associated renal vasculitis: 2-year results of a randomised trial. Ann Rheum Dis. 2015;74:1178–82.
112. Specks U, Merkel PA, Seo P, et al. Efficacy of remission-induction regimens for ANCA-associated vasculitis. N Engl J Med. 2013;369:417–27.
113. Westwell-Roper C, Lubieniecka JM, Brown KL, et al. Clinical practice variation and need for pediatric-specific treatment guidelines among rheumatologists caring for children with ANCA-associated vasculitis: an international clinician survey. Pediatr Rheumatol Online J. 2017;15:61.

114. Holle JU, Dubrau C, Herlyn K, et al. Rituximab for refractory granulomatosis with polyangiitis (Wegener's granulomatosis): comparison of efficacy in granulomatous versus vasculitic manifestations. Ann Rheum Dis. 2012;71:327–33.
115. Charles P, Bienvenu B, Bonnotte B, et al. Rituximab: recommendations of the French Vasculitis Study Group (FVSG) for induction and maintenance treatments of adult, antineutrophil cytoplasm antibody-associated necrotizing vasculitides. Presse Med. 2013;42:1317–30.
116. Cartin-Ceba R, Diaz-Caballero L, Al-Qadi MO, et al. Diffuse alveolar hemorrhage secondary to antineutrophil cytoplasmic antibody-associated vasculitis: predictors of respiratory failure and clinical outcomes. Arthritis Rheumatol. 2016;68:1467–76.
117. Uechi E, Okada M, Fushimi K. Effect of plasma exchange on in-hospital mortality in patients with pulmonary hemorrhage secondary to antineutrophil cytoplasmic antibody-associated vasculitis: a propensity-matched analysis using a nationwide administrative database. PLoS One. 2018;13:e0196009.
118. Walsh M, Casian A, Flossmann O, et al. Long-term follow-up of patients with severe ANCA-associated vasculitis comparing plasma exchange to intravenous methylprednisolone treatment is unclear. Kidney Int. 2013;84:397–402.
119. Walsh M, Catapano F, Szpirt W, et al. Plasma exchange for renal vasculitis and idiopathic rapidly progressive glomerulonephritis: a meta-analysis. Am J Kidney Dis. 2011;57:566–74.
120. Walsh M, Merkel PA, Peh CA, et al. Plasma exchange and glucocorticoid dosing in the treatment of anti-neutrophil cytoplasm antibody associated vasculitis (PEXIVAS): protocol for a randomized controlled trial. Trials. 2013;14:73.
121. Pagnoux C, Mahr A, Hamidou MA, et al. Azathioprine or methotrexate maintenance for ANCA-associated vasculitis. N Engl J Med. 2008;359:2790–803.
122. Langford CA, Talar-Williams C, Barron KS, Sneller MC. A staged approach to the treatment of Wegener's granulomatosis: induction of remission with glucocorticoids and daily cyclophosphamide switching to methotrexate for remission maintenance. Arthritis Rheum. 1999;42:2666–73.
123. Metzler C, Miehle N, Manger K, et al. Elevated relapse rate under oral methotrexate versus leflunomide for maintenance of remission in Wegener's granulomatosis. Rheumatology (Oxford). 2007;46:1087–91.
124. Hiemstra TF, Walsh M, Mahr A, et al. Mycophenolate mofetil vs azathioprine for remission maintenance in antineutrophil cytoplasmic antibody-associated vasculitis: a randomized controlled trial. JAMA. 2010;304:2381–8.
125. Reinhold-Keller E, Fink CO, Herlyn K, Gross WL, De Groot K. High rate of renal relapse in 71 patients with Wegener's granulomatosis under maintenance of remission with low-dose methotrexate. Arthritis Rheum. 2002;47:326–32.
126. Mahr A, Katsahian S, Varet H, et al. Revisiting the classification of clinical phenotypes of anti-neutrophil cytoplasmic antibody-associated vasculitis: a cluster analysis. Ann Rheum Dis. 2013;72:1003–10.
127. Karras A, Pagnoux C, Haubitz M, et al. Randomised controlled trial of prolonged treatment in the remission phase of ANCA-associated vasculitis. Ann Rheum Dis. 2017;76:1662–8.
128. Miloslavsky EM, Lu N, Unizony S, et al. Myeloperoxidase-antineutrophil cytoplasmic antibody (ANCA)-positive and ANCA-negative patients with granulomatosis with polyangiitis (Wegener's): distinct patient subsets. Arthritis Rheumatol. 2016;68:2945–52.
129. Pagnoux C, Springer J. Editorial: classifying antineutrophil cytoplasmic antibody (ANCA)-associated vasculitides according to ANCA type or phenotypic diagnosis: salt or pepper? Arthritis Rheumatol. 2016;68:2837–40.
130. Schirmer JH, Wright MN, Herrmann K, et al. Myeloperoxidase-antineutrophil cytoplasmic antibody (ANCA)-positive granulomatosis with polyangiitis (Wegener's) is a clinically distinct subset of ANCA-associated vasculitis: a retrospective analysis of 315 patients from a German vasculitis referral center. Arthritis Rheumatol. 2016;68:2953–63.
131. McGregor JG, Hogan SL, Hu Y, Jennette CE, Falk RJ, Nachman PH. Glucocorticoids and relapse and infection rates in anti-neutrophil cytoplasmic antibody disease. Clin J Am Soc Nephrol. 2012;7:240–7.

132. Cartin-Ceba R, Golbin JM, Keogh KA, et al. Rituximab for remission induction and maintenance in refractory granulomatosis with polyangiitis (Wegener's): ten-year experience at a single center. Arthritis Rheum. 2012;64:3770–8.
133. Jones RB, Ferraro AJ, Chaudhry AN, et al. A multicenter survey of rituximab therapy for refractory antineutrophil cytoplasmic antibody-associated vasculitis. Arthritis Rheum. 2009;60:2156–68.
134. Smith RM, Jones RB, Guerry MJ, et al. Rituximab for remission maintenance in relapsing antineutrophil cytoplasmic antibody-associated vasculitis. Arthritis Rheum. 2012;64:3760–9.
135. Roubaud-Baudron C, Pagnoux C, Meaux-Ruault N, et al. Rituximab maintenance therapy for granulomatosis with polyangiitis and microscopic polyangiitis. J Rheumatol. 2012;39:125–30.
136. Alberici F, Smith RM, Jones RB, et al. Long-term follow-up of patients who received repeat-dose rituximab as maintenance therapy for ANCA-associated vasculitis. Rheumatology (Oxford). 2015;54:1153–60.
137. Guillevin L, Pagnoux C, Karras A, et al. Rituximab versus Azathioprine for Maintenance in ANCA-Associated Vasculitis. N Engl J Med. 2014;371:1771–80.
138. Gopaluni S, Smith RM, Lewin M, et al. Rituximab versus azathioprine as therapy for maintenance of remission for anti-neutrophil cytoplasm antibody-associated vasculitis (RITAZAREM): study protocol for a randomized controlled trial. Trials. 2017;18:112.
139. Charles P, Terrier B, Perrodeau E, et al. Comparison of individually tailored vs systematic rituximab regimens to maintain ANCA-associated vasculitis remissions: results of a prospective, randomized–controlled, phase 3 trial. Arthritis Rheumatol. 2017;69:Abst 2754.
140. Unizony S, Villarreal M, Miloslavsky EM, et al. Clinical outcomes of treatment of anti-neutrophil cytoplasmic antibody (ANCA)-associated vasculitis based on ANCA type. Ann Rheum Dis. 2016;75:1166–9.
141. Azar L, Springer J, Langford CA, Hoffman GS. Rituximab with or without a conventional maintenance agent in the treatment of relapsing granulomatosis with polyangiitis (Wegener's): a retrospective single-center study. Arthritis Rheumatol. 2014;66:2862–70.
142. de Groot K, Reinhold-Keller E, Tatsis E, et al. Therapy for the maintenance of remission in sixty-five patients with generalized Wegener's granulomatosis. Methotrexate versus trimethoprim/sulfamethoxazole. Arthritis Rheum. 1996;39:2052–61.
143. Stegeman CA, Tervaert JW, de Jong PE, Kallenberg CG. Trimethoprim-sulfamethoxazole (co-trimoxazole) for the prevention of relapses of Wegener's granulomatosis. Dutch Co-Trimoxazole Wegener Study Group. N Engl J Med. 1996;335:16–20.
144. Cohen Tervaert JW. Trimethoprim-sulfamethoxazole and antineutrophil cytoplasmic antibodies-associated vasculitis. Curr Opin Rheumatol. 2018;30:388.
145. Zycinska K, Wardyn KA, Zielonka TM, Krupa R, Lukas W. Co-trimoxazole and prevention of relapses of PR3-ANCA positive vasculitis with pulmonary involvement. Eur J Med Res. 2009;14(Suppl 4):265–7.
146. Pagnoux C, Hogan SL, Chin H, et al. Predictors of treatment resistance and relapse in anti-neutrophil cytoplasmic antibody-associated small-vessel vasculitis: comparison of two independent cohorts. Arthritis Rheum. 2008;58:2908–18.
147. Finkielman JD, Merkel PA, Schroeder D, et al. Antiproteinase 3 antineutrophil cytoplasmic antibodies and disease activity in Wegener granulomatosis. Ann Intern Med. 2007;147:611–9.
148. Kemna MJ, Damoiseaux J, Austen J, et al. ANCA as a predictor of relapse: useful in patients with renal involvement but not in patients with nonrenal disease. J Am Soc Nephrol. 2015;26:537–42.
149. Fussner LA, Hummel AM, Schroeder DR, et al. Factors determining the clinical utility of serial measurements of antineutrophil cytoplasmic antibodies targeting proteinase 3. Arthritis Rheumatol. 2016;68:1700–10.
150. Walsh M, Flossmann O, Berden A, et al. Risk factors for relapse of antineutrophil cytoplasmic antibody-associated vasculitis. Arthritis Rheum. 2012;64:542–8.

151. Stegeman CA. Anti-neutrophil cytoplasmic antibody (ANCA) levels directed against proteinase-3 and myeloperoxidase are helpful in predicting disease relapse in ANCA-associated small-vessel vasculitis. Nephrol Dial Transplant. 2002;17:2077–80.
152. de Groot K, Rasmussen N, Bacon PA, et al. Randomized trial of cyclophosphamide versus methotrexate for induction of remission in early systemic antineutrophil cytoplasmic antibody-associated vasculitis. Arthritis Rheum. 2005;52:2461–9.
153. Hu W, Liu C, Xie H, Chen H, Liu Z, Li L. Mycophenolate mofetil versus cyclophosphamide for inducing remission of ANCA vasculitis with moderate renal involvement. Nephrol Dial Transplant. 2008;23:1307–12.
154. Jayne DR, Chapel H, Adu D, et al. Intravenous immunoglobulin for ANCA-associated systemic vasculitis with persistent disease activity. QJM. 2000;93:433–9.
155. Crickx E, Machelart I, Lazaro E, et al. Intravenous immunoglobulin as an immunomodulating agent in antineutrophil cytoplasmic antibody-associated vasculitides: a French nationwide study of ninety-two patients. Arthritis Rheumatol. 2016;68:702–12.
156. McAdoo SP, Bedi R, Tarzi R, Griffith M, Pusey CD, Cairns TD. Ofatumumab for B cell depletion therapy in ANCA-associated vasculitis: a single-centre case series. Rheumatology (Oxford). 2016;55:1437–42.
157. Jayne DRW, Bruchfeld AN, Harper L, et al. Randomized trial of C5a receptor inhibitor avacopan in ANCA-associated vasculitis. J Am Soc Nephrol. 2017;28:2756–67.
158. Langford CA, Monach PA, Specks U, et al. An open-label trial of abatacept (CTLA4-Ig) in non-severe relapsing granulomatosis with polyangiitis (Wegener's). Ann Rheum Dis. 2014;73:1376–9.
159. Jayne D, Blockmans D, Luqmani R, et al. Efficacy and Safety of Belimumab and Azathioprine for Maintenance of Remission in Antineutrophil Cytoplasmic Antibody-Associated Vasculitis: A Randomized Controlled Study. Arthritis Rheumatol. 2019;71:952–63.
160. Berti A, Cavalli G, Campochiaro C, et al. Interleukin-6 in ANCA-associated vasculitis: rationale for successful treatment with tocilizumab. Semin Arthritis Rheum. 2015;45:48–54.
161. Sakai R, Kondo T, Kikuchi J, et al. Corticosteroid-free treatment of tocilizumab monotherapy for microscopic polyangiitis: a single-arm, single-center, clinical trial. Mod Rheumatol. 2016;26:900–7.
162. Trial U-CC. Clinical trial of tocilizumab versus cyclophosphamide for microscopic polyangiitis and granulomatosis with polyangiitis. 01 May 2017 edn. UMIN-CTR Clinical Trial portal. 2018.
163. Kusunoki Y, Nakazawa D, Shida H, et al. Peptidylarginine deiminase inhibitor suppresses neutrophil extracellular trap formation and MPO-ANCA production. Front Immunol. 2016;7:227.
164. Nishide M, Nojima S, Ito D, et al. Semaphorin 4D inhibits neutrophil activation and is involved in the pathogenesis of neutrophil-mediated autoimmune vasculitis. Ann Rheum Dis. 2017;76:1440–8.
165. Booth A, Harper L, Hammad T, et al. Prospective study of TNF alpha blockade with infliximab in anti-neutrophil cytoplasmic antibody-associated systemic vasculitis. J Am Soc Nephrol. 2004;15:717–21.
166. de Menthon M, Cohen P, Pagnoux C, et al. Infliximab or rituximab for refractory Wegener's granulomatosis: long-term follow up. A prospective randomised multicentre study on 17 patients. Clin Exp Rheumatol. 2011;29:S63–71.
167. Silva F, Seo P, Schroeder DR, et al. Solid malignancies among etanercept-treated patients with granulomatosis with polyangiitis (Wegener's): long-term follow up of a multicenter longitudinal cohort. Arthritis Rheum. 2011;63:2495–503.
168. Walsh M, Chaudhry A, Jayne D. Long-term follow-up of relapsing/refractory anti-neutrophil cytoplasm antibody associated vasculitis treated with the lymphocyte depleting antibody alemtuzumab (CAMPATH-1H). Ann Rheum Dis. 2008;67:1322–7.
169. Shen J, Gill J, Shangguan M, Sampaio MS, Bunnapradist S. Outcomes of renal transplantation in recipients with Wegener's granulomatosis. Clin Transplant. 2011;25:380–7.

170. Avina-Zubieta JA, Mai A, Amiri N, et al. Risk of myocardial infarction and stroke in patients with granulomatosis with polyangiitis (Wegener's): a population-based study. Arthritis Rheumatol. 2016;68:2752–9.
171. Tan JA, Dehghan N, Chen W, Xie H, Esdaile JM, Avina-Zubieta JA. Mortality in ANCA-associated vasculitis: a meta-analysis of observational studies. Ann Rheum Dis. 2017;76:1566–74.
172. Charlier C, Henegar C, Launay O, et al. Risk factors for major infections in Wegener granulomatosis: analysis of 113 patients. Ann Rheum Dis. 2009;68:658–63.
173. Kostianovsky A, Charles P, Alves JF, et al. Immunogenicity and safety of seasonal and 2009 pandemic A/H1N1 influenza vaccines for patients with autoimmune diseases: a prospective, monocentre trial on 199 patients. Clin Exp Rheumatol. 2012;30:S83–9.
174. Pagnoux C, Mahendira D, Laskin CA. Fertility and pregnancy in vasculitis. Best Pract Res Clin Rheumatol. 2013;27:79–94.
175. Heijl C, Harper L, Flossmann O, et al. Incidence of malignancy in patients treated for anti-neutrophil cytoplasm antibody-associated vasculitis: follow-up data from European Vasculitis Study Group clinical trials. Ann Rheum Dis. 2011;70:1415–21.

Microscopic Polyangiitis 8

Renato Alberto Sinico, Filippo Maria Sala,
Maria Rosa Pozzi, Paolo Fabbrini, and Federico Pieruzzi

8.1 Introduction

Microscopic polyangiitis (MPA) is defined as a necrotizing small vessel vasculitis (i.e., capillaries, venules, or arterioles) with no or few immune-deposits in which necrotizing glomerulonephritis (GN) is very common and pulmonary capillaritis often occurs. It can be differentiated from granulomatosis with polyangiitis (GPA) because granulomatous inflammation is absent and necrotizing arteritis involving small and medium arteries may be present [1, 2].

It is classified among the so-called anti-neutrophil cytoplasmic antibody (ANCA)-associated vasculitis (AAV) along with GPA and eosinophilic granulomatosis polyangiitis (EGPA) [1, 2]. Anti-neutrophil cytoplasmic antibodies are usually directed against myeloperoxidase (MPO) in MPA giving rise to a perinuclear pattern (P-ANCA) by indirect immunofluorescence on ethanol-fixed neutrophils [3, 4]. In a minority of patients, ANCA recognizes as antigenic target proteinase 3 (PR3) that gives a granular cytoplasmic neutrophil fluorescence with central interlobular accentuation (C-ANCA) [3, 4].

R. A. Sinico (✉) · F. M. Sala · P. Fabbrini · F. Pieruzzi
Renal Unit, Department of Medicine and Surgery, Università degli Studi di Milano Bicocca, ASST-Monza, Ospedale San Gerardo, Milano/Monza, Italy
e-mail: renato.sinico@unimib.it; f.sala40@campus.unimib.it; federico.pieruzzi@unimib.it

M. R. Pozzi
Rheumatology Unit, ASST Monza—San Gerardo Hospital, Monza, Italy
e-mail: m.pozzi@asst-monza.it

R. A. Sinico, L. Guillevin (eds.), *Anti-Neutrophil Cytoplasmic Antibody (ANCA) Associated Vasculitis*, Rare Diseases of the Immune System,
https://doi.org/10.1007/978-3-030-02239-6_8

8.2 Historical Notes

MPA was temporally the last type of vasculitis, included within the AAV group, that was recognized as a distinct entity. Until then, it was considered a variant of polyarteritis nodosa (PAN). A clinical form distinct from classical PAN was first noted by F. Wohlwill in 1923; he described a form of periarteritis nodosa whose lesions were only microscopically identifiable [5]. In 1948, Davson et al compared cases of classical PAN and its variant that they defined as microscopic form of periarteritis nodosa [6]. In their work, they described the presence of glomerular renal lesions and the absence of medium-sized vessels involvement as in the classical form. This form did not correspond to the criteria for PAN identified by Kussmaul and Maier in 1889. In the same year, Zeek described the pulmonary involvement in hypersensitivity angiitis that separated this form of vasculitis from PAN [7]. Interestingly, he already reported with detailed images fundamental histological features that differentiated MPA from PAN, such as necrotizing glomerulonephritis and pulmonary arteritis.

In 1954, Goodman and Churg described the similarities between MPA, GPA, and EGPA [8]. However, it was only in 1985 that MPA was recognized as a disease entity when Savage et al described a case series of 34 patients with prominent renal involvement [9].

The current definition of microscopic polyangiitis was proposed during the International Chapel Hill Consensus Conference Nomenclature of Vasculitides in 1994 [1].

8.3 Epidemiology

AAVs are rare diseases with an annual incidence ranging from 12 to 20 cases per million population and a prevalence of 4.6 to 18.4 cases per 100,000 individuals [10]. There is a geographic variation in AAVs with a higher incidence of GPA in northern Europe and Australia, and a higher frequency of MPA in southern Europe and in Asia [11–15]. The incidence of ANCA-associated vasculitis in the Midlands of the UK was estimated at 23.1 per million person-years [16]. In particular, the incidence rates of GPA, MPA, and EGPA were 8.2 per million (95% CI: 5.8, 11.3), 13.4 per million (95% CI: 10.3, 17.2), and 1.5 per million (95% CI: 0.6, 3.1), respectively [16]. Worth of note, the age- and sex-adjusted incidence of ANCA-associated vasculitis in the black and minority ethnic and the white populations was similar [16]. A recent study from Minnesota has found an annual incidence rate of MPA of 16 per million population vs. 13 per million for GPA [17]. MPA may affect any age; however, most of the patients are usually >50 years old with a slight male prevalence [11–13]. Recent data seem to indicate an increasing age of patients [18–20] (Table 8.1). This is probably due to the wider availability of ANCA testing and to a greater awareness of the disease especially in the elderly.

Epidemiological data in children are scarce because most of the pediatric reports are based on single-center and national retrospective cohort studies and

Table 8.1 Main clinical features of MPA in some of the largest published series

Reference	Hogan [21]	Guillevin [22]	Ahn [23]	Sugijama [24]	Sada [25]	Furuta 1 [19]	Furuta 2 [19]	Schirmer [20]
Year of publication	1996	1999	2012	2013	2014	2014	2014	2016
No. of cases (RLV/MPA)	107 (38/69)	85	55	697	78 (33/45)	147 (17/130)	312 (35/277)	144 (2/142)
Age years (mean ± SD)	57 ± 18	56.8 ± 14.6	59.29 ± 13.60	69.4 ± 0.4	71.1 ± 10.0	64.8	71.0	59.3 ± 14.4
Range	2–92	16–86	–	–	–	15–89	16–94	18–86
M:F ratio	58:49 (1.18)	47:38 (1.24)	33:22 (1.5)	299:398 (0.75)	35/43 (0.81)	81:66 (1.23)	142:170 (0.84)	65:79 (0.82)
General (fever, weight loss) %	–	47 (55.3%)	43 (78.2%)	560 (80.3%)	56 (71.8%)	124 (84.4%)	234 (75.0%)	132 (91.7%)
Renal	107 (100%)	67 (78.8%)	41 (74.5%)	606 (86.9%)	71 (91.0%)	121 (82.3%)	271 (86.9%)	117 (81.3%)
Pulmonary	38 (36%)	21 (24.7%)	23 (41.8%)	514 (73.7%)	30 (38.5%)	51 (34.7%)	157 (52.5%)	76 (52.8%)
Pulmonary hemorrhage	–	10 (11.8%)	4 (7.3%)	79 (11.3%)	9 (11.5%)	30 (20.4%)	33 (10.6%)	37 (25.7%)
Fibrosing interstitial lung disease	–	–	13 (23.6%)	–	37 (47.4%)	25 (17.0%)	116 (37.1%)	22 (15.3%)
Cutaneous	13 (12%)	53 (62.4%)	28 (50.9%)	247 (35.4%)	16 (20.5%)	36 (24.5%)	35 (11.2%)	26 (18.1%)
Gastrointestinal	9 (8%)	26 (30.6%)	11 (20.0%)	71 (10.2%)	0 (0.0%)	4 (2.7%)	13 (4.2%)	7 (4.9%)
Cardiac	–	15 (17.6%)	2 (3.8%)	100 (14.3%)	6 (7.7%)	6 (4.1%)	9 (2.9%)	11(7.6%)
ENT	14 (13%)	1 (1.2%)	15 (27.3%)	98 (14.1%)	7 (9.0%)	20 (13.6%)	38 (12.2%)	3 (2.1%)
Ocular/mucous membrane	2 (2%)	1 (1.2%)	0 (0.0%)	91 (13.1%)	9 (11.5%)	22 (15.0%)	21 (6.7%)	20 (13.9%)
Nervous system	9 (8%)	49 (57.6%)	24 (43.6%)	315 (45.2%)	33 (42.3%)	29 (19.7%)	92 (29.5%)	61 (42.4%)°°
ANCA positivity (IIF or ELISA)	107 (100%)	74.5%	–	697 (100%)	78 (100%)	132 (89.8%)	301(96.5%)	144(100%)
PR3-ANCA/c-ANCA	37 (35%)	5 (13.1%)	0 (0.0%)	49 (7.0)	2 (2.6%)	33 (22.4%)	10 (3.2%)	6 (4.2%)
MPO-ANCA/p-ANCA	68 (65%)	33 (86.8%)	38 (69.1%)	677 (97.1)	76 (97.4%)	102 (69.4%)	299 (95.8%)	138 (95.8%)
Double positive	0 (0.0%)	–	–	–	0 (0.0%)	3 (2.0%)	8 (2.6%)	0 (0.0%)
Negative	0 (0.0%)	13 (25.5%)	–	–	1(1.3%)	15 (10.2%)	11 (3.5%)	0 (0.0%)

RLV renal limited vasculitis, *MPA* microscopic polyangiitis, *ENT* ear, nose and throat

also because vasculitis in children is extremely rare [26]. The annual incidence of AAV reported in a retrospective multicenter French study including 66 children, the largest cohort in Europe, was ~0.5 per million children [27]. Higher incidence rates of up to 6.39 cases/million children/year were reported in a Canadian study [28]. A population-based study from southern Sweden has found an annual incidence rate per million children of 1.4 (0–2.8) for each of GPA and MPA [29]. Unlike in adults, where AAVs occur more frequently in male than in female patients, childhood AAVs are more common in female subjects and their onset peaks in the early second decade, with a median age at diagnosis of approximately 11–14 years [26].

8.4 Pathogenesis

Pathogenesis of ANCA-associated vasculitis is the topic of another chapter of this book. In brief, clinical and experimental animal data support the hypothesis that ANCA can activate neutrophils and cause vasculitis, especially if there is a concurrent synergistic proinflammatory stimulus (reviewed in [30, 31]). This is particularly true for MPO-ANCA (and MPA) since most of the experimental models have succeeded only with anti-MPO antibodies [32]. Environmental factors, including silica, infection especially with *Staphylococcus aureus*, and drugs, have been considered important in the development of ANCA [30, 31]. How ANCAs are generated is not known. However, studies suggest that molecular mimicry and responses to complementary peptides may be initiating events for ANCAs production [30]. A genetic background has long been suspected for AAVs. A recent genome-wide association study has confirmed that the pathogenesis of ANCA-associated vasculitis has a genetic component, and has demonstrated a genetic distinction between GPA and MPA that is associated with ANCA specificity [33].

8.5 Clinical Presentation

MPA can have a wide range of presentation ranging from indolent renal-limited disease to acute pulmo-renal syndrome [11–13]. Acute presentation manifesting principally with diffuse alveolar hemorrhage (DAH), rapidly progressive glomerulonephritis (RPGN), or motor mononeuritis multiplex can lead to dysfunction of one or more organs. In most cases, however, the disease begins with insidious non-specific symptoms, usually prodromal constitutional symptoms such as low-grade fever, arthralgia, weight loss, and discomfort that lead within a few weeks or months to an acute phase with involvement of one or more organs. General symptoms are present in 55.3–91.7% of patients in the largest case series [19–25] (Table 8.1).

8.6 Renal Involvement

The kidneys are the organs most frequently affected, up to 90–100% in some series (Table 8.1) [19–25]. The main clinical presentation is represented by rapidly progressive glomerulonephritis (RPGN) [34, 35]. RPGN is characterized clinically by a rapid decrease in the glomerular filtration rate (GFR) of at least 50% over a short period, from a few days to 3 months and, histologically, by extensive glomerular crescent formation. Other features include microscopic hematuria with often erythrocyte casts, and usually non-nephrotic proteinuria [34, 35]. Quite often RPGN is so severe to cause dialysis dependence at diagnosis in almost 60% of patients [34, 35]. With improvement in early diagnosis, a minor but significant number of patients may have just urinary abnormalities, microscopic hematuria and proteinuria, with serum creatinine within the normal range. A small but significant percentage of patients, especially those with MPA (14% in our series), may have a more indolent course and present, at diagnosis, with chronic renal insufficiency [34].

The histological lesions are represented by necrosis of capillary loops, extracapillary proliferation with crescent formation, periglomerular and interstitial infiltrates, and necrotizing arteritis [34, 35]. Crescents can involve only a part of the glomerular tuft or can be circumferential with collapse of the glomerular tuft. They can be florid or fibrous according to the stage of the disease [34, 35]. When such lesions are present in the context of a paucity of immune deposits, they become diagnostic [34].

Chronic damage is significantly higher in MPA than in GPA [36–39]. Moreover, MPO-ANCA-positive patients have significantly higher percentage of globally sclerosed glomeruli, whereas PR3-ANCA-positive patients show more glomeruli with active lesions and arteritis [38, 39]. This difference has been explained by a delayed establishment of diagnosis in MPA compared to patients with GPA and/or by a different pathogenesis of renal lesions [38].

In a subgroup of patients, kidney, apparently, is the only organ/system involved and pauci-immune crescentic necrotizing glomerulonephritis is considered a renal-limited form of MPA [21, 34, 35].

8.7 Lung Involvement

Pulmonary involvement ranges from 25% to more than 70% (Table 8.1) and often represents the most frequent clinical sign that leads patients to medical supervision [11]. Two main types of lung involvement can be identified. The first is a direct consequence of the acute capillaritis, typically presenting in an acute phase of the disease, and the second is interstitial lung disease (ILD) [40, 41]. Interestingly, in the majority of these patients, pulmonary fibrosis occurs concurrently or predates the diagnosis of ANCA vasculitis [40–43]. Diffuse alveolar hemorrhage (DAH) is reported at presentation in 20% to 50% generally associated with RPGN (pulmonary renal syndrome) [40–43]. Hemoptysis is experienced by the patients in variable degrees [40]. Overt lung hemorrhage, requiring mechanical ventilation, happens in up to a third of subjects with DAH in AAV. However, the typical triad (hemoptysis, anemia, and dyspnea) is not always detected and DAH should be suspected when severe anemia or rapidly decreasing hemoglobin values are present [44]. Focal or more often diffuse infiltrates with ground-glass opacities and consolidation are the most frequent radiological findings but are not specific [44, 45]. Bronchoscopy with bronchoalveolar lavage is diagnostic but it cannot always be performed [44]. The mortality rate of MPA patients with pulmonary hemorrhage is 8.65 times greater than that of MPA patients without pulmonary hemorrhage [46]. In a recent large series from Mayo Clinic, eight out of 73 patients (11%) died during hospitalization [47]. The most important predictor of respiratory failure in patients with DAH secondary to AAV was the degree of hypoxemia upon presentation [47].

ILD can present either as usual interstitial pneumonia or as nonspecific interstitial pneumonia [40]. Two main different subsets of patients can be recognized: one with lung disease presenting after other organs have been affected by MPA, another as MPA with ILD since diagnosis recognition [40]. A higher mortality has been found associated with fibrosing interstitial lung disease in MPA [20].

Recently, a few studies have shown that bronchiectasis is a highly prevalent preexisting respiratory condition in patients with anti-MPO AAV ranging from 16% to 37.9% [48, 49]. Which implication has this finding for the pathogenesis of the disease is not known yet.

8.8 Skin Involvement

Cutaneous manifestations are found in 12–62% of patients [19–25] (Table 8.1).

The most frequent skin lesion is palpable purpura. Other manifestations in decreasing order of discovery are: cutaneous ulcers, livedo reticularis, nodules, and the rarest vasculitic urticaria [24]. Skin biopsies often show leukocytoclastic vasculitis, with fibrinoid necrosis, neutrophilic infiltration of the small vessels in the dermis, and nuclear dust [50].

8.9 Gastrointestinal

Gastrointestinal (GI) involvement, characterized by abdominal pain and GI bleeding, has been reported in 2–30% of patients [19–25] (Table 8.1). Because of perforation, patients may undergo hemicolectomy or small intestine resection.

In a recent series from Sweden, fourteen (6.5%) of 216 consecutive patients with GPA/MPA had GI manifestations. Abdominal pain and GI bleeding were the most common symptoms. Radiology was important for detection of GI disease, while endoscopy failed to support the diagnosis in many patients [51].

Despite its low frequency, GI involvement is associated with poorer outcome [52].

8.10 Nervous System

Nervous system (NS) involvement is described in 20–58% of patients [19, 20, 22–25] (Table 8.1). The most frequent and typical NS manifestation is peripheral neuropathy [53–55]. Vasculitic neuropathies are usually but not always painful and tend to produce sensory motor or sensory symptoms. Deficits are typically multifocal or asymmetric, but distal symmetric polyneuropathy can occur [53–55]. Vasculitic peripheral neuropathy typically results from ischemic axonal injury. Evaluation requires laboratory tests, electrodiagnostic studies, and nerve or nerve/muscle biopsy. Electrodiagnostic studies in vasculitic neuropathy typically show asymmetric or non-length-dependent patterns of axonal neuropathy [53–55].

The EUVAS group has reported the incidence and prevalence of peripheral neuropathy in a series of 506 patients with AAV enrolled in therapeutical trials. Forty (8%) of 506 patients had vasculitic neuropathy at baseline and a further eight patients developed active vasculitic neuropathy at a later time point [56]. The presence of motor (or motor-sensory) neuropathy at baseline was identical between MPA [16 (7%) out of 237] and granulomatosis with polyangiitis [19 (7%) out of 269], $P = 0.94$. Pure sensory neuropathy was reported in 5 (2%) out of 269 patients with granulomatosis with polyangiitis, but not in any of the patients with MPA, $P = 0.065$. Cranial nerve palsy was more common in granulomatosis with polyangiitis [45 (17%) out of 269] compared with MPA [18 (8%) out of 237], $P = 0.002$ [56].

Central nervous system (CNS) disease is an uncommon complication and affects probably less than 10% of patients [57]. CNS involvement is more frequently observed in GPA than in MPA. In MPA, most reported cases are CNS vasculitis, responsible for cerebral infarcts and subarachnoid hemorrhages [57–59]. Diagnosis relies on imaging, mainly MRI angiography [57].

8.11 Eye

Eye involvement is present in a minority of patients [19, 20, 22–25] (Table 8.1). The most frequent ocular manifestations include episcleritis, scleritis, iridocyclitis, and conjunctivitis. Retinal involvement is rare but also documented. These symptoms are caused by a vasculitic involvement of the vessels of the choroidal membrane, retina, and conjunctiva. Ocular involvement can be the first vasculitic manifestation of the disease, usually misdiagnosed [60].

8.12 ENT

ENT manifestations affecting the upper airways and the ear, although not specific for MPA, are reported in significant percentages: up to 27% of the cases in some studies [19, 20, 22–25]. The percentage range is narrower in the most recent cohorts validated by the EMA algorithm and appears to be slightly more common in Asian patients. Sinusitis is the most typical symptom of this group along with otitis media frequently associated with hearing loss. Otitis media ANCA vasculitis (OMAAV) has been recently described not only concomitant with PR3-ANCA but also with MPO-ANCA.

MPO-ANCA positive otitis media predominantly presents as otitis media with effusion and is frequently associated with hearing loss due to the autoimmune inflammatory process in the internal ear. OMAVV can be associated with facial palsy and pachymeningitis in MPA patients [61].

8.13 Heart

Cardiac involvement is described in 3.8–17.6% of patients [19, 20, 22–25] and may have different forms, including coronary vessels vasculitis, pericarditis, myocarditis, endocarditis, myocardial infarction, and subendocardial vasculitis [11, 22]. The most commonly reported manifestations are pericardial effusion and chronic heart failure [11].

8.14 Diagnosis

When MPA is suspected, a complete clinical history should be collected and an exhaustive physical examination performed. Further investigations should be aimed, on the one hand, to evaluate organ/system involvement and, on the other, to correctly classify the patient on an etiologic/pathogenetic point of view.

An initial set of laboratory tests should include complete blood count, inflammatory markers such as erythrocyte sedimentation rate (ESR) and C-reactive protein (CPR), renal function, and urinary sediment. The clinical picture should dictate further investigations; for instance, paresthesia should suggest performing electromyography in order to confirm or exclude neuropathy, cough, and/or shortness of breath, CT scan and lung function test, urinary abnormalities, kidney biopsy, and so on.

Anti-neutrophil cytoplasmic antibodies have a crucial role in diagnosing AAVs and are detected in up to 80–90% of patients with active MPA [3, 4]. According to the 1999 international consensus on ANCA testing, indirect immunofluorescence (IIF) should be used to screen for ANCAs, and samples containing ANCAs should then be tested by immunoassays for proteinase 3 (PR3)-ANCAs and myeloperoxidase (MPO)-ANCAs [3, 4]. New guidelines for ANCA testing have been developed based on a recent European multicenter study, and according to the revised 2017 international consensus recommendations, testing for ANCA in small vessel vasculitis can be done by PR3- and MPO-ANCA immunoassays, without the categorical need for IIF [62]. Antigen specificity (PR3 or MPO) does not effectively differentiate among the different AAVs; however, C-ANCA/PR3-ANCA are mainly found in GPA, while P-ANCA/MPO-ANCA are more prevalent in MPA (65–97%) [19–25] (Table 8.1) and EGPA [3, 4, 62]. Recent developments have shown that ANCA specificity is more closely associated with disease phenotype and prognosis than clinical diagnosis. In particular, as expected, patients with kidney-limited disease or any form of vasculitis without radiographic or histologic proof of granulomatous inflammation were more likely to have MPO-ANCA, and those with the most compelling evidence for necrotizing granulomatous inflammation were most likely to have PR3-ANCA [3].

The presence of determined clinical findings plus specific laboratory tests allows to correctly classifying the vast majority of patients.

There are no validated diagnostic/classification criteria for MPA. MPA is usually defined according to the Chapel Hill Consensus Conference [1] and classified using the European Medicines Agency (EMA) algorithm [63]. Classification of the ANCA-associated vasculitides remains controversial. Existing systems, developed by the American College of Rheumatology (ACR) in 1990, the CHCC in 1994, all have deficiencies, especially when applied to unselected patients. The ACR system did not include ANCA or microscopic polyangiitis, and the CHCC (1994) included MPA but not ANCA. To partly overcome these limitations, the European Medicines Agency (EMA) has developed a stepwise algorithm to categorize patients with GPA, MPA, EGPA, and PAN into single clinically relevant categories. The ACR and Lanham criteria for EGPA and ACR criteria for GPA are applied first, as these are considered to be the most specific. Surrogate markers for GPA are included to distinguish GPA from MPA. MPA is classified using the CHCC definition and surrogate markers for renal vasculitis. This algorithm has been shown to perform better than the previous ones with an increased sensitivity [63]. To summarize, a patient with a clinical diagnosis of primary small vessel vasculitis and/or pauci-immune necrotizing glomerulonephritis is diagnosed as having MPA if no criteria for EGPA or GPA are satisfied [63].

8.15 Pathology

Histologically, MPA is characterized by necrotizing vasculitis of small vessels (arterioles, capillaries, venules) and lack or paucity of immune deposits within the vessel wall [1, 10–13]. Kidney is the most studied organ: as said before, the typical lesions are represented by necrosis of capillary loops, extracapillary proliferation with crescent formation, and periglomerular and interstitial infiltrates in the context of a paucity of immune deposits, the so-called "pauci-immune necrotizing crescentic glomerulonephritis" [1, 10–13]. Capillaritis with fibrinoid necrosis is the typical finding in the lungs where, in contrast with GPA, granulomatous inflammation is absent [40]. The histopathological pattern of MPA in skin lesions is represented by leukocytoclastic vasculitis [50].

8.16 Prognosis and Outcome

Untreated MPA has an unfavorable course with a patient survival of less than 20% at 5 years [11–13]. Even if the frequency of relapses is lower in MPA in comparison with GPA, patient survival is, on the contrary, lower for MPA than for GPA and EGPA (27.5 vs. 13%) [11, 64, 65].

Factors independently related to death are the presence and severity of renal involvement, cardiac symptoms, gastrointestinal involvement, and age over 65 years [64, 65]. ENT symptoms, affecting patients with WG and CSS, are associated with a lower relative risk of death [64, 65].

8.17 Treatment

Therapy of AAV will be covered in another chapter of this book. However, some guidelines on the treatment of MPA will be given.

Patients with serum creatinine lower than 500 μmol/l (5.7 mg/dl) should be treated with prednisone and cyclophosphamide for 3–6 months until remission is reached [66]. Oral and pulse cyclophosphamide have been shown to be equivalent in terms of clinical response [67]. Cyclophosphamide pulses are, however, associated with less episodes of leukopenia and the cumulative dose of the drug is inferior to that found in the oral cyclophosphamide-treated patients [67]. Long-term follow-up of CYCLOPS study has shown that pulse cyclophosphamide is associated with a higher relapse risk than daily oral cyclophosphamide. However, this is not associated with increased mortality or long-term morbidity [68].

Once that disease is into remission (usually within 3–6 months), azathioprine is as effective as cyclophosphamide and more effective than mycophenolate/mofetil to maintain remission [66]. How long to continue maintenance therapy is not known.

Patients with renal involvement with a serum creatinine higher than 500 μmol per liter (5.7 mg/dl) and/or lung hemorrhage should be treated with a course of plasma exchange (7 sessions in 2 weeks) in addition to prednisone and oral cyclophosphamide. In a randomized controlled trial, plasma exchange (PLEX) was shown to be more effective than methylprednisolone pulses (IV MeP) in terms of renal function recovery [69]. However, although short-term results with PLEX were encouraging, the long-term benefits remain unclear since, after a median of almost 4 years follow-up, there was no evidence of a net difference between PLEX and IV MeP in clinical outcomes [70].

In a larger unpublished trial presented at the last ERA/EDTA meeting, an additive effect of plasma exchange on the cumulative end point of ESRD and death was not confirmed raising doubts on its utility [71].

While rituximab has been shown in a *post hoc* analysis to be superior to cyclophosphamide to induce remission in patients with PR3-AAV (GPA), the same drug was found to be as effective as cyclophosphamide in MPO-AAV (MPA) [72, 73]. Therefore, rituximab can be used instead of cyclophosphamide in MPA, especially in younger patients in order to preserve fertility.

Preliminary results from small pilot studies indicate that mycophenolate mofetil is effective for induction and maintenance of remission in microscopic polyangiitis with mild-to-moderate renal involvement [74, 75].

8.18 Conclusions

MPA is a severe chronic relapsing disease with a particular predilection for kidney and lung. It is classified among the so-called AAV and it can be distinguished from GPA for the absence of granulomatous inflammation and from EGPA for the absence of asthma and eosinophilia.

ANCA, usually P-ANCA with specificity for MPO, are found in 80–90% of cases.

Renal involvement is characterized by pauci-immune necrotizing crescentic glomerulonephritis. Even though there are no qualitative differences in glomerular lesions in patients with MPA or with GPA, chronic damage is significantly higher in MPA (and/or MPO-ANCA-positive patients) than in GPA (and/or PR3-ANCA-positive patients).

Two main types of lung involvement can be identified: alveolar hemorrhage that is a direct consequence of acute necrotizing capillaritis, and interstitial lung disease that often occurs concurrently or predates the diagnosis of ANCA vasculitis and, therefore, cannot be considered a direct consequence of vasculitis.

Even if the frequency of relapses is lower in MPA in comparison with GPA, patient outcome is worse. Age over 65 years old, renal, gastrointestinal, and cardiac involvement are associated with poorer prognosis.

References

1. Jennette JC, Falk RJ, Andrassy K, et al. Nomenclature of systemic vasculitides. Proposal of an international consensus conference. Arthritis Rheum. 1994;37(2):187–92.
2. Jennette JC, Falk RJ, Bacon PA, et al. 2012 revised international chapel hill consensus conference nomenclature of vasculitides. Arthritis Rheum. 2012;65:1–11.
3. Sinico RA, Radice A. Antineutrophil cytoplasmic antibodies (ANCA) testing: detection methods and clinical application. Clin Exp Rheumatol. 2014;32(3 Suppl 82):S112–7.
4. Csernok E, Moosig F. Current and emerging techniques for ANCA detection in vasculitis. Nat Rev Rheumatol. 2014;10:494–501.
5. Wohlwill F. Über die nur mikroskopisch erkennbare Form der Periarteriitis nodosa. Virchows Arch Path Anat. 1923;246:377–411.
6. Davson J, Bal J, Plat R. The kidney in periarteritis nodosa. Q J Med. 1948;17:175–202.
7. Zeek PM, Smith CC, Weeter JC. Studies on periarteritis nodosa; the differentiation between the vascular lesions of periarteritis nodosa and of hypersensitivity. Am J Pathol. 1948;24(4):889–917.
8. Godman GC, Churg J. Wegener's granulomatosis: pathology and review of the literature. AMA Arch Pathol. 1954;58(6):533–53.
9. Savage CO, Winearls CG, Evans DJ, Rees AJ, Lockwood CM. Microscopic polyarteritis: presentation, pathology and prognosis. Q J Med. 1985;56(220):467–83.
10. Jennette JC, Falk RJ. Small-vessel vasculitis. N Engl J Med. 1997;337:1512–23.
11. Villiger PM, Guillevin L. Microscopic polyangiitis: clinical presentation. Autoimmun Rev. 2010;9(12):812–9.
12. Kallenberg CG. The diagnosis and classification of microscopic polyangiitis. J Autoimmun. 2014;48-49:90–3.
13. Greco A, De Virgilio A, Rizzo MI, et al. Microscopic polyangiitis: advances in diagnostic and therapeutic approaches. Autoimmun Rev. 2015;14(9):837–44.

14. Fujimoto S, Watts RA, Kobayashi S, et al. Comparison of the epidemiology of anti-neutrophil cytoplasmic antibody-associated vasculitis between Japan and the U.K. Rheumatology (Oxford). 2011;50(10):1916–20.
15. Scott DGI, Watts RA. Epidemiology and clinical features of systemic vasculitis. Clin Exp Nephrol. 2013;17(5):607–10.
16. Pearce FA, Lanyon PC, Grainge MJ, et al. Incidence of ANCA-associated vasculitis in a UK mixed ethnicity population. Rheumatology (Oxford). 2016;55(9):1656–63.
17. Berti A, Cornec D, Crowson CS, Specks U, Matteson EL. The epidemiology of Antineutrophil cytoplasmic autoantibody-associated Vasculitis in Olmsted County, Minnesota: a twenty-year US population-based study. Arthritis Rheumatol. 2017;69(12):2338–50.
18. Ahn JK, Hwang JW, Lee J, Jeon CH, Cha HS, Koh EM. Clinical features and outcome of microscopic polyangiitis under a new consensus algorithm of ANCA-associated vasculitides in Korea. Rheumatol Int. 2012;32(10):2979–86.
19. Furuta S, Chaudhry AN, Hamano Y, et al. Comparison of phenotype and outcome in microscopic polyangiitis between Europe and Japan. J Rheumatol. 2014;41(2):325–33.
20. Schirmer JH, Wright MN, Vonthein R, et al. Clinical presentation and long-term outcome of 144 patients with microscopic polyangiitis in a monocentric German cohort. Rheumatology (Oxford). 2016;55(1):71–9.
21. Hogan SL, Nachman PH, Wilkman S, et al. Prognostic markers in patients with antineutrophil cytoplasmic autoantibody-associated microscopic polyangiitis and glomerulonephritis. J Am Soc Nephrol. 1996;7(1):23–32.
22. Guillevin L, Durand-Gasselin B, Cevallos R, et al. Microscopic polyangiitis: clinical and laboratory findings in eighty-five patients. Arthritis Rheum. 1999;42(3):421–30.
23. Ahn JK, Hwang JW, Lee J, et al. Clinical features and outcome of microscopic polyangiitis under a new consensus algorithm of ANCA-associated vasculitides in Korea. Rheumatol Int. 2012;32(10):2979–86.
24. Sugiyama K, Sada K, Kurosawa M, et al. Current status of the treatment of microscopic polyangiitis and granulomatosis with polyangiitis in Japan. Clin Exp Nephrol. 2013;17(1): 51–8.
25. Sada K, Yamamura M, Harigai M, et al. Classification and characteristics of Japanese patients with antineutrophil cytoplasmic antibody-associated vasculitis in a nationwide, prospective, inception cohort study. Arthritis Res Ther. 2014;16(2):R101.
26. Calatroni M, Oliva E, Gianfreda D, et al. ANCA-associated vasculitis in childhood: recent advances. Ital J Pediatr. 2017;43(1):46.
27. Sacri AS, Chambaraud T, Ranchin B, et al. Clinical characteristics and outcomes of childhood-onset ANCA-associated vasculitis: a French nationwide study. Nephrol Dial Transplant. 2015;30(Suppl 1):i104–12.
28. Grisaru S, Yuen GW, Miettunen PM, Hamiwka LA. Incidence of Wegener's granulomatosis in children. J Rheumatol. 2010;37(2):440–2.
29. Mossberg M, Segelmark M, Kahn R, Englund M, Mohammad AJ. Epidemiology of primary systemic vasculitis in children: a population-based study from southern Sweden. Scand J Rheumatol. 2018;7:1–8.
30. Jennette JC, Falk RJ, Gasim AH. Pathogenesis of antineutrophil cytoplasmic autoantibody vasculitis. Curr Opin Nephrol Hypertens. 2011;20(3):263–70.
31. Kallenberg CG. Pathogenesis of ANCA-associated vasculitides. Ann Rheum Dis. 2011;70(Suppl. 1):i59–63.
32. Salama AD, Little MA. Animal models of antineutrophil cytoplasm antibody associated vasculitis. Curr Opin Rheumatol. 2012;24(1):1–7.
33. Lyons PA, Rayner TF, Trivedi S, et al. Genetically distinct subsets within ANCA-associated vasculitis. N Engl J Med. 2012;367(3):214–23.
34. Sinico RA, Di Toma L, Radice A. Renal involvement in anti-neutrophil cytoplasmic autoantibody associated vasculitis. Autoimmun Rev. 2013;12:477–82.
35. Binda V, Moroni G, Messa P. ANCA-associated vasculitis with renal involvement. J Nephrol. 2018;31(2):197–208.

36. Rutgers A, Sanders JS, Stegeman CA, Kallenberg CG. Pauci-immune necrotizing glomerulonephritis. Rheum Dis Clin N Am. 2010;36(3):559–72.
37. Bajema IM. Pathological classification of anti-neutrophil cytoplasmic antibody (ANCA)-associated glomerulonephritis. Clin Exp Immunol. 2011;164(Suppl. 1):14–6.
38. Hauer HA, Bajema IM, Van Houwelingen HC, et al. Determinants of outcome in ANCA-associated glomerulonephritis: a prospective clinico-histopathological analysis of 96 patients. Kidney Int. 2002;62(5):1732–42.
39. Day CJ, Howie AJ, Nightingale P, et al. Prediction of ESRD in pauci-immune necrotizing glomerulonephritis: quantitative histomorphometric assessment and serum creatinine. Am J Kidney Dis. 2010;55(2):250–8.
40. Flores-Suárez LF, Alba MA, Mateos-Toledo H, Ruiz N. Pulmonary involvement in systemic vasculitis. Curr Rheumatol Rep. 2017;19(9):56.
41. Alba MA, Flores-Suárez LF, Henderson AG, et al. Interstital lung disease in ANCA vasculitis. Autoimmun Rev. 2017;16(7):722–9.
42. García-Nava M, Mateos-Toledo H, Guevara-Canseco APG, Infante-González CE, Reyes-Nava DA, Estrada-Castro E. Early interstitial lung disease in microscopic polyangiitis: case report and literature review. Reumatol Clin. 2018;14(2):106–8.
43. Talarico R, Barsotti S, Elefante E, Baldini C, Tani C, Mosca M. Systemic vasculitis and the lung. Curr Opin Rheumatol. 2017;29(1):45–50.
44. Krause ML, Cartin-Ceba R, Specks U, Peikert T. Update on diffuse alveolar hemorrhage and pulmonary vasculitis. Immunol Allergy Clin N Am. 2012;32(4):587–600.
45. Feragalli B, Mantini C, Sperandeo M, et al. The lung in systemic vasculitis: radiological patterns and differential diagnosis. Br J Radiol. 2016;89(1061):20150992.
46. Hogan SL, Nachman PH, Wilkman AS, Jennette JC, Falk R. Prognostic markers in patients with antineutrophil cytoplasmic autoantibody-associated microscopic polyangiitis and glomerulonephritis. J Am Soc Nephrol. 1996;7(1):23–32.
47. Cartin-Ceba R, Diaz-Caballero L, Al-Qadi MO, et al. Diffuse alveolar Hemorrhage secondary to Antineutrophil cytoplasmic antibody-associated Vasculitis: predictors of respiratory failure and clinical outcomes. Arthritis Rheumatol. 2016;68(6):1467–76.
48. Néel A, Espitia-Thibault A, Arrigoni PP, et al. Bronchiectasis is highly prevalent in anti-MPO ANCA-associated vasculitis and is associated with a distinct disease presentation. Semin Arthritis Rheum. 2018;48(1):70–6.
49. Tashiro H, Takahashi K, Tanaka M, et al. Characteristics and prognosis of microscopic polyangiitis with bronchiectasis. J Thorac Dis. 2017;9(2):303–9.
50. Marzano AV, Vezzoli P, Berti E. Skin involvement in cutaneous and systemic vasculitis. Autoimmun Rev. 2013;12(4):467–76.
51. Eriksson P, Segelmark M, Hallböök O. Frequency, diagnosis, treatment, and outcome of gastrointestinal disease in Granulomatosis with Polyangiitis and microscopic Polyangiitis. J Rheumatol. 2018;45(4):529–37.
52. Guillevin L, Pagnoux C, Seror R, et al. The five-factor score revisited: assessment of prognoses of systemic necrotizing vasculitides based on the French Vasculitis study group (FVSG) cohort. Medicine (Baltimore). 2011;90(1):19–27.
53. Collins MP, Arnold WD, Kissel JT. The neuropathies of vasculitis. Neurol Clin. 2013;31(2):557–95.
54. Gwathmey KG, Burns TM, Collins MP, Dyck PJ. Vasculitic neuropathies. Lancet Neurol. 2014;13(1):67–82.
55. Hadden RDM, Collins MP, Živković SA, et al. Vasculitic peripheral neuropathy: case definition and guidelines for collection, analysis, and presentation of immunisation safety data. Vaccine. 2017;35(11):1567–78.
56. Suppiah R, Hadden RD, Batra R, et al. Peripheral neuropathy in ANCA-associated vasculitis: outcomes from the European Vasculitis Study Group trials. Rheumatology (Oxford). 2011;50(12):2214–22.
57. Graf J. Central nervous system disease in antineutrophil cytoplasmic antibodies-associated vasculitis. Rheum Dis Clin N Am. 2017;43:573–8.

58. Han S, Rehman HU, Jayaratne PS, Carty JE. Microscopic polyangiitis complicated by cerebral haemorrhage. Rheumatol Int. 2006;26:1057–60.
59. Sassi SB, Ghorbel IB, Mizouni H, Houman MH, Hentati F. Microscopic polyangiitis presenting with peripheral and central neurological manifestations. Neurol Sci. 2011;32:727–9.
60. Kubal AA, Perez VL. Ocular manifestations of ANCA-associated vasculitis. Rheum Dis Clin N Am. 2010;36(3):573–86.
61. Harabuchi Y, Kishibe K, Tateyama K, et al. Clinical features and treatment outcomes of otitis media with antineutrophil cytoplasmic antibody (ANCA)-associated vasculitis (OMAAV): a retrospective analysis of 235 patients from a nationwide survey in Japan. Mod Rheumatol. 2017;27(1):87–94.
62. Bossuyt X, Cohen Tervaert JW, Arimura Y, et al. Position paper: revised 2017 international consensus on testing of ANCAs in granulomatosis with polyangiitis and microscopic polyangiitis. Nat Rev Rheumatol. 2017;13(11):683–92.
63. Watts R, Lane S, Hanslik T, et al. Development and validation of a consensus methodology for the classification of the ANCA-associated vasculitides and polyarteritis nodosa for epidemiological studies. Ann Rheum Dis. 2007;66:222–7.
64. Mukhtyar C, Flossmann O, Hellmich B, et al. Outcomes from studies of antineutrophil cytoplasm antibody associated vasculitis: a systematic review by the European league against rheumatism systemic vasculitis task force. Ann Rheum Dis. 2008;67(7):1004–10.
65. Solans-Laqué R, Fraile G, Rodriguez-Carballeira M, et al. Clinical characteristics and outcome of Spanish patients with ANCA-associated vasculitides: impact of the vasculitis type, ANCA specificity, and treatment on mortality and morbidity. Medicine (Baltimore). 2017;96(8):e6083.
66. Jayne D, Rasmussen N, Andrassy K, et al. A randomized trial of maintenance therapy for vasculitis associated with antineutrophil cytoplasmic autoantibodies. N Engl J Med. 2003;349(1):36–44.
67. de Groot K, Harper L, Jayne DR, et al. Pulse versus daily oral cyclophosphamide for induction of remission in antineutrophil cytoplasmic antibody-associated vasculitis: a randomized trial. Ann Intern Med. 2009;150(10):670–80.
68. Harper L, Morgan MD, Walsh M, et al. EUVAS investigators. Pulse versus daily oral cyclophosphamide for induction of remission in ANCA-associated vasculitis: long-term follow-up. Ann Rheum Dis. 2012;71(6):955–60.
69. Jayne DR, Gaskin G, Rasmussen N, et al. Randomized trial of plasma exchange or high-dosage methylprednisolone as adjunctive therapy for severe renal vasculitis. J Am Soc Nephrol. 2007;18(7):2180–8.
70. Walsh M, Casian A, Flossmann O, et al. European Vasculitis Study Group (EUVAS). Long-term follow-up of patients with severe ANCA-associated vasculitis comparing plasma exchange to intravenous methylprednisolone treatment is unclear. Kidney Int. 2013;84(2):397–402.
71. Walsh M, Merkel P, Peh CA, et al. The effect of plasma exchange on end stage renale disease and death in patients with severe ANCA associated vasculitis. Nephrol Dial Transpl. 2018;33(Suppl 1):i636.
72. Unizony S, Villarreal M, Miloslavsky EM, et al. RAVE-ITN research group. Clinical outcomes of treatment of anti-neutrophil cytoplasmic antibody (ANCA)-associated vasculitis based on ANCA type. Ann Rheum Dis. 2016;75(6):1166–9.
73. Stone JH, Merkel PA, Spiera R, et al. Rituximab versus cyclophosphamide for ANCA-associated vasculitis. N Engl J Med. 2010;363(3):221–32.
74. Silva F, Specks U, Kalra S, et al. Mycophenolate mofetil for induction and maintenance of remission in microscopic polyangiitis with mild to moderate renal involvement—a prospective, open-label pilot trial. Clin J Am Soc Nephrol. 2010;5(3):445–53.
75. Han F, Liu G, Zhang X, et al. Effects of mycophenolate mofetil combined with corticosteroids for induction therapy of microscopic polyangiitis. Am J Nephrol. 2011;33(2):185–92.

Part II

Vasculitis/Organs Involvement

9 ANCA-Associated Vasculitis—ENT Involvement

Trimarchi Matteo, Galli Andrea, and Roberto Teggi

9.1 Introduction

Antineutrophil cytoplasmic antibody (ANCA)-associated vasculitis (AAV) are idiopathic, immunologically mediated diseases predominantly affecting small vessels throughout the body (capillaries, venules arterioles, and small arteries), which are pathogenetically associated with pauci-immune vasculitis and with either proteinase 3-ANCA (PR3-ANCA or c-ANCA) or myeloperoxidase-ANCA (MPO-ANCA or p-ANCA) [1]. AAV are typically characterized by necrotizing, granulomatous inflammation of the upper and lower respiratory tract and focal or proliferative glomerulonephritis in combination with other eventual vasculitis-related manifestations; long-term prognosis is poor if adequate treatment is not promptly established [2].

The 2012 revised Chapel Hill Consensus Conference (CHCC) defined microscopic polyangiitis (MPA), granulomatosis with polyangiitis (GPA, formerly Wegener's granulomatosis), eosinophilic granulomatosis with polyangiitis (EGPA, also known as Churg-Strauss syndrome), and single-organ manifestations (e.g., acute renal-limited disease known as pauci-immune necrotizing crescentic

T. Matteo (✉)
Otorhinolaryngology—Head and Neck Surgery Department, San Raffaele Hospital, Milan, Italy

ENT—Head and Neck Surgery Department, IRCCS San Raffaele, Milan, Italy

Department of Otorhinolaryngology, San Raffaele Hospital, Vita-Salute University, Milan, Italy
e-mail: trimarchi.matteo@hsr.it

G. Andrea · R. Teggi
Otorhinolaryngology—Head and Neck Surgery Department, San Raffaele Hospital, Milan, Italy

ENT—Head and Neck Surgery Department, IRCCS San Raffaele, Milan, Italy
e-mail: galli1.andrea@hsr.it; teggi.roberto@hsr.it

R. A. Sinico, L. Guillevin (eds.), *Anti-Neutrophil Cytoplasmic Antibody (ANCA) Associated Vasculitis*, Rare Diseases of the Immune System,
https://doi.org/10.1007/978-3-030-02239-6_9

glomerulonephritis, NCGN) as the main clinic-pathological variants within the AAV spectrum [3]. PR3-ANCA cases are more frequent than MPO-ANCA in GPA, whereas MPO-ANCA-positive patients are more common in MPA, EGPA, and renal-limited pauci-immune NCGN [4].

It is often difficult to consider each entity by itself due to the overall rarity of AAV and the frequent overlap of clinical and pathological factors: most trials, indeed, have recruited patients from the entire spectrum, especially GPA and MPA [5]. However, recognizing minor phenotypes is nowadays mandatory, not only for epidemiological issues, but also because each has a different clinical course, with the obvious therapeutic implications [6].

MPA is defined as a pauci-immune small-vessel vasculitis (SVV), potentially affecting any organ or tissue, in the absence of evidences for GPA or EGPA [7]. Its reported prevalence ranges from 2.7 to 94 cases per million [8], with southern Europe more affected than northern (11.6/million in Spain against 2.7/million in Norway) [9]: mean age at onset is between 50 and 60 years, with a slight male predominance (male:female ratio 1.8:1) [10].

Initial single-organ involvement with or without subsequent systemic spread is typical MPA course. Common clinical features are purpura (determined by dermal venulitis), hemorrhagic pulmonary alveolar capillaritis, NCGN, and mononeuritis multiplex as a consequence of epineural arteritis [1]. ENT and eye manifestations are not considered as typical clinical symptoms of MPA, in contrast to GPA and EGPA. However, such findings are not so uncommon: different series report their presence in 9% [11], 20% [12], and 30% [13] of MPA patients, especially in association with chronic rhinosinusitis [10] or sensorineural hearing loss [14].

GPA, formerly known as Wegener's granulomatosis [15], is also a SVV that is pathologically identical to MPA, except for the presence of necrotizing granulomatous inflammation that can affect vessels or appear exclusively in extravascular tissues [1]. This peculiar extravascular necrosis, in the absence of clearly identifiable vessels, is known as "pathergic granulomatosis" [16]. Such granulomatous inflammation commonly involves the upper or lower respiratory tract, even though it can occur anywhere (e.g., skin, orbit meninges), and is usually very different from that observed in cases with mycobacteriosis, sarcoidosis, or fungal infections [16]. In addition to necrotizing granulomatous lesions and pathological-related vasculitis, GPA is typically defined by focal or proliferative glomerulonephritis [17].

Single-organ GPA, lacking clear systemic involvement, may also occur, frequently as isolated head and neck granulomatous manifestations [18]: classic otorhinolaryngologic symptoms may define the initial clinical picture in many GPA patients, since the upper respiratory tract is involved in 70–100% of cases [19]. These localized forms, in the same way of single-organ EGPA, are less often associated with ANCA-positivity and their course is often unpredictable in terms of systemic progression [1, 20].

The prevalence of GPA is about 5 cases per 100,000 in Europe, with northern counties more commonly involved. Mean age at diagnosis is 40 years (range: 8–99); both sexes seem equally affected [21, 22].

EGPA, also known as Churg–Strauss syndrome, is a condition at the crossroads between SVV and hypereosinophilic disorders. It is generally characterized by a non-vasculitis prodrome of asthma and/or allergic rhinitis, subsequent blood hypereosinophilia with single-organ eosinophilic inflammation (e.g., pneumonia, gastroenteritis), and a final systemic stage defined by SVV and glomerulonephritis [7]. ANCA-positive patients usually develop peripheral neuropathy, glomerulonephritis, and purpura due to prevalent SVV, while myocardial involvement, lung infiltrates, and gastrointestinal symptoms are easily detectable within the ANCA-negative subset [23, 24].

Both vasculitis and glomerulonephritis are substantially indistinguishable from those occurring in GPA and MPA, except for the number of eosinophils detectable within inflammatory lesions; the same applies for "pathergic granulomatosis" in comparison to GPA [1].

Head and neck manifestations are typical of the first stage of the disease, when recurrent or chronic rhinosinusitis with/without nasal polyps are commonly encountered; sinonasal granulomas, recalcitrant endonasal crusting, and otological or orbital involvement are less frequently part of the clinical picture [25, 26].

The estimated prevalence of EGPA is of 10.7–14 cases per million [27], with a mean age of onset of 38–54 years [28].

Other than the AAV spectrum, the so-called cocaine-induced midline destructive lesions (*CIMDL*) are emerging pathologies caused by habitual cocaine insufflation frequently presenting with clinical, endoscopic, serological, and histopathological features resembling those of systemic vasculitis, especially GPA [29]. Their incidence is increasing with the widespread illicit use of the drug, whose most common route of administration is the intranasal one by inhalation [30]. In these conditions, patients may display focal/diffuse destruction of the osteocartilagineous nasal framework, positive ANCA tests, and leukocytoclastic vasculitis with fibrinoid necrosis, in a pattern significantly mimicking a localized-form of GPA [31]. Differential diagnosis between CIMDL and sinonasal GPA is thus particularly challenging, as patients do not readily admit their drug abuse: in these settings, blood, urine, and hair evaluation for cocaine metabolites is mandatory to confirm addiction and rule out a misleading diagnosis [29]. Though difficult, clinicians must recognize these peculiar manifestations in order to provide appropriate treatment [32].

Since head and neck involvement in AAV is quite common and occasionally the first and isolated sign of active disease, otorhinolaryngologists become essential members of the multidisciplinary team approaching these conditions. We now review the most common ENT manifestations of AAV, according to the phenotype of vasculitis involved (Table 9.1). The CIMDL spectrum is also analyzed due to its large and troublesome similarity to the sinonasal, localized-form of GPA.

9.2 Microscopic Polyangiitis (MPA)

MPA is primarily a cause of pulmonary–renal syndrome (i.e., pulmonary capillaritis with glomerulonephritis), a group of disorders including Goodpasture's disease [9]. ENT manifestations are not considered a typical feature, in contrast to the GPA and

Table 9.1 Summary of head and neck involvement in course of antineutrophil cytoplasmic antibody-associated vasculitis, stratified for peculiar vasculitis phenotypes according to Revised International Chapel Hill Consensus Conference [3], and cocaine-induced midline destructive lesions (CIMDL)

	MPA	GPA	EGPA	CIMDL
Sinonasal	• Chronic rhinosinusitis with or without nasal polyps	• Crusting rhinitis • Chronic rhinosinusitis with or without nasal polyps • Midline destructive lesions – Nasal septum perforation – Saddle-nose deformity • Naso-lacrimal duct obstruction	• Allergic rhinitis • Chronic rhinosinusitis with or without nasal polyps • Crusting rhinitis • Midline destructive lesions – Nasal septum perforation	• Crusting rhinitis • Midline destructive lesions – Nasal septum perforation – Saddle-nose deformity • Naso-lacrimal duct obstruction
Ear	• Sensorineural hearing loss with tinnitus	• Otitis media with effusion • Chronic suppurative otitis media • Facial nerve palsy • Sensorineural hearing loss with tinnitus • Vertigo	• Otitis media with effusion • Chronic suppurative otitis media • Sensorineural hearing loss with tinnitus	• Otitis media with effusion • Sudden hearing loss
Larynx		• Laryngo-tracheal ulcers • Subglottic stenosis		
Salivary		• Sialadenitis of submandibular/parotid gland		
Oral cavity		• Ulcerative stomatitis • "Strawberry" gingival hyperplasia • Oro-antral fistula • Osteo-necrosis of hard palate		• Oro-antral fistula • Osteo-necrosis of hard/soft palate
Orbit		• Episcleritis • Uveitis • Retinal vasculitis and thrombosis • Orbital granulomatous mass • Orbital cellulitis • Lacrimal sac involvement	• Orbital granulomatous mass	• Orbital cellulitis

EGPA phenotypes; however, head and neck involvement has been documented in 9%, 20%, and 30% of MPA cases in three major series [11–13]. Chronic rhinosinusitis is the most common condition [33] along with sensorineural hearing loss with tinnitus [14].

9.3 Granulomatosis with Polyangiitis (GPA)

The nasal cavity and paranasal sinuses are the most commonly affected sites within the head and neck area in GPA patients (85–100%) [22, 34]. Interestingly, the nose is the only diseased site in 30% of cases [35]. In active nasal disease, the nasal mucosa displays copious crusting, diffuse hemorrhages, swelling, and purulent secretions due to superimposed bacterial infection (e.g., *S. aureus*, *P. aeruginosa*), conditions that may lead to nasal obstruction, hyposmia/anosmia, cacosmia, recurrent epistaxis, nasal pain, and finally to chronic rhinosinusitis with or without nasal polyps [18].

Mucosal granulomatous inflammation primarily affects the turbinates and nasal septum, especially at the locus Valsalvae (Fig. 9.1a): vasculitic involvement at Kiesselbach's plexus can cause transmural necrosis of the underlying cartilage and consequent septal perforation [18, 22]. Although distressing for patients, this finding is not necessarily synonymous of an active disease state [36]. A deeper involvement of nasal framework by vasculitic and "pathergic granulomatosis" process can determine the collapse of its cartilaginous midvault, resulting in a depressed appearance of the nose, the so-called "saddle-nose" deformity [37]: this condition generally develops in 10–25% of patients with blown nasal GPA [22].

Endonasal mucosal swelling and/or granulomatous destructive lesions can also lead to nasolacrimal duct obstruction (NLDO) or direct lacrimal sac involvement, with epiphora as a possible initial sign of disease [38]. Further extension

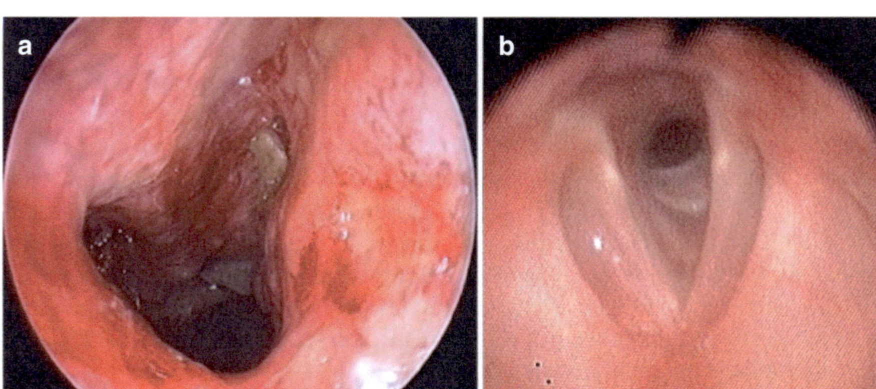

Fig. 9.1 GPA-related endonasal granulomatous inflammation affecting anterior mucosa of nasal septum and turbinates (**a**); subglottic stenosis markedly reducing laryngo-tracheal respiratory space (**b**)

of inflammation to the paranasal sinuses is the result of prolonged active disease, occurring in 50% of patients with nasal GPA [35]. Sinus imaging (CT or MRI) does not allow distinguishing GPA-related inflammation from non-specific inflammation/infection occurring during clinical relapses, but it can help in the chronic stage by noting long-term sequelae of the disease, such as the scar tissue frequently filling maxillary sinuses and the progressive ossification of the paranasal cavities [39]. Moreover, narrow-band imaging (NBI) endoscopy can be helpful in the diagnostic process to detect peculiar vascular patterns and guide physicians toward a biopsy diagnosis of GPA [40].

Otologic manifestations are commonly reported during the clinical course of GPA, with a prevalence reported in the range between 19% and 61%. Otologic disorders may be part of the initial presentation in about 33% of cases [41, 42].

The external ear is less frequently involved, with ulcerated lesions (in a clinical picture resembling perichondritis or acute external otitis) being the most common manifestations; these lesions are poorly responsive to antibiotic or local steroids [43].

Since Eustachian tube dysfunction resulting from nasopharyngeal involvement is a common finding in GPA patients, unilateral or bilateral serous or, less frequently, purulent otitis media is the most recurrent otologic feature of the disease. More rarely otitis media may be caused by granulomatous involvement of the middle ear itself, which in turn leads to mastoiditis and chronic otitis media [21, 44]. Different authors underline how GPA should be considered within potential differential diagnoses in this context, especially in otitis that are poorly responsive to therapy and/or whenever a discrepancy between otoscopic findings and severity of the hearing loss is noticed: in these cases surgical intervention (i.e. exploratory tympanotomy with or without concurrent tympanoplasty) should be performed, at least with diagnostic purpose and in a minimally invasive fashion [21, 45].

Progressive sensorineural hearing loss, initially high pitched and associated with tinnitus, has been reported in around one-third of GPA cases [46]. Its pathogenesis remains unclear: hearing loss may be related to the toxic action of inflammatory by-products released in the middle ear that can act beyond it against the inner portion of the organ through the round window [21, 36]. As far as this hypothesis is concerned, a case of a rapidly progressive hearing loss occurring during chronic otitis media with effusion has been reported [47]: in this patient, T1-weighted gadolinium-enhanced ear MRI demonstrated bilateral enhancement of the basal turn of the cochlea, a possible expression of cochleitis related to the above-mentioned mechanism [47]. Similar involvement of the vestibule can lead to acute onset of vertigo [36]. Other suggested pathogeneses are vasculitis of the vasa nervorum of the VIII cranial nerve, deposition of immune complexes within the inner ear, and pressure on the acoustic nerve by granulomatous lesions [17, 21, 36, 46, 48, 49]. The same processes, in a small percentage of GPA patients, can lead to VII cranial nerve palsy, with or without concurrent middle ear disorder [46].

Recently, a stand-alone nosological entity has been advocated by the Japanese Otorhinolaryngology Society with proper diagnostic criteria: *otitis media ANCA-associated vasculitis* (OMAAV) [50]. This proposal derives from the evidence that exclusive otitis media refractory to antibiotics or tympanostomy tube with findings suggestive for GPA but formally inconclusive (e.g., serological MPO-ANCA positivity) could represent an independent disease. Whether or not this hypothesis is true is still controversial, since granulomas do exist in the middle ear of these patients, destroying ossicles as they grow up: OMAAV may indeed be considered as a peculiar, localized form of GPA [50].

Oral lesions in GPA patients are uncommon findings, occurring in about 5–10% of cases. Their incidence as presenting manifestations of the disease is even more infrequent (around 2%) [51, 52]. When observed, such include non-specific deep ulcers of tongue, cheek, and palate mucosa (i.e., ulcerative stomatitis) as well as "strawberry" gingival hyperplasia, an exophytic gingival swelling of reddish purple color with petechiae that commonly originates in the interdental papillae. This latter is an obvious pathognomonic sign of GPA, although its occurrence is quite rare [53, 54]. However, recognition of this typical condition is crucial for timely diagnosis [53]. Moreover, sinonasal involvement in the form of granulomatous destructive lesions can evolve downward as osteonecrosis of the hard palate and/or oro-antral fistula, although these findings favor a diagnosis of CIMDL over GPA [55].

Sialoadenitis of major salivary glands (i.e., parotid, submandibular) is another rare manifestation of GPA, and rarely its presenting symptom: enlargement of the glands with pain and signs of acute/subacute inflammation are indeed sometimes noticed within GPA patients [56, 57]. Salivary involvement is nonetheless non-specific and may even mimic malignancies: when this is the presenting condition, a diagnosis of GPA is uncertain until more common features arise or it is demonstrated histopathologically [18].

Laryngo-tracheal involvement is reported in 15–55% of GPA patients, and rarely as a presenting condition [58–61]. Mucosal ulcers are found in 25% of cases, more commonly than subglottic stenosis (16%) (Fig. 9.1b) [62]: many of these lesions, however, become heavily symptomatic, causing progressively hoarseness, cough, wheezing, and dyspnea; in acute settings, urgent tracheostomy becomes mandatory to ensure airway patency [58, 59, 63]. Subglottic stenosis often requires invasive approaches in the course of GPA treatment, depending on its type and localization: translesional injection of corticosteroids, endoscopic pneumatic dilation, laser ablation with radial incisions, stenting (preferring silastic to metal wire mesh ones), or even tracheal resection with reanastomosis [62, 64]. In any case, non-medical treatment should be delayed after the healing of acute inflammatory phase, minimizing additional surgical injury to laryngo-tracheal tissues [18].

Ocular and orbital manifestations may occur in about 50–60% of GPA patients; these can even remain as stand-alone symptoms, especially in limited forms of GPA [22]. Episcleritis is found in up to 16–38% of cases [51]; other possible findings are uveitis, retinal ischemia, and optic neuropathy [22, 51].

Orbital inflammation can also be noticed within GPA subjects, typically affecting both sides, with proptosis, diplopia, visual loss, and periorbital cellulitis as symptoms [51, 65]. Inflammation is generally the result of sinonasal disease whenever it diffusely involves orbital tissues, but may arise as discrete granulomatous mass similar to presentations of pseudotumor or lymphoma [22].

9.4 Eosinophilic Granulomatosis with Polyangiitis (EGPA)

The prodromal phase of EGPA may last months to years and is usually characterized by constitutional symptoms, such as arthralgia, myalgia, malaise, fever, and weight loss, accompanied by asthma (96–100%) and upper respiratory tract involvement (47–93%) [25, 26]. This latter feature generally includes a simple allergic rhinitis, with diffuse mucosal swelling and distressing serous rhinorrhea, but also wider inflammation of the sinonasal tract with chronic rhinosinusitis (62–77%) with or without nasal polyps (Fig. 9.2) [25, 26].

Clear granulomatous destructive lesions, as observed in GPA patients, are less common in EGPA: as a consequence, recalcitrant crusting rhinitis with typical foul-smelling discharge, recurrent epistaxis, septal perforation, nasal framework collapse, and orbital pseudotumor are rarer findings in these patients [25, 26].

Otologic manifestations of EGPA, seen in about 50% of patients, occur more frequently in early stages and include both sensorineural and conductive hearing loss, otitis media with effusion, and chronic suppurative otitis media [25, 26, 66]. According to two recently published papers, sensorineural and conductive deficit has been detected in 12–14% and 12–17% of subjects, respectively [67, 68]. The latter is mainly caused by effusion in the middle ear or chronic suppurative inflammation [67, 68].

Vestibular impairment is a sporadic finding: BPPV is observed in 9% of EGPA patients, and unspecified dizziness in 11.8% [68].

As far as otologic pathogenesis is concerned, ear involvement has been correlated to vasculitic involvement of middle ear mucosa rather than as a consequence of extended nasal disease [67, 68].

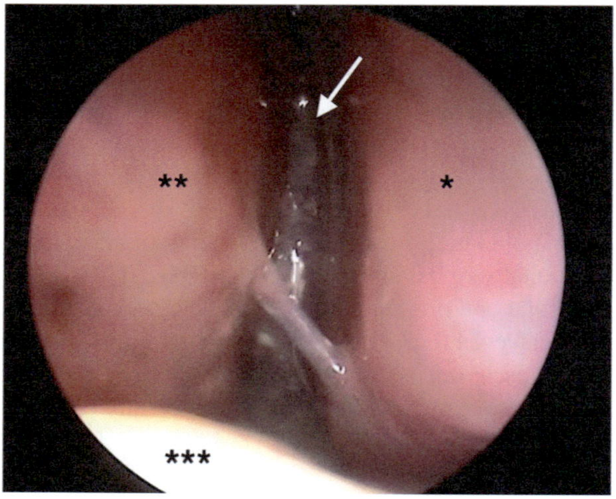

Fig. 9.2 Chronic rhinosinusitis with nasal polyposis extending beyond middle meatus and completely obstructing left nasal cavity in an EGPA patient. * inferior turbinate; ** nasal septum with cartilaginous spur; *** floor of the nasal cavity

9.5 Cocaine-Induced Midline Destructive Lesion (CIMDL)

Long-lasting nasal obstruction, epistaxis, and moderate-to-severe facial pain are the most common symptoms referred by CIMDL patients. Endoscopic examination frequently reveals diffuse necrotizing ulcerative lesions, extensive crusting, and septal perforation (Fig. 9.3a) [31]. More severe cases are characterized by broader osteocartilagineous destruction (e.g., "saddle-nose" deformity), which extends to the lateral wall of the nose (i.e., middle and superior turbinates), to the orbit (producing proptosis and diplopia), and to the hard and soft palate (causing dysphagia and disturbing nasal reflux). Recurrent superimposed bacterial infections are also typical, triggering distressing cacosmia (Fig. 9.3b) [31].

Systemic symptoms (e.g., malaise, fever, weight loss, arthralgia) are usually absent at presentation [29]. Concurrent enlargement of palatine and pharyngeal tonsils is a common finding, as well as signs of otitis media (with effusion), which is a direct consequence of prolonged nasal involvement [29, 31].

Secondary acquired NLDO is also noticeable in cocaine abusers, with epiphora and recurrent dacryocystitis as leading manifestations [69]. Widespread intranasal destruction is commonly found in these patients, with loss of the head of the inferior turbinate and consequent exposure of the nasal valve of the nasolacrimal duct to snorted cocaine effects [70]. Even orbital cellulitis is potentially detectable [70].

A few recent papers have even described sudden hearing loss following cocaine abuse, which is frequently unilateral [71, 72] and possibly related to decreased cochlear blood flow [73] or, on the contralateral side, to direct action of the drug on hair cells, since cocaine has been demonstrated to be a fast K^+-channel blocker [74].

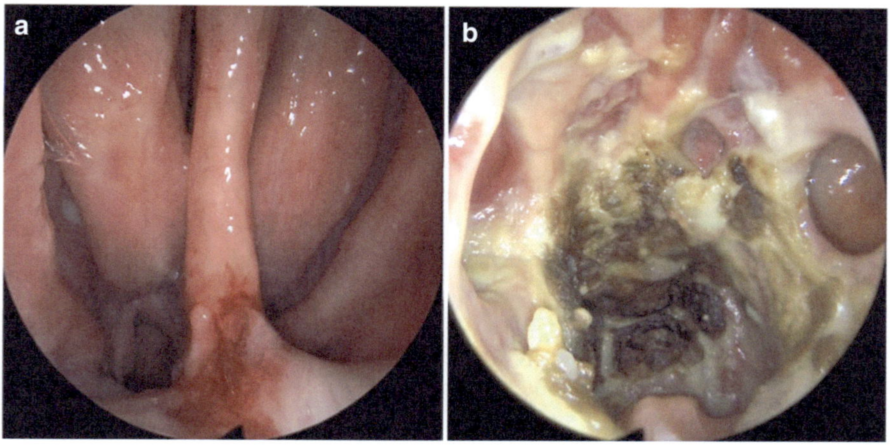

Fig. 9.3 Cocaine-induced septal perforation (**a**) and more severe endonasal osteocartilagineous destruction with superimposed ulcerative lesions and crusting (**b**)

Table 9.2 Differential diagnosis in head and neck midline granulomatous lesions (in bold the most common etiologies)

Infection	Inflammation	Neoplasm
Bacterial	**GPA**	**NK-T cell lymphoma**
Tuberculosis	**EGPA**	**Squamous cell carcinoma**
Leprosy	MPA	Rhabdomyosarcoma
Tertiary syphilis	**Sarcoidosis**	Adenoid cystic carcinoma
Rhinoscleroma	**CIMDL**	Basal cell carcinoma
Actinomicosis	Eosinophilic granulomatosis	Esthesioneuroblastoma
Fungal	Inflammatory bowel disease	Lymphomatoid granulomatosis
Aspergillosis	Relapsing polychondritis	Necrotizing sialometaplasia
Zygomycosis	Behcet's disease	
Dermatacietes	Systemic lupus erythematosus	
Rhinosporidiosis	Mixed connective tissue disease	
Blastomycosis	Giant cell granuloma	
Histoplasmosis	Post-surgical	
Sporotrichosis	Toxic agents	
Coccidioidomycosis		
Protozoal		
Leishmaniasis		
Brachycera		

Proper diagnosis of CIMDL is based upon clinical history, documentation of drug abuse, and exclusion of other potential etiologies (Table 9.2) [30]. Although multiple biopsy specimens and samples are very useful to rule out infections (e.g., tuberculosis, tertiary syphilis, leishmaniasis, mucormycosis), neoplasms (e.g., lymphoproliferative disorders, squamous cell carcinoma), and many inflammatory conditions (e.g., sarcoidosis), it may not be adequate to differentiate CIMDL from a sinonasal limited form of GPA, especially in the absence of extravascular changes such as stromal granulomas with giant cells, microabscesses, and deeply located necrosis [31, 32]. A high apoptotic cell index determined by a commercially available in situ terminal deoxynucleotidyl transferase-mediated dUTP-dygoxygenin nick end labeling (TUNEL) cell death detection kit on tissue specimens may be helpful for distinguishing CIMDL from nasal GPA on individual basis [75].

Serologic differentiation between these two conditions is sometimes easier: given that almost all CIMDL patients have circulating ANCAs, these antibodies primarily target human neutrophil elastase (HNE), producing a p-ANCA staining pattern, without reacting against myeloperoxidase (MPO) [76]. Instead, GPA patients most often show c-ANCA staining pattern addressing proteinase 3 (PR3) and more rarely MPO-targeting p-ANCA one or even ANCA-negative serology [77]. In any case, in CIMDL, the immune response is generally directed against multiple antigens at the same time, while in GPA patients toward a single one [77].

Moreover, downward evolution of nasal granulomatous destructive lesions (e.g., osteonecrosis of the hard and/or soft palate, oro-antral fistula) is a clinical finding that favors a diagnosis of CIMDL over localized GPA (Fig. 9.4) [55].

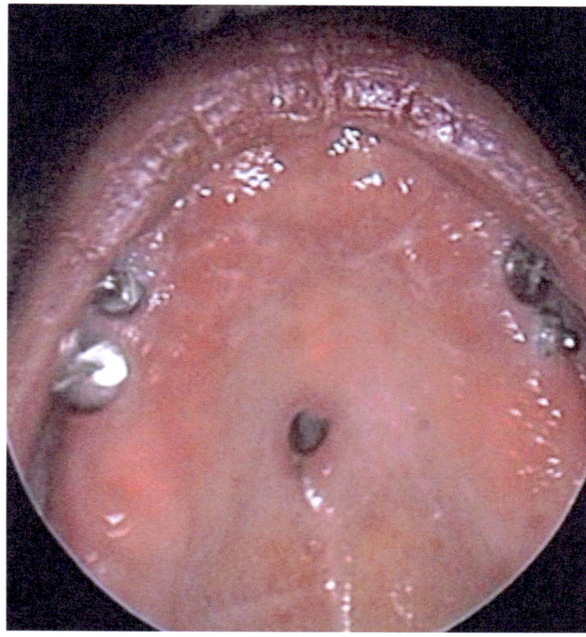

Fig. 9.4 Midline oro-nasal fistula resulting from downward evolution of cocaine-induced endonasal granulomatous destructive lesion

9.6 Conclusion

As detailed herein, head and neck involvement in the course of AAV is a quite frequent finding, and not uncommonly a first and stand-alone sign of active disease. This is particularly true for GPA and EGPA, especially in limited forms of disease: this renders the otorhinolaryngologist a key figure in the multidisciplinary team approaching these conditions, mainly in the diagnostic phase. Correlation with other concurrent clinical symptoms and biochemical findings, when present, is essential to rule out a potentially misleading diagnosis. In particular, discrimination between CIMDL and sinonasal localized GPA is often challenging, owing to their large similarity and the reluctance of patients in admitting cocaine addiction: this must always be kept in mind in diagnostic algorithms.

References

1. Jennette JC, Falk RJ, Hu P, Xiao H. Pathogenesis of antineutrophil cytoplasmic autoantibody-associated small-vessel vasculitis. Annu Rev Pathol. 2013;8:139–60.
2. Berden A, Goceroglu A, Jayne D, et al. Diagnosis and management of ANCA associated vasculitis. BMJ. 2012;344:e26.
3. Jennette JC, Falk RJ, Bacon PA, et al. 2012 revised international Chapel Hill consensus conference nomenclature of Vasculitides. Arthritis Rheum. 2013;65(1):1–11.

4. Fujimoto S, Watts RA, Kobayashi S, et al. Comparison of the epidemiology of anti-neutrophil cytoplasmic antibody-associated vasculitis between Japan and the U.K. Rheumatology (Oxford). 2011;50(10):1916–20.
5. Hellmich B, Flossmann O, Gross WL, et al. EULAR recommendations for conducting clinical studies and/or clinical trials in systemic vasculitis: focus on anti-neutrophil cytoplasm antibody-associated vasculitis. Ann Rheum Dis. 2007;66(5):605–17.
6. Hoffman GS, Langford CA. Are there different forms of life in the antineutrophil cytoplasmic antibody universe? Ann Intern Med. 2005;143(9):683–5.
7. Jennette JC, Falk RJ. Small-vessel vasculitis. N Engl J Med. 1997;337(21):1512–23.
8. Chung SA, Seo P. Microscopic polyangiitis. Rheum Dis Clin N Am. 2010;36(3):545–58.
9. Greco A, De Virgilio A, Rizzo MI, et al. Microscopic polyangiitis: advances in diagnostic and therapeutic approaches. Autoimmun Rev. 2015;14(9):837–44.
10. Guillevin L, Durand-Gasselin B, Cevallos R, et al. Microscopic polyangiitis: clinical and laboratory findings in eighty-five patients. Arthritis Rheum. 1999;42(3):421–30.
11. Savage CO, Winearls CG, Evans DJ, Rees AJ, Lockwood CM. Microscopic polyarteritis: presentation, pathology and prognosis. Q J Med. 1985;56(220):467–83.
12. Adu D, Howie AJ, Scott DG, Bacon PA, McGonigle RJ, Micheal J. Polyarteritis and the kidney. Q J Med. 1987;62(239):221–37.
13. Serra A, Cameron JS, Turner DR, et al. Vasculitis affecting the kidney: presentation, histopathology and long-term outcome. Q J Med. 1984;53(210):181–207.
14. Veldman J. Immune-mediated sensorineural hearing loss. Auris Nasus Larynx. 1998;25(3):309–17.
15. Falk RJ, Gross WL, Guillevin L, et al. Granulomatosis with polyangiitis (Wegener's): an alternative name for Wegener's granulomatosis. Arthritis Rheum. 2011;63(4):863–4.
16. Mark EJ, Matsubara O, Tan-Liu NS, Fienberg R. The pulmonary biopsy in the early diagnosis of Wegener's (pathergic) granulomatosis: a study based on 35 open lung biopsies. Hum Pathol. 1988;19(9):1065–71.
17. Kornblut AD, Wolff SM, deFries HO, Fauci AS. Wegener's granulomatosis. Laryngoscope. 1980;90(9):1453–65.
18. Trimarchi M, Sinico RA, Teggi R, Bussi M, Specks U, Meroni PL. Otorhinolaryngological manifestations in granulomatosis with polyangiitis (Wegener's). Autoimmun Rev. 2013;12(4):501–5.
19. Hartl DM, Aidan P, Brugiere O, Sterkers O. Wegener's granulomatosis presenting as a recurrence of chronic otitis media. Am J Otolaryngol. 1998;19(1):54–60.
20. Sinico RA, Di Toma L, Maggiore U, et al. Renal involvement in Churg-Strauss syndrome. Am J Kidney Dis. 2006;47(5):770–9.
21. Takagi D, Nakamaru Y, Maguchi S, Furuta Y, Fukuda S. Otologic manifestations of Wegener's granulomatosis. Laryngoscope. 2002;112(9):1684–90.
22. Gubbels SP, Barkhuizen A, Hwang PH. Head and neck manifestations of Wegener's granulomatosis. Otolaryngol Clin N Am. 2003;36(4):685–705.
23. Sinico RA, Di Toma L, Maggiore U, et al. Prevalence and clinical significance of antineutrophil cytoplasmic antibodies in Churg-Strauss syndrome. Arthritis Rheum. 2005;52(9):2926–35.
24. Sable-Fourtassou R, Cohen P, Mahr A, et al. Antineutrophil cytoplasmic antibodies and the Churg-Strauss syndrome. Ann Intern Med. 2005;143(9):632–8.
25. Baldini C, Talarico R, Della Rossa A, Bombardieri S. Clinical manifestations and treatment of Churg-Strauss syndrome. Rheum Dis Clin N Am. 2010;36(3):527–43.
26. Papadimitraki ED, Kyrmizakis DE, Kritikos I, Boumpas DT. Ear-nose-throat manifestations of autoimmune rheumatic diseases. Clin Exp Rheumatol. 2004;22(4):485–94.
27. Mahr A, Guillevin L, Poissonnet M, Ayme S. Prevalences of polyarteritis nodosa, microscopic polyangiitis, Wegener's granulomatosis, and Churg-Strauss syndrome in a French urban multiethnic population in 2000: a capture-recapture estimate. Arthritis Rheum. 2004;51(1):92–9.

28. Sinico RA, Bottero P. Churg-Strauss angiitis. Best Pract Res Clin Rheumatol. 2009;23(3):355–66.
29. Trimarchi M, Bussi M, Sinico RA, Meroni P, Specks U. Cocaine-induced midline destructive lesions - an autoimmune disease? Autoimmun Rev. 2013;12(4):496–500.
30. Seyer BA, Grist W, Muller S. Aggressive destructive midfacial lesion from cocaine abuse. Oral Surg Oral Med Oral Pathol Oral Radiol Endod. 2002;94(4):465–70.
31. Trimarchi M, Gregorini G, Facchetti F, et al. Cocaine-induced midline destructive lesions: clinical, radiographic, histopathologic, and serologic features and their differentiation from Wegener granulomatosis. Medicine (Baltimore). 2001;80(6):391–404.
32. Trimarchi M, Nicolai P, Lombardi D, et al. Sinonasal osteocartilaginous necrosis in cocaine abusers: experience in 25 patients. Am J Rhinol. 2003;17(1):33–43.
33. Metaxaris G, Prokopakis EP, Karatzanis AD, et al. Otolaryngologic manifestations of small vessel vasculitis. Auris Nasus Larynx. 2002;29(4):353–6.
34. Greco A, Marinelli C, Fusconi M, et al. Clinic manifestations in granulomatosis with polyangiitis. Int J Immunopathol Pharmacol. 2016;29(2):151–9.
35. McDonald TJ, DeRemee RA. Wegener's granulomatosis. Laryngoscope. 1983;93(2):220–31.
36. Rasmussen N. Management of the ear, nose, and throat manifestations of Wegener granulomatosis: an otorhinolaryngologist's perspective. Curr Opin Rheumatol. 2001;13(1):3–11.
37. Wojciechowska J, Krajewski W, Krajewski P, Krecicki T. Granulomatosis with Polyangiitis in otolaryngologist practice: a review of current knowledge. Clin Exp Otorhinolaryngol. 2016;9(1):8–13.
38. Kwan AS, Rose GE. Lacrimal drainage surgery in Wegener's granulomatosis. Br J Ophthalmol. 2000;84(3):329–31.
39. Muhle C, Reinhold-Keller E, Richter C, et al. MRI of the nasal cavity, the paranasal sinuses and orbits in Wegener's granulomatosis. Eur Radiol. 1997;7(4):566–70.
40. Trimarchi M, Bozzolo E, Pilolli F, et al. Nasal mucosa narrow band imaging in granulomatosis with polyangiitis (Wegener granulomatosis): a preliminary study. Am J Rhinol Allergy. 2015;29(3):170–4.
41. Langford CA, Hoffman GS. Rare diseases.3: Wegener's granulomatosis. Thorax. 1999;54(7):629–37.
42. Nicklasson B, Stangeland N. Wegener's granulomatosis presenting as otitis media. J Laryngol Otol. 1982;96(3):277–80.
43. Illum P, Thorling K. Otological manifestations of Wegener's granulomatosis. Laryngoscope. 1982;92(7 Pt 1):801–4.
44. Moussa AE, Abou-Elhmd KA. Wegener's granulomatosis presenting as mastoiditis. Ann Otol Rhinol Laryngol. 1998;107(7):560–3.
45. Wierzbicka M, Szyfter W, Puszczewicz M, Borucki L, Bartochowska A. Otologic symptoms as initial manifestation of wegener granulomatosis: diagnostic dilemma. Otol Neurotol. 2011;32(6):996–1000.
46. Holle JU, Gross WL. Neurological involvement in Wegener's granulomatosis. Curr Opin Rheumatol. 2011;23(1):7–11.
47. Teszler CB, Williams MT, Belange G, Ayache D. Labyrinthitis related to Wegener granulomatosis: magnetic resonance imaging findings. Otol Neurotol. 2008;29(5):721–2.
48. Dagum P, Roberson JB Jr. Otologic Wegener's granulomatosis with facial nerve palsy. Ann Otol Rhinol Laryngol. 1998;107(7):555–9.
49. Fenton JE, O'Sullivan TJ. The otological manifestations of Wegener's granulomatosis. J Laryngol Otol. 1994;108(2):144–6.
50. Kobari Y, Nagasawa T. Otitis media with ANCA-associated vasculitis: a new concept and the associated criteria. Intern Med. 2017;56(24):3365–7.
51. Fauci AS, Haynes BF, Katz P, Wolff SM. Wegener's granulomatosis: prospective clinical and therapeutic experience with 85 patients for 21 years. Ann Intern Med. 1983;98(1):76–85.

52. Knecht K, Mishriki YY. More than a mouth ulcer. Oral ulcer due to Wegener's granulomatosis. Postgrad Med. 1999;105(5):200, 3.
53. Patten SF, Tomecki KJ. Wegener's granulomatosis: cutaneous and oral mucosal disease. J Am Acad Dermatol. 1993;28(5. Pt 1):710–8.
54. Knight JM, Hayduk MJ, Summerlin DJ, Mirowski GW. "Strawberry" gingival hyperplasia: a pathognomonic mucocutaneous finding in Wegener granulomatosis. Arch Dermatol. 2000;136(2):171–3.
55. Trimarchi M, Bondi S, Della Torre E, Terreni MR, Bussi M. Palate perforation differentiates cocaine-induced midline destructive lesions from granulomatosis with polyangiitis. Acta Otorhinolaryngol Ital. 2017;37(4):281–5.
56. Specks U, Colby TV, Olsen KD, DeRemee RA. Salivary gland involvement in Wegener's granulomatosis. Arch Otolaryngol Head Neck Surg. 1991;117(2):218–23.
57. Ah-See KW, McLaren K, Maran AG. Wegener's granulomatosis presenting as major salivary gland enlargement. J Laryngol Otol. 1996;110(7):691–3.
58. Daum TE, Specks U, Colby TV, et al. Tracheobronchial involvement in Wegener's granulomatosis. Am J Respir Crit Care Med. 1995;151(2 Pt 1):522–6.
59. Gluth MB, Shinners PA, Kasperbauer JL. Subglottic stenosis associated with Wegener's granulomatosis. Laryngoscope. 2003;113(8):1304–7.
60. Hoffman GS, Thomas-Golbanov CK, Chan J, Akst LM, Eliachar I. Treatment of subglottic stenosis, due to Wegener's granulomatosis, with intralesional corticosteroids and dilation. J Rheumatol. 2003;30(5):1017–21.
61. Cordier JF, Valeyre D, Guillevin L, Loire R, Brechot JM. Pulmonary Wegener's granulomatosis. A clinical and imaging study of 77 cases. Chest. 1990;97(4):906–12.
62. Lebovics RS, Hoffman GS, Leavitt RY, et al. The management of subglottic stenosis in patients with Wegener's granulomatosis. Laryngoscope. 1992;102(12 Pt 1):1341–5.
63. McDonald TJ, Neel HB 3rd, DeRemee RA. Wegener's granulomatosis of the subglottis and the upper portion of the trachea. Ann Otol Rhinol Laryngol. 1982;91(6 Pt 1):588–92.
64. Utzig MJ, Warzelhan J, Wertzel H, Berwanger I, Hasse J. Role of thoracic surgery and interventional bronchoscopy in Wegener's granulomatosis. Ann Thorac Surg. 2002;74(6):1948–52.
65. Haynes BF, Fishman ML, Fauci AS, Wolff SM. The ocular manifestations of Wegener's granulomatosis. Fifteen years experience and review of the literature. Am J Med. 1977;63(1):131–41.
66. Greco A, Rizzo MI, De Virgilio A, et al. Churg-Strauss syndrome. Autoimmun Rev. 2015;14(4):341–8.
67. Nakamaru Y, Takagi D, Suzuki M, et al. Otologic and Rhinologic manifestations of eosinophilic granulomatosis with polyangiitis. Audiol Neurootol. 2016;21(1):45–53.
68. Seccia V, Fortunato S, Cristofani-Mencacci L, et al. Focus on audiologic impairment in eosinophilic granulomatosis with polyangiitis. Laryngoscope. 2016;126(12):2792–7.
69. Allard FD, Yee EU, Freitag SK. Dacryocystitis secondary to intranasal cocaine abuse: a case report and literature review. Orbit. 2013;32(6):405–8.
70. Alexandrakis G, Tse DT, Rosa RH Jr, Johnson TE. Nasolacrimal duct obstruction and orbital cellulitis associated with chronic intranasal cocaine abuse. Arch Ophthalmol. 1999;117(12):1617–22.
71. Iqbal N. Hearing loss in amphetamine users. J Psychoactive Drugs. 2002;34(4):401–7.
72. Ciorba A, Bovo R, Prosser S, Martini A. Considerations on the physiopathological mechanism of inner ear damage induced by intravenous cocaine abuse: cues from a case report. Auris Nasus Larynx. 2009;36(2):213–7.
73. Nicoucar K, Sakbani K, Vukanovic S, Guyot JP. Intralabyrinthine haemorrhage following cocaine consumption. Acta Otolaryngol. 2005;125(8):899–901.
74. Bauman JL, DiDomenico RJ. Cocaine-induced channelopathies: emerging evidence on the multiple mechanisms of sudden death. J Cardiovasc Pharmacol Ther. 2002;7(3):195–202.
75. Trimarchi M, Miluzio A, Nicolai P, Morassi ML, Bussi M, Marchisio PC. Massive apoptosis erodes nasal mucosa of cocaine abusers. Am J Rhinol. 2006;20(2):160–4.

76. Wiesner O, Russell KA, Lee AS, et al. Antineutrophil cytoplasmic antibodies reacting with human neutrophil elastase as a diagnostic marker for cocaine-induced midline destructive lesions but not autoimmune vasculitis. Arthritis Rheum. 2004;50(9):2954–65.
77. Peikert T, Finkielman JD, Hummel AM, et al. Functional characterization of antineutrophil cytoplasmic antibodies in patients with cocaine-induced midline destructive lesions. Arthritis Rheum. 2008;58(5):1546–51.

Lung Involvement in ANCA-Associated Vasculitis

10

Marta Casal Moura and Ulrich Specks

10.1 Introduction

This chapter focuses on the clinical presentation, diagnostic evaluation, and specific management issues associated with the various aspects of pulmonary parenchymal and tracheobronchial involvement of GPA and MPA. We emphasize the pulmonologist's perspective and refer to general treatment recommendations of GPA and MPA only briefly when necessary. Diagnosis and management of EGPA is covered elsewhere in this book.

10.2 Necrotizing Granulomatous Inflammation of the Lung

Disease manifestations caused by necrotizing granulomatous inflammation are the hallmark and disease-defining feature of GPA, setting GPA apart from MPA and EGPA [1]. In the lung, the pathognomonic histopathologic features of GPA include neutrophilic microabscesses, fibrinoid necrosis, palisading histiocytes, and giant cells forming a granulomatous inflammation pattern that is often called "geographic necrosis" [2]. Areas involved with this type of necrotizing granulomatous inflammation may encroach on vessel walls or contain focal vasculitis, thrombosis, and fibrous obliteration of vascular lumina. Other more non-specific histopathologic features have also been reported to occur rarely in GPA, including organizing pneumonia, bronchocentric inflammation, and occasionally prominent eosinophils in the inflammatory infiltrates [3, 4].

M. C. Moura · U. Specks (✉)
Thoracic Disease Research Unit, Division of Pulmonary and Critical Care Medicine, Mayo Clinic, Rochester, MN, USA
e-mail: CasalMoura.Marta@mayo.edu; specks.ulrich@mayo.edu

R. A. Sinico, L. Guillevin (eds.), *Anti-Neutrophil Cytoplasmic Antibody (ANCA) Associated Vasculitis*, Rare Diseases of the Immune System,
https://doi.org/10.1007/978-3-030-02239-6_10

Radiographic correlates of the necrotizing granulomatous inflammation are solitary or multiple pulmonary nodules or mass lesions with or without cavitation or non-specific pulmonary infiltrates that are radiographically indistinguishable from pneumonia (Fig. 10.1). A peribronchial distribution of the inflammatory lesions can often be seen by computed tomography (Fig. 10.1) [5]. Fibrotic changes are usually not a radiographic feature associated with GPA, but rather with MPO-ANCA associated MPA (see below).

The differential diagnosis of these lesions is broad, particularly when they are the only disease manifestations in a given patient [5]. Infections, including fungal infections, such as histoplasmosis, coccidioidomycosis and, to a lesser degree, blastomycosis are endemic in certain defined areas of the world. Nocardia infections can occur in immunocompetent patients and mimic the pulmonary presentation of GPA [6, 7]. Cryptogenic organizing pneumonia can be radiographically indistinguishable from GPA limited to the lung. This differentiation is further complicated by the fact that organizing pneumonia has been described as a rare histopathologic occurrence in GPA [4]. Malignancy, including metastatic disease and lymphoproliferative disorders, can cause multiple bilateral pulmonary nodules and therefore also needs to be considered in the differential diagnosis. Particularly, lymphomatoid granulomatosis, a rare angiocentric and angiodestructive, Epstein Barr virus-related T-cell-rich B-cell lymphoma can mimic GPA because, like GPA, it often affects different extra-pulmonary organs [8, 9].

Microbiologic studies and cytology performed on sputum samples or samples obtained during bronchoscopy procedures are usually helpful in the differential diagnostic evaluation. Transbronchial biopsies can provide tissue samples that are supportive of a diagnosis of GPA in about 50% of patients who have other supportive clinical features or ANCA [10]. Tissue samples obtained by transbronchoscopic biopsy are diagnostic by themselves in up to a quarter of patients [10]. A CT-guided

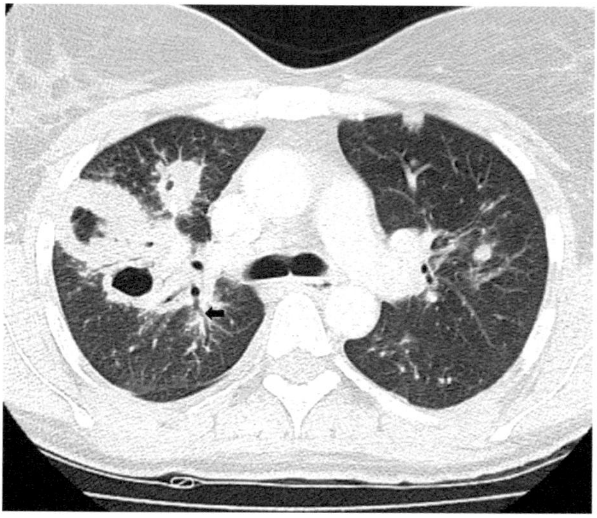

Fig. 10.1 Necrotizing granulomatous lung lesions of GPA. Typical computed tomography cut from a 67-year-old woman with GPA showing multiple bilateral nodules and cavitating mass lesions as well as peribronchial inflammation (black arrow)

core needle biopsy is preferred to transbronchial biopsies when the lesions are very peripheral. A video-assisted thoracoscopic lung biopsy has the highest diagnostic yield for GPA, but it is also associated with the highest morbidity and should therefore be used very judiciously.

The pulmonary parenchymal lesions caused by the necrotizing granulomatous inflammation may be asymptomatic, and they may not lead to measurable impairment of lung function. Consequently, they may be a serendipitous radiographic finding in newly diagnosed patients. For the same reason, any screening for disease activity during follow-up of patients with AAV must include chest imaging even if the patient does not endorse any respiratory symptoms.

Cough and minor hemoptysis are symptoms that may be associated with such lesions having access to subsegmental bronchi. The development of cavitation as a consequence of necrotizing granulomatous inflammation also signals involvement of a draining airway. Air-fluid levels within cavitary lesions are usually a sign of bacterial superinfection and should prompt a careful microbiologic evaluation and appropriate antibiotic therapy.

The disease manifestations caused by necrotizing granulomatous inflammation usually progress more slowly than capillaritis-related disease manifestations (see below), are not life-threatening, and they rarely cause irreversible lung damage. Therefore, patients who only have these disease manifestations are categorized for treatment stratification as having "non-severe" disease, implying that the combination of glucocorticoids with weekly methotrexate should be tried as first-line remission induction therapy [11]. Patients who fail this regimen usually respond well to the combination of glucocorticoids and rituximab [12, 13]. Sometimes, if the overall pulmonary disease burden is deemed extensive, treatment following the recommendations for "severe" disease using the combination of glucocorticoids with cyclophosphamide or rituximab may be appropriate [11]. Since most of the patients with such "severe" disease are PR3-ANCA-positive and have a very highly likelihood of relapse, management with rituximab from the get-go may be preferable.

10.3 Tracheobronchial Inflammation of GPA

In GPA, tracheobronchial involvement (Fig. 10.2) has been reported in 15–55% of cases, but it is usually not a feature of MPA [14]. Patients with tracheobronchial disease, including subglottic inflammation and subsequent stenosis, most commonly have PR3-ANCA, but may have MPO-ANCA or be ANCA-negative. The tracheobronchial inflammation is thought to be the result of necrotizing granulomatous inflammation, but confirmation by biopsy is rare. Therefore, we acknowledge that, whether tracheobronchial involvement is reported as a feature of GPA or MPA in cohort reports depends on the clinician's acceptance and application of different disease definitions and clinical surrogates of GPA-defining necrotizing granulomatous inflammation [15–17].

One characteristic feature of the tracheobronchial inflammation of GPA is its localized or patchy distribution throughout the airway with affected areas

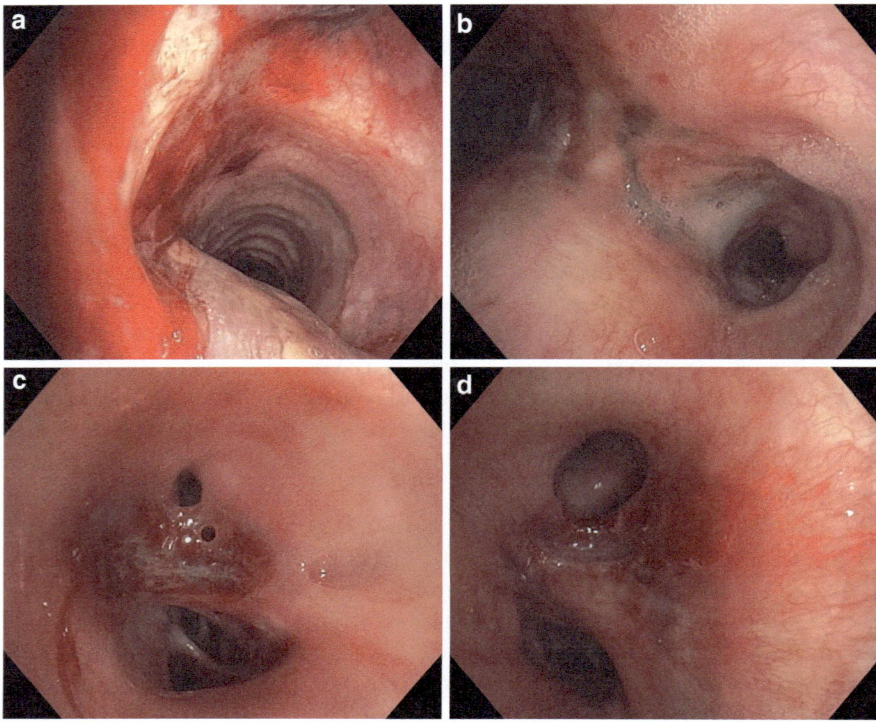

Fig. 10.2 Tracheobronchial involvement of GPA. (Panel **a**) Significant erythema and friable mucosa in the immediate subglottic region. (Panel **b**) Scarring of the main carina which is significantly broadened, but the entrance to the right main stem bronchus is widely patent. (Panel **c**) Anterior segment of the right lower lobe occluded by a web with two pin holes. The other segments appeared normal. (Panel **d**) The bronchoscopically introduced microknife was used to make a couple of cuts in the anterior segment of the right lower lobe leading to significant improvement of the lumen (**d**)

right next to entirely normal appearing airways. The subglottic region is most commonly involved, but airway inflammation may occur at any level of the tracheobronchial tree from the trachea down to the subsegmental airways. The inflammation of affected airways can consist of mucosal erythema, edematous swelling, friability, ulcerations, or so-called cobble-stoning. The inflammation is often circumferential. If it is transmural, it is detectable by CT imaging of the chest. If the cartilage of the airways is damaged by the inflammation, tracheo- or bronchomalacia with significant expiratory dynamic airway collapse may be the result. Alternatively, the acute inflammation as well as subsequent scarring occurring with immunosuppressive therapy can cause stenosis of the affected airway or complete occlusion.

The differential diagnosis of the tracheobronchial inflammation of GPA may be difficult in patients who do not have other typical organ manifestations of GPA or typical PR3- or MPO-ANCA. Relapsing polychondritis [18], inflammatory bowel disease [19, 20], and sarcoidosis [21] should be considered as alternative diagnoses in such patients, and infections, particularly with fungal organisms, should be ruled out.

Symptoms that can occur as the result of airway inflammation of GPA include cough, streaky hemoptysis, stridor, localized wheezes, and dyspnea. Early inflammatory lesions remain often undetected because they do not cause significant airway obstruction. The presence and degree of stridor, localized wheezes, or dyspnea depend on the localization and severity of large airway obstruction.

The diagnostic approach is determined by the degree of suspicion for the presence of airway inflammation as well as by the symptoms of the patient. Pulmonary function testing, bronchoscopic inspection of the airways, as well as three-dimensional reconstruction of computed tomography images are important components of the diagnostic evaluation [14]. Inspiratory and expiratory flow-volume tracings allow the detection of airway stenoses and an estimate of their functional severity. When assessing and following airway stenosis in patients with GPA, measurements of the maximum voluntary ventilation during pulmonary function testing or of the peak expiratory flow, using a peak flow meter, are very useful for determining the degree of airflow limitation. Serial pulmonary function testing during follow-up is helpful in assessing the effects of medical therapy or of bronchoscopic interventions on airway patency. Pulmonary function testing is indicated for any patient with GPA who has respiratory symptoms such cough, dyspnea, or hemoptysis. It should also be pursued in any patient who has radiographic abnormalities of the pulmonary parenchyma or the airways, regardless of the presence or absence of symptoms.

Bronchoscopic inspection of the airways is indicated for patients with respiratory symptoms, abnormalities on pulmonary function testing, or on chest imaging studies. Bronchoscopy is indispensable for (1) the assessment and mapping of inflammatory lesions in the tracheobronchial tree, (2) planning of any therapeutic interventions, (3) to obtain specimens for microbiologic studies, and (4) to assess the effect of therapy on the airways. The so-called "virtual bronchoscopy" or three-dimensional reconstruction of CT images of the airways plays a significant role in the planning of dilation procedures or stent placement as it is important to assess airway patency distal to tight stenosis that cannot accommodate a pediatric bronchoscope [22].

The treatment of tracheobronchial involvement of GPA often poses specific challenges. First, tracheobronchial inflammation may be more resistant to systemic immunosuppressive therapy compared to other disease manifestations. Second, symptoms of progressive airway obstruction may be the result of scarring or damage rather than of persistent inflammation, explaining their resistance to immunosuppressive therapy and calling for other interventions, such as dilation procedures or stent placements for airway stenosis or the application of continuous positive airway pressure (CPAP) treatment in patients with tracheo- or bronchomalacia. Third, localized persistent infections with organisms such as *Staphylococcus aureus* or *Pseudomonas aeruginosa* may be persistent "antigenic drivers" of the autoimmune inflammation unless addressed with appropriate antimicrobial therapy. For this reason, potential pathogens identified by bronchoscopic sampling of the airway secretions are treated based on antimicrobial susceptibility results in our practice. Finally, to suppress airway inflammation while minimizing cumulative systemic glucocorticoid exposure, we also advocate for the use of high-dose inhaled glucocorticoids in patients with tracheobronchial disease.

10.4 Pulmonary Capillaritis and Diffuse Alveolar Hemorrhage

GPA and MPA represent the most common causes of capillaritis of the lung leading to diffuse alveolar hemorrhage (DAH) [23] (Fig. 10.3). About a quarter of patients with GPA or MPA will present with or experience DAH during the course of their disease [13, 24]. By contrast, DAH occurs rarely (0–10%) in EGPA, where it seems to be linked to the presence of MPO-ANCA [25–27]. The clinical presentation of DAH is non-specific, consisting of various degrees of dyspnea, hypoxemia, diffuse alveolar filling defects detectable by chest imaging studies, and anemia. Cough may not be a prominent feature, and hemoptysis is absent as presenting feature in a third of patients with DAH [28, 29].

If suspected, DAH should be confirmed or ruled out. This is usually accomplished by bronchoscopy with bronchoalveolar lavage (BAL). At the same time, the BAL procedure offers the opportunity to collect specimens for detailed microbiologic studies

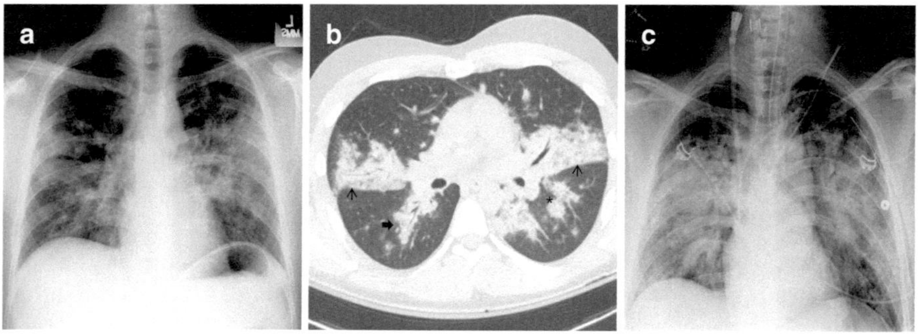

Fig. 10.3 Diffuse alveolar hemorrhage. (Panel **a**) Chest roentgenogram of a 20-year-old man with known GPA, PR3-ANCA-positive, presenting with cough, fever, malaise, and arthralgias, but without hemoptysis, to the emergency department on Day 1. Hemoglobin is 11.0 g/dL and oxygen saturation on room air is 94%. The patient is given antibiotics and dismissed for further outpatient evaluation the next day. (Panel **b**) Computed tomography is performed the next day (day 2) showing typical features of diffuse alveolar hemorrhage, including dense infiltrates and consolidation with air bronchograms, partially respecting lobar borders (thin arrows). Nodules (star) and peribronchial inflammation (bold arrow) are radiographic features that point toward GPA as underlying cause of the hemorrhage. The patient is admitted to the intensive care unit. (Panel **c**) Rapid progression of hemorrhage by day 3. Hemoglobin is now 8.0 g/dL, and the patient is intubated and receives mechanical ventilation. This patient also suffered bilateral pneumothoraces requiring placement of chest tubes. This case illustrates how quickly patients with diffuse alveolar hemorrhage can progress from a relatively indolent clinical presentation to respiratory failure requiring intensive care

for the identification or exclusion of an infection. If the bleeding originates with the alveolar space, successively returned BAL aliquots turn bloodier. In contrast, if the bleeding source is in the large airways, the first returned aliquot is the bloodiest, and subsequent aliquots of return become clearer. A negative BAL does not rule out that the diffuse alveolar filling defect on chest imaging is caused by DAH or capillaritis as the bleeding may have stopped by the time the BAL is performed. However, in that case, at least 20% of alveolar macrophages should stain positive for iron deposits, which is a well-accepted BAL criterion for alveolar hemorrhage [30]. However, this criterion is not entirely specific for DAH as up to a third of patients with diffuse alveolar damage may also have more than 20% hemosiderin-laden macrophages in their BAL fluid [31]. In very acute situations, iron-laden alveolar macrophages may not yet be detectable, as it is assumed to take a minimum of 24–48 h for the macrophages to engulf the hemoglobin and turn positive on iron stains; this is based on a study in mice in which hemosiderin was first detectable in alveolar macrophages on day 3 following intranasal blood instillation [32]. The percentage of hemosiderin-laden macrophages was not identified as a predictor of progression to respiratory failure in DAH caused by AAV, but the presence of greater than 30% neutrophils on the BAL differential cell count was an independent risk factor for development of respiratory failure, probably because it is an indirect marker for the severity of the interstitial inflammation [28]. Bronchoscopy and BAL should only be performed in clinical setting where the level of care can easily be escalated, as the procedure may result in temporary acute worsening of the patient's respiratory status requiring a higher level of respiratory support including intubation and mechanical ventilation.

The differential diagnosis of DAH related to AAV depends on when it occurs in the patient's disease course. If DAH is the first presentation of the disease, all other possible causes of DAH need to be considered until the diagnosis of AAV is substantiated. Once respiratory support is assured and adequate oxygenation has been secured, the first decision to make is whether and when to initiate therapy with high-dose glucocorticoids (usually in the form of 1–3 pulses of 500–1000 mg of intravenous methyl-prednisolone). This decision depends on whether an immunologic cause of the DAH is suspected or not. Any combination of the four factors, including the presence of (1) respiratory symptoms exceeding 11 days prior to presentation, (2) constitutional symptoms such as fatigue and/or weight loss, (3) arthralgias or arthritis, and (4) proteinuria of greater than 1 g per liter, has been identified as having a very high positive predictive value for an immunologic cause of DAH, which should prompt the institution of glucocorticoid therapy [33, 34].

The diagnosis of a specific immunologic cause of DAH including GPA, MPA, or EGPA can usually be established when the complete clinical context is considered in conjunction with specific serological testing for the specific autoimmune conditions that can cause alveolar hemorrhage. A lung biopsy is usually not necessary and is associated with a very unfavorable risk-to-benefit ratio. If tissue confirmation is needed for a diagnosis of GPA or MPA, it can usually be obtained in a safer manner from other organs such as skin, nose and sinuses, or kidneys. A kidney biopsy may also provide additional valuable prognostic information, which a lung biopsy cannot [35–37].

If DAH is suspected in an established patient with GPA or MPA because of the clinical presentation of dyspnea, hypoxemia, and radiographic alveolar filling defects, the differential diagnosis includes infection, particularly if the patient is being treated with immunosuppressive agents, drug toxicity, and other unrelated co-morbidities. Again, bronchoscopy with BAL is indicated in such patients.

DAH is a severe disease manifestation of GPA and MPA, which can rapidly progress to respiratory failure threatening the patient's life. Mortality rates reported in the largest most recent series range from about 10% to 25% [28, 38]. If patients survive the original episode of DAH, their response to treatment is similar to that of patients with all other disease manifestations of GPA and MPA in aggregate [13, 28]. In most cases, the lung parenchyma also recovers without significant loss in lung function [28, 39]. Early detection of DAH and prompt implementation of definitive therapy is the key to curb the early mortality associated with DAH caused by GPA or MPA.

A multivariate analysis conducted in a cohort of 73 patients with DAH caused by GPA or MPA has identified three risk factors portending a high likelihood of progression to respiratory failure requiring ventilatory support. They include an oxygen saturation measured by pulse oximetry (SpO_2) to fraction of inspired oxygen (FiO_2) ratio of <450 (OR 74, 95% CI 9–180) measured at the time of first presentation, a C-reactive protein level >25 mg/dL (OR 7.4, 95% CI 1.7–48), and the presence of >30% neutrophils on the differential cell count of the BAL fluid (OR 6.4, 95% CI 1.6–34) [28]. Consequently, the SpO_2:FiO_2 ratio should be determined in any patient with vasculitis presenting with dyspnea or with a pulmonary infiltrate even in the absence of dyspnea or hemoptysis, so that the appropriate level of care can be chosen for the implementation of further diagnostic and therapeutic interventions.

Patients with DAH caused by GPA or MPA respond well to standard therapy for severe disease manifestations. The response of patients with DAH to the application of 1–3 daily pulses of 1 g of intravenous methyl-prednisolone followed by oral prednisone in combination with either rituximab (RTX) or cyclophosphamide (CYC) was equivalent to that of the entire trial cohort in the RAVE trial [13]. An analysis of a large single-center cohort (n = 73) showed similar early response rates and hospital survival in patients treated with RTX or CYC. Complete remission, defined as a Birmingham Vasculitis Activity score of 0 and complete discontinuation of prednisone by 6 months, was superior in patients treated with RTX compared to those treated with CYC (89% versus 68%, $p = 0.02$), even in the subset of patients who required mechanical ventilation ($n = 31$, 83% with RTX versus 42% with CYC, $p = 0.02$), a group of patients that was excluded from enrollment into the RAVE trial [28].

The addition of plasma exchange (PLEX) to standard immunosuppressive therapy has been advocated to curb the early mortality associated with DAH in the setting of AAV based on a single report of 20 patients treated with PLEX and surviving the initial hospitalization [40]. However, a larger single-center cohort analysis of 73 patients, 32 of which were treated with PLEX, did not identify any benefit derived from PLEX after adjustment for the disease severity and treatment (RTX versus CYC) [28]. Results from a large multicenter randomized controlled trial comparing

PLEX to no PLEX in AAV also showed no benefit of PLEX in the subset of patients with DAH [41]. Consequently, the addition of PLEX to standard immunosuppressive therapy can no longer be advocated.

10.5 Interstitial Lung Disease and ANCA with or Without MPA

An association between fibrotic interstitial lung disease (ILD) and MPO-ANCA and MPA is increasingly recognized but remains poorly understood [42–44]. Case reports and case series from all over the world have documented interstitial lung disease in patients who are ANCA-positive. MPO-ANCA is the predominant ANCA type encountered in the context of interstitial lung disease. In contrast, PR3-ANCA occurs rarely. The patients with PR3-ANCA may or may not have abnormal markers of inflammation or typical signs of vasculitis (MPA) in other organs. Careful review and analysis of these reports indicate that in the majority of cases, the interstitial lung disease either has radiographic and histopathologic features of nonspecific interstitial pneumonitis (NSIP) (Fig. 10.4a, b) or of usual interstitial pneumonia (UIP) (Fig. 10.4c, d). However, atypical features including follicular bronchiolitis have also been reported. The available reports suggest the following common themes:

1. Patients who are MPO-ANCA-positive with ILD have a 25% chance of subsequently developing clinical features of MPA [45, 46]. This progression to MPA has been documented for MPO-ANCA, but has not been observed for PR3-ANCA [45].
2. The lung disease seems to precede the development of frank MPA. This is most clearly documented for lung fibrosis with radiographic patterns of UIP [43].
3. Patients who present with a radiographic pattern of NSIP show a response to immunosuppressive therapy of their ILD, whereas patients with UIP appear unresponsive to immunosuppressive therapy, and the lung continues to decline as expected for idiopathic pulmonary fibrosis.
4. Patients with overt manifestations of MPA, with or without alveolar hemorrhage superimposed on their ILD, show a clinical response to immunosuppressive therapy of the vasculitis disease manifestations as expected for MPA. If overt MPA is present, the ILD may respond to immunosuppressive therapy if the fibrosis has features of cellular NSIP. However, if the patient's lung fibrosis is of the UIP variety, no response to immunosuppression can be expected for the pulmonary fibrosis. It remains unclear, whether such patients with UIP would benefit from treatment with anti-fibrotic agents.

Based on these observations, pulmonologists at Mayo Clinic have adopted the empiric clinical management approach to patients with MPO-ANCA and ILD summarized in Table 10.1. This clinical approach assures that patients who have overt features of MPA receive appropriate therapy for severe disease manifestations of

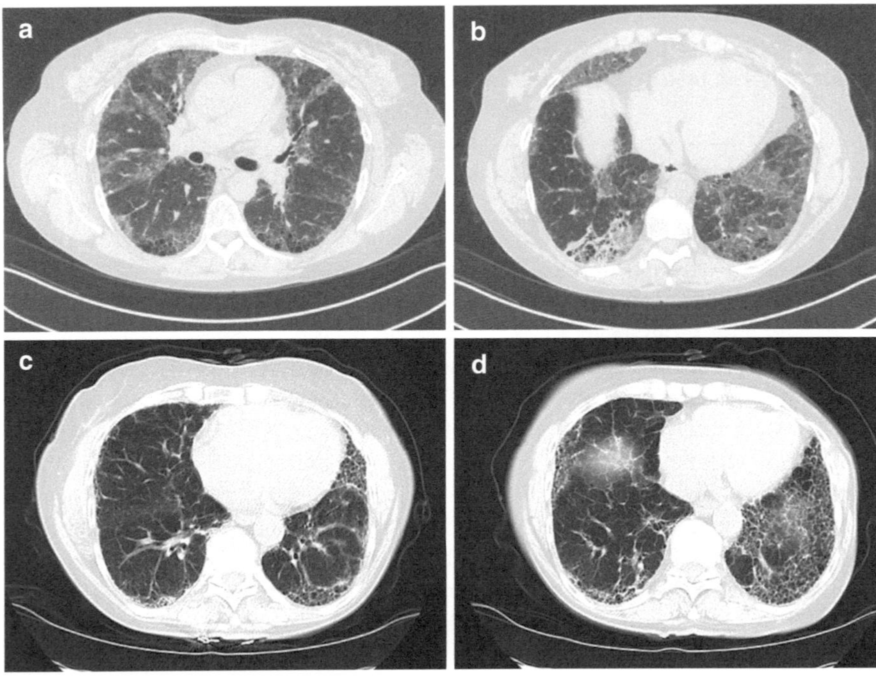

Fig. 10.4 Interstitial lung disease associated with MPO-ANCA. (Panel **a** and **b**) Chest computed tomography cuts from a 49-year-old patient with a 4-year history of MPO-ANCA-positive interstitial lung disease showing bilateral diffuse ground-glass infiltrates in the upper and lower lobes. Cystic scarring is also seen in the lower lobes posteriorly with some traction bronchiectases. These features are consistent with nonspecific interstitial pneumonitis. The cystic fibrotic lesions are too large to be called honeycombing. Two years following the diagnosis of interstitial lung disease, the patient developed mononeuritis multiplex and glomerulonephritis despite receiving low-dose prednisone and mycophenolate mofetil. (Panel **c** and **d**). Chest computed tomography cuts obtained from a 76-year-old lady who presented with cough and shortness of breath, an elevated sedimentation rate and C-reactive protein, and a positive MPO-ANCA test result, but without any other organ symptomatology. The images show fibrotic changes, including honeycombing and traction bronchiectases with a lower lung predominance and peripheral distribution and complete absence of ground-glass infiltrates; these features are typical for usual interstitial pneumonia (UIP). Review of old chest X-rays revealed the presence of fibrotic changes in the lower lungs dating back 4 years. She never developed any signs or symptoms of MPA, and died 5 years later of an "acute exacerbation of IPF"

ANCA vasculitis in the form of remission induction therapy with glucocorticoids and cyclophosphamide or rituximab following the principles and guidelines of therapy for AAV [11].

Also, patients who present with an NSIP pattern will receive a trial of immunosuppressive therapy, even if no other organ disease manifestations of MPA are apparent. Since this immunosuppressive therapy is generally regarded as effective remission maintenance therapy for AAV, it may prevent the development of overt MPA in other organs while also preventing progression of the lung disease to irreversible fibrosis.

Table 10.1 Management of patients with MPO-ANCA and interstitial lung disease

Fibrosis pattern	Elevated markers of inflammation (ESR, DAH)	Extrapulmonary signs of vasculitis or DAH	Management
UIP	No	No	Observe and monitor for microhematuria[b]
UIP	Yes	No	Observe and monitor for microhematuria[a]
UIP	Yes	Yes	Treat for MPA[a,b]
NSIP	No	No	GCS plus MMF or AZA
NSIP	Yes	No	GCS plus MMF or AZA
NSIP	Yes	Yes	Treat for MPA[a]

[a]Standard immunosuppressive therapy following standard guidelines for MPA
[b]Consider anti-fibrotic therapy for UIP following guidelines for idiopathic pulmonary fibrosis
AZA azathioprine, *CRP* C-reactive protein, *DAH* diffuse alveolar hemorrhage, *ESR* erythrocyte sedimentation rate, *GCS* glucocorticoids, *MPA* microscopic poliangiitis, *MMF* mycophenolate mofetil, *NSIP* non-specific interstitial pneumonia, *UIP* usual interstitial pneumonia

At this point, we have not seen any beneficial effect of lung fibrosis of the UIP pattern in patients with MPO-ANCA, with or without features of MPA. Therefore, we do not believe that immunosuppressive therapy is beneficial or indicated in such patients in the absence of other overt features of MPA. However, since a sizable proportion of such patients will develop MPA later, and the development of renal disease can be slow and indolent, yet lead to irreversible renal insufficiency, we monitor patients for the development of glomerulonephritis by screening the urine for microhematuria at least on a monthly basis. This way, the development of glomerulonephritis is detected early, and effective therapy can be initiated before severe renal damage occurs. At the same time, such patients with UIP are not exposed to immunosuppressive therapy that could even be detrimental as shown in a randomized controlled trial of idiopathic pulmonary fibrosis [47]. As the UIP seems to precede disease manifestations of MPA in most patients, we do not consider the lung fibrosis a priori a disease manifestation of MPA, but rather a pre-existing comorbidity, and anti-fibrotic therapy may be an appropriate option for such patients with UIP.

10.6 Conclusion

Pulmonary parenchymal or tracheobronchial involvement is common in ANCA-associated vasculitis. The clinical presentation and symptoms including the severity of the disease depend on the underlying type of inflammation, on the affected tissue compartments, and on the ANCA-type and the clinical syndrome in which they occur. A conceptual separation into four main categories, including, (1) pulmonary parenchymal disease manifestations caused by the necrotizing granulomatous inflammation of GPA, (2) tracheobronchial inflammation often leading to airway compromise in the context of GPA, (3) diffuse alveolar hemorrhage as an acute and severe disease manifestation caused by capillaritis in GPA or MPA, and (4) an association of interstitial lung disease and fibrosis with MPO-ANCA and MPA, is practical for clinicians, as such a categorization allows a systematic differential diagnostic approach and therapy that is appropriately targeted to individual patients.

References

1. Jennette JC, Falk RJ, Bacon PA, et al. 2012 revised International Chapel Hill Consensus Conference Nomenclature of Vasculitides. Arthritis Rheum. 2013;65(1):1–11.
2. Colby TV, Specks U. Wegener's granulomatosis in the 1990s--a pulmonary pathologist's perspective. Monogr Pathol. 1993;36:195–218.
3. Travis WD, Hoffman GS, Leavitt RY, Pass HI, Fauci AS. Surgical pathology of the lung in Wegener's granulomatosis. Review of 87 open lung biopsies from 67 patients. Am J Surg Pathol. 1991;15(4):315–33.
4. Travis WD. Common and uncommon manifestations of Wegener's granulomatosis. Cardiovasc Pathol. 1994;3(3):217–25.
5. Martinez F, Chung JH, Digumarthy SR, et al. Common and uncommon manifestations of Wegener granulomatosis at chest CT: radiologic-pathologic correlation. Radiographics. 2012;32(1):51–69.
6. Gibb W, Williams A. Nocardiosis mimicking Wegener's granulomatosis. Scand J Infect Dis. 1986;18(6):583–5.
7. Singh A, Chhina D, Soni RK, Kakkar C, Sidhu US. Clinical spectrum and outcome of pulmonary nocardiosis: 5-year experience. Lung India. 2016;33(4):398–403.
8. Wechsler RJ, Steiner RM, Israel HL, Patchefsky AS. Chest radiograph in lymphomatoid granulomatosis: comparison with Wegener granulomatosis. AJR Am J Roentgenol. 1984;142(1):79–83.
9. Roschewski M, Wilson WH. Lymphomatoid granulomatosis. Cancer J. 2012;18(5):469–74.
10. Daum TE, Specks U, Colby TV, et al. Tracheobronchial involvement in Wegener's granulomatosis. Am J Respir Crit Care Med. 1995;151(2 Pt 1):522–6.
11. Yates M, Watts R, Bajema I, et al. Validation of the EULAR/ERA-EDTA recommendations for the management of ANCA-associated vasculitis by disease content experts. RMD Open. 2017;3(1):e000449.
12. Seo P, Specks U, Keogh KA. Efficacy of rituximab in limited Wegener's granulomatosis with refractory granulomatous manifestations. J Rheumatol. 2008;35(10):2017–23.
13. Stone JH, Merkel PA, Spiera R, et al. Rituximab versus cyclophosphamide for ANCA-associated vasculitis. N Engl J Med. 2010;363(3):221–32.
14. Polychronopoulos VS, Prakash UB, Golbin JM, Edell ES, Specks U. Airway involvement in Wegener's granulomatosis. Rheum Dis Clin North Am. 2007;33(4):755–75. vi.
15. Jennette JC, Falk RJ, Andrassy K, et al. Nomenclature of systemic vasculitides. Proposal of an international consensus conference. Arthritis Rheum. 1994;37(2):187–92.
16. Watts R, Lane S, Hanslik T, et al. Development and validation of a consensus methodology for the classification of the ANCA-associated vasculitides and polyarteritis nodosa for epidemiological studies. Ann Rheum Dis. 2007;66(2):222–7.
17. Lionaki S, Blyth ER, Hogan SL, et al. Classification of antineutrophil cytoplasmic autoantibody vasculitides: the role of antineutrophil cytoplasmic autoantibody specificity for myeloperoxidase or proteinase 3 in disease recognition and prognosis. Arthritis Rheum. 2012;64(10):3452–62.
18. Ernst A, Rafeq S, Boiselle P, et al. Relapsing polychondritis and airway involvement. Chest. 2009;135(4):1024–30.
19. Chiu K, Wright JL. Large and small airway disease related to inflammatory bowel disease. Arch Pathol Lab Med. 2017;141(3):470–3.

20. Camus P, Colby TV. The lung in inflammatory bowel disease. Eur Respir J. 2000;15(1):5–10.
21. Polychronopoulos VS, Prakash UBS. Airway involvement in sarcoidosis. Chest. 2009;136(5):1371–80.
22. Summers RM, Aggarwal NR, Sneller MC, et al. CT virtual bronchoscopy of the central airways in patients with Wegener's granulomatosis. Chest. 2002;121(1):242–50.
23. Niles JL, Böttinger EP, Saurina GR, et al. The syndrome of lung hemorrhage and nephritis is usually an ANCA-associated condition. Arch Intern Med. 1996;156(4):440–5.
24. Hoffman GS, Kerr GS, Leavitt RY, et al. Wegener granulomatosis: an analysis of 158 patients. Ann Intern Med. 1992;116(6):488–98.
25. Keogh KA, Specks U. Churg-Strauss syndrome: clinical presentation, antineutrophil cytoplasmic antibodies, and leukotriene receptor antagonists. Am J Med. 2003;115(4):284–90.
26. Sinico RA, Di Toma L, Maggiore U, et al. Prevalence and clinical significance of antineutrophil cytoplasmic antibodies in Churg-Strauss syndrome. Arthritis Rheum. 2005;52(9):2926–35.
27. Comarmond C, Pagnoux C, Khellaf M, et al. Eosinophilic granulomatosis with polyangiitis (Churg-Strauss): clinical characteristics and long-term followup of the 383 patients enrolled in the French Vasculitis Study Group cohort. Arthritis Rheum. 2013;65(1):270–81.
28. Cartin-Ceba R, Diaz-Caballero L, Al-Qadi MO, et al. Diffuse alveolar hemorrhage secondary to antineutrophil cytoplasmic antibody-associated vasculitis: predictors of respiratory failure and clinical outcomes. Arthritis Rheumatol. 2016;68(6):1467–76.
29. Lara AR, Schwarz MI. Diffuse alveolar hemorrhage. Chest. 2010;137(5):1164–71.
30. De Lassence A, Fleury-Feith J, Escudier E, Beaune J, Bernaudin JF, Cordonnier C. Alveolar hemorrhage. Diagnostic criteria and results in 194 immunocompromised hosts. Am J Respir Crit Care Med. 1995;151(1):157–63.
31. Maldonado F, Parambil JG, Yi ES, Decker PA, Ryu JH. Haemosiderin-laden macrophages in the bronchoalveolar lavage fluid of patients with diffuse alveolar damage. Eur Respir J. 2009;33(6):1361–6.
32. Epstein CE, Elidemir O, Colasurdo GN, Fan LL. Time course of hemosiderin production by alveolar macrophages in a murine model. Chest. 2001;120(6):2013–20.
33. de Prost N, Parrot A, Cuquemelle E, Picard C, Cadranel J. Immune diffuse alveolar hemorrhage: a retrospective assessment of a diagnostic scale. Lung. 2013;191(5):559–63.
34. Picard C, Cadranel J, Porcher R, et al. Alveolar haemorrhage in the immunocompetent host: a scale for early diagnosis of an immune cause. Respiration. 2010;80(4):313–20.
35. Berden AE, Ferrario F, Hagen EC, et al. Histopathologic classification of ANCA-associated glomerulonephritis. J Am Soc Nephrol. 2010;21(10):1628–36.
36. Berti, A., Cornec-Le Gall E, Cornec D, et al., Incidence, prevalence, mortality and chronic renal damage of anti-neutrophil cytoplasmic antibody-associated glomerulonephritis in a 20-year population-based cohort. Nephrol Dial Transplant. 2018.
37. Sethi S, VD D'A, Nast CC, et al. A proposal for standardized grading of chronic changes in native kidney biopsy specimens. Kidney Int. 2017;91(4):787–9.
38. de Prost N, Parrot A, Picard C, et al. Diffuse alveolar haemorrhage: factors associated with in-hospital and long-term mortality. Eur Respir J. 2010;35(6):1303–11.
39. Lauque D, Cadranel J, Lazor R, et al. Microscopic polyangiitis with alveolar hemorrhage. A study of 29 cases and review of the literature. Groupe d'Etudes et de Recherche sur les Maladies "Orphelines" Pulmonaires (GERM"O"P). Medicine (Baltimore). 2000;79(4):222–33.
40. Klemmer PJ, Chalermskulrat W, Reif MS, Hogan SL, Henke DC, Falk RJ. Plasmapheresis therapy for diffuse alveolar hemorrhage in patients with small-vessel vasculitis. Am J Kidney Dis. 2003;42(6):1149–53.
41. Walsh M, Merkel PA, Jayne D. The effects of plasma exchange and reduced-dose glucocorticoids during remission-induction for treatment of severe ANCA-associated vasculitis [abstract]. Arthritis Rheumatol. 2018;70(Suppl 10)
42. Katsumata Y, Kawaguchi Y, Yamanaka H. Interstitial lung disease with ANCA-associated vasculitis. Clin Med Insights Circ Respir Pulm Med. 2015;9(Suppl 1):51–6.

43. Alba MA, Flores-Suárez LF, Henderson AG, et al. Interstital lung disease in ANCA vasculitis. Autoimmun Rev. 2017;16(7):722–9.
44. Borie R, Crestani B. Antineutrophil cytoplasmic antibody-associated lung fibrosis. Semin Respir Crit Care Med. 2018;39(4):465–70.
45. Kagiyama N, Takayanagi N, Kanauchi T, Ishiguro T, Yanagisawa T, Sugita Y. Antineutrophil cytoplasmic antibody-positive conversion and microscopic polyangiitis development in patients with idiopathic pulmonary fibrosis. BMJ Open Respir Res. 2015;2(1):e000058.
46. Hozumi H, Oyama Y, Yasui H, et al. Clinical significance of myeloperoxidase-anti-neutrophil cytoplasmic antibody in idiopathic interstitial pneumonias. PLoS One. 2018;13(6):e0199659.
47. Idiopathic Pulmonary Fibrosis Clinical Research Network, et al. Prednisone, azathioprine, and N-acetylcysteine for pulmonary fibrosis. N Engl J Med. 2012;366(21):1968–77.

11 Kidney Involvement

Renato Alberto Sinico, Fabio Pagni, Vincenzo L'Imperio, Valentina Binda, Paolo Fabbrini, Federico Pieruzzi, and Gabriella Moroni

11.1 Introduction

The term vasculitides encompasses a group of inflammatory disorders that may affect the kidney by damaging its blood supply. Virtually any size or type of vessel may be involved; involvement of glomerular capillaries leads to necrotizing glomerulitis, while involvement of larger arteries can cause renal infarction and ischemia. Although the kidney may be affected by many types of systemic vasculitis, renal involvement is particularly frequent in some forms of small-vessel systemic necrotizing vasculitis that are considered primary, such as granulomatosis with polyangiitis (GPA), microscopic polyangiitis (MPA), and eosinophilic granulomatosis with polyangiitis (EGPA), collectively called antineutrophil cytoplasmic autoantibody (ANCA)-associated vasculitis (AAV) [1].

Renal involvement is of particular importance in AAV because of its frequency and impact on prognosis. With the exception of EGPA, where kidney involvement is not a prominent feature [2], renal involvement is present in about 70% of patients with granulomatosis with polyangiitis, and in almost 100% of patients with microscopic polyangiitis [1].

R. A. Sinico (✉) · P. Fabbrini · F. Pieruzzi
Renal Unit, Department of Medicine and Surgery, ASST Monza—San Gerardo Hospital, University of Milano-Bicocca, Monza, Italy
e-mail: renato.sinico@unimib.it; federico.pieruzzi@unimib.it

F. Pagni · V. L'Imperio
Department of Medicine and Surgery, Section of Pathology, ASST Monza—San Gerardo Hospital, University of Milano-Bicocca, Monza, Italy
e-mail: fabio.pagni@unimib.it; v.limperio@campus.unimib.it

V. Binda · G. Moroni
Renal Unit, Fondazione IRCCS Ca' Granda Ospedale Maggiore Policlinico, Milan, Italy
e-mail: valentina.binda@policlinico.mi.it; gmoroni@policlinico.mi.it

R. A. Sinico, L. Guillevin (eds.), *Anti-Neutrophil Cytoplasmic Antibody (ANCA) Associated Vasculitis*, Rare Diseases of the Immune System,
https://doi.org/10.1007/978-3-030-02239-6_11

Moreover, the presence and severity of kidney involvement are associated with poorer prognosis (both patient and renal survival) [1].

11.2 Clinical Presentation

The main clinical presentation of renal involvement in AAV is represented by rapidly progressive glomerulonephritis (RPGN). RPGN is characterized clinically by a rapid decrease in the glomerular filtration rate (GFR) of at least 50% over a short period, from a few days to 3 months, and histologically, by extensive glomerular crescent formation. Other features include microscopic hematuria with often erythrocyte casts, and usually non-nephrotic proteinuria [1]. Quite often RPGN is so severe to cause dialysis dependence at diagnosis in almost 60% of patients [1]. With improvement in early diagnosis, a minor but significant number of patients may have urinary abnormalities, microscopic hematuria, and proteinuria, with serum creatinine within the normal range. A small but significant percentage of patients, especially those with MPA (14% in our series), may have a more indolent course and present, at diagnosis, with chronic renal insufficiency [1].

RPGN is one of the clinical presentations of glomerular diseases. It is one of the most dramatic and must be considered as a medical emergency.

RPGNs are classified according to their pathogenesis and immunofluorescence patterns [1, 3]. Type 1 is caused by the deposition of autoantibodies to glomerular basement membrane (GBM) and is characterized by linear deposits of immunoglobulin G. When lung involvement is present, the association of RPGN (due to antiglomerular basement membrane antibody) and pulmonary hemorrhage is named Goodpasture's syndrome. Type 2 RPGNs are due to the deposition of immune complexes and are characterized by granular deposits of immunoglobulin and/or complement in the glomerulus. RPGN that we see in AAV is classified as type 3 or pauci-immune because immune deposits are absent or scanty and its pathogenesis is ANCA related. Type 3 RPGN accounts for more than 50% of all RPGNs, especially in older ages [4]. RPGNs are characterized by extracapillary proliferation (the so-called crescents) that is very similar in all the three types and can be distinguished from each other on the basis of the immunofluorescence pattern [1, 3, 5].

Renal vasculitis can occur at any age, but is seen particularly frequently in middle-aged and elderly subjects [1]. The median age at presentation is between 55 and 65 years in the majority of studies, being significantly greater for MPA [1].

Because of the high prevalence of renal involvement in AAV, urinary sediment as well as renal function tests (serum creatinine, glomerular filtration rate, and proteinuria) should be performed at diagnosis and at follow-up in all patients. Kidney biopsy has a fundamental role in AAV, not only for diagnosis, but also for prognosis, and can be used to guide treatment. The gold standard for diagnosis remains renal biopsy [1, 3].

11.3 Pathology

The basic lesions are represented by necrosis of capillary loops, extracapillary proliferation with crescent formation, periglomerular and interstitial infiltrates, necrotizing arteritis, and absence or paucity of immune deposits (Fig. 11.1a–g).

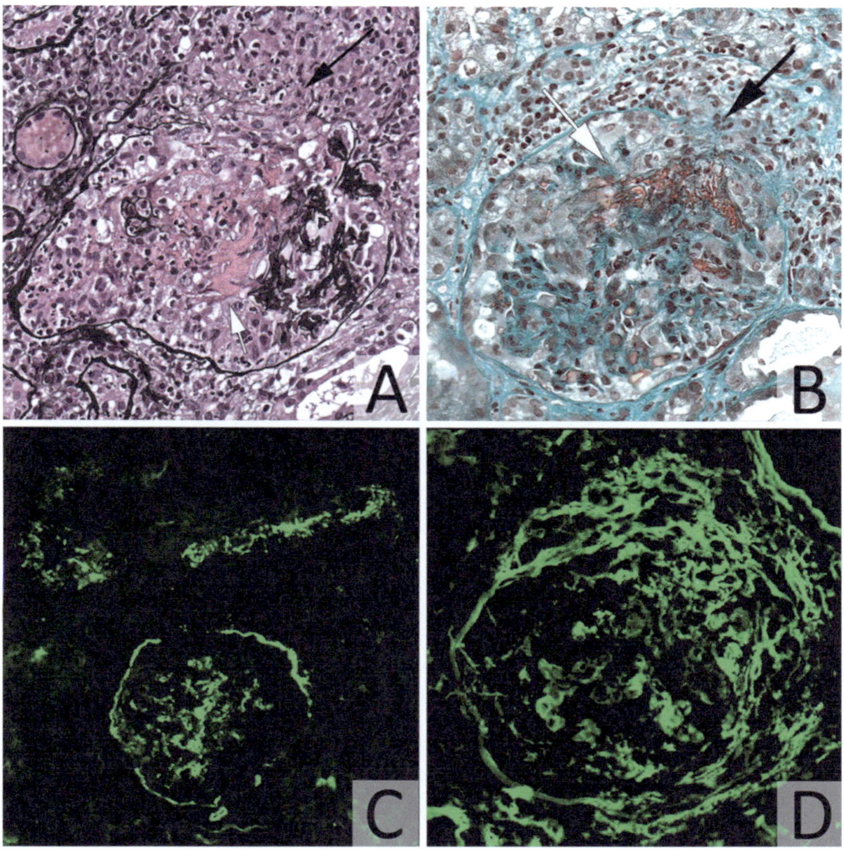

Fig. 11.1 Histopathologic features of ANCA-associated glomerulonephritis. During the active phase of the disease glomeruli can show extracapillary hypercellularity with the formation of cellular crescents and fibrinoid necrosis (**a**, white arrow, Jones methenamine silver stain), with consequent collapse of the glomerular tuft at the hilar pole and disruption of the Bowman capsule due to the inflammatory process (**a** and **b**, black arrow). Masson's trichrome stain can highlight fibrinoid necrosis as fuchsinophilic material in the context of glomeruli (**b**, white arrow) and, occasionally, in small vessels wall (**e**). Immunofluorescence generally shows granular deposits composed of C3 in the glomerular tuft, Bowman capsule, and vessel wall (**c**), and intense positivity to fibrinogen in cellular crescents and in fibrinoid necrosis (**d**). During the resolving/chronic phase of the disease, inflammatory lesions are replaced by glomerular scarring with segmental sclerosis of the tuft and formation of fibrous crescent (**f**, black arrow, PAS stain). Finally, some cases of ANCA-associated glomerulonephritis can be accompanied by an intense plasma cells-rich tubulointerstitial nephritis (**g**, white arrow, Jones) characterized by the peculiar prevalence of IgG4-mounting plasma cells (**h**, IgG4 immunohistochemistry). In these cases, the differential diagnosis with IgG4-related renal disease is mandatory

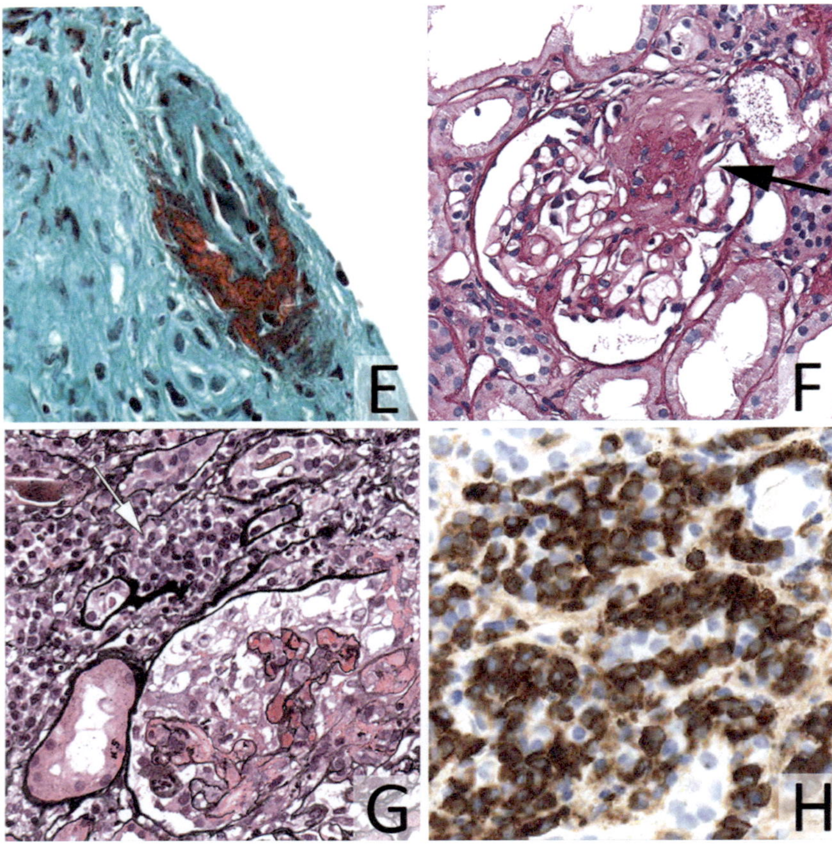

Fig. 11.1 (continued)

Capillaritis appears as fibrinoid necrosis of capillary loop (Fig. 11.1b) and is usually (but not invariably) accompanied by extracapillary proliferation with crescent formation (Fig. 11.1a). Crescents can involve only a part of the glomerular tuft or can be circumferential with collapse of the glomerular tuft. They can be florid or fibrous according to the stage of the disease. Usually, there are important interstitial and periglomerular infiltrates which can be massive. Necrotizing arteritis is present in less than 20% of biopsy specimens (Fig. 11.1e). These lesions, although characteristics, are not pathognomonic. However, when such lesions are present in the contest of a paucity of immune deposits they become diagnostic [1, 5]. Crescents (and necrosis) can involve less than 50% of glomeruli (focal forms) or more (diffuse), and the lesions can be restricted to a part of the glomerular tuft (segmental) or involve all the glomerulus (global). Interstitium and tubuli can also be involved, to a various degree, with important lymphoplasmacellular infitrates. In some cases, IgG4+ plasma cells are increased in the tissue biopsies and the association of AAV and IgG4-related disease has been described as a new overlap syndrome (Fig. 11.1h) [6, 7].

The extension and the stage of the lesions determine the severity of the clinical manifestations [8].

On the basis of the extension of the lesions and their characteristics (active or sclerotic), the European Vasculitis Study Group (EUVAS) has proposed a histopathological classification for ANCA-associated glomerulonephritis [8]. The classification scheme has four general categories of lesions named focal, crescentic, sclerotic, and mixed. The first three categories are based on the predominance of normal glomeruli, glomeruli with cellular crescents, and globally sclerotic glomeruli, respectively. The mixed category represents a heterogeneous phenotype and comprises those biopsies in which none of the aforementioned features is dominant [9–13]. Preliminary results have shown that the proposed classification system is of prognostic value for 1- and 5-year renal outcomes.

Subsequent studies agreed about the best prognosis of the focal class [9–14] and many about the sclerotic class as having the worst prognosis. The difference in survival between crescentic and mixed forms, on the contrary, varies in different studies [9–16].

Even though there are not qualitative differences in glomerular lesions in patients with GPA or with MPA, chronic damage is significantly higher in MPA (and/or MPO-ANCA-positive patients) than in GPA (and/or PR3-ANCA-positive patients) [5, 17]. Moreover, MPO-ANCA-positive patients have significantly higher percentage of globally sclerosed glomeruli, whereas PR3-ANCA-positive patients show more glomeruli with active lesions and arteritis [17]. This difference has been explained by a delayed establishment of diagnosis in MPA compared to patients with GPA and/or by a different pathogenesis of renal lesions [17].

Necrotizing crescentic glomerulonephritis in AAV is defined as pauci-immune because of the absence or paucity of significant immunoglobulin deposits. However, a subgroup of patients (18%) has substantial deposition of immunoglobulin in the mesangium and/or along the glomerular basement membrane [18]. Such deposits are found even in a higher percentage (54%) of cases by electron microscopy [19]. The presence of immune deposits is associated with a significantly greater degree of proteinuria [18, 19].

11.4 Clinical and Pathological Correlations

The prognostic significance of histological characteristics at kidney biopsy is still controversial. In addition to the proposed histological classification, there are other recognized factors correlating with poorer renal outcomes. Among the prognostic clinical features identified, some are associated with renal survival and others are associated with poor patient survival.

Generally, the percentage of normal glomeruli is the strongest predictor of glomerular filtration rate (GFR) at diagnosis, with higher GFR in those patients whose biopsy had shown the highest percentages of normal glomeruli [1, 17]. Other parameters which are correlated with serum creatinine are: percentage of glomeruli with cellular crescents, percentage of globally sclerosed glomeruli, extent of interstitial infiltrates, interstitial fibrosis, and tubular lesions [1, 17]. No correlation is usually found between renal function and fibrinoid necrosis or with the presence of arteritis [17].

11.5 Prognosis and Prognostic Factors

Untreated necrotizing and crescentic glomerulonephritis has an unfavorable course leading in a few weeks or months to end-stage renal disease (ESRD). Even if the prognosis has improved in the last years with the introduction of corticosteroids and cyclophosphamide as treatment of choice, a significant percentage of patients still require renal replacement therapy because of progressive disease. In a recently published large series, 14% and 18% of patients required permanent dialysis and 23% and 40% had died in 1 and 5 years, respectively. The presence and severity of renal involvement at diagnosis have an important impact on both renal and patient survival [20, 21].

Among predictors of renal outcome, a number of clinical and histological determinants have been identified. They can be summarized, pooling data from different large cohorts of patients, as follows: older age, female gender, serum creatinine for clinical predictors, and chronic lesions (glomerulosclerosis, interstitial fibrosis, and tubular atrophy) for histological parameters [reviewed in 1]. Other predictors are treatment resistance and relapses [21]. Considering diagnosis, MPA and renal-limited vasculitis tend to have a worse prognosis because of older age and because of more chronic lesions at kidney biopsy [11, 14, 17, 20, 21].

Including clinical and histological features, at multivariate analysis, Moroni et al. [11] found that serum creatinine ($p = 0.009$, relative ratio [RR] 1.11 for every mg of serum creatinine, 95% CI 1.03–1.21), presence of arterial hypertension ($p = 0.006$, RR 5.54, 95% CI 1.6–18.8), and less than 20% of normal glomeruli ($p = 0.022$, RR 3.05, 95% CI 1.17–7.93) emerged as the independent predictors of development of ESRD.

11.6 Renal Involvement in EPGA

EPGA is considered one of the so-called ANCA-associated systemic vasculitis because of its clinical and pathologic features that overlap with those of the other AAV, GPA, and MPA [1]. However, these two diseases differ from EGPA clinically, by the absence of asthma, and pathologically, by the absence of eosinophilia and eosinophil-rich tissue infiltrates [22]. Moreover, although ANCA are consistently found in 75–95% of patients with active GPA and MPA [23], the prevalence of ANCA in EGPA is much lower [24, 25]. Indeed, ANCA, usually P-ANCA/MPO-ANCA, are present in only about 40% of patients [24, 25].

Renal disease is often an overlooked feature of EGPA. Although less frequent and severe than in the other ANCA-associated vasculitides, renal manifestations occur in 25% of EGPA patients and range from isolated urinary abnormalities to rapidly progressive glomerulonephritis; some patients have chronic renal failure at diagnosis [2]. The most typical picture is pauci-immune focal and segmental necrotizing glomerulonephritis, with or without crescents, which usually involve less than 50% of the glomeruli. Tubulointerstitial nephritis with eosinophilic predominance is found only occasionally; a few patients have mesangial glomerulonephritis or focal segmental sclerosis [2].

Patients with necrotizing crescentic glomerulonephritis and, in general, patients with clinical signs of glomerular involvement have a higher prevalence of ANCA positivity [2, 24–26].

Renal flares are rare, and long-term prognosis and outcome are generally good [2]. Nonetheless, kidney disease is an adverse prognostic factor for EGPA patients; the largest study accurately assessing renal involvement in EGPA demonstrated a (albeit not statistically significant) higher 5-year mortality rate in patients with than in those without renal involvement [2]; previous studies also showed that particularly proteinuria >1 g/24 h was a strong predictor of mortality in EGPA [27].

11.7 Treatment of Renal Involvement

Therapy of AAV will be covered in another chapter of this book. However, some guidelines on the specific aspects of treatment of necrotizing crescentic glomerulonephritis will be given. EUVAS has categorized renal AAV patients in two subgroups according to the presence and severity of kidney involvement [28]. Randomized controlled trials have been conducted in order to obtain evidence-based recommendations [29–31].

Patients with serum creatinine lower than 500 μmol/l (5.7 mg/dl) should be treated with prednisone and cyclophosphamide for 3–6 months until remission is reached [29]. Oral and pulse cyclophosphamide have been shown to be equivalent in terms of clinical response [31]. Cyclophosphamide pulses are, however, associated with less episodes of leukopenia and the cumulative dose of the drug is inferior to that found in the oral cyclophosphamide-treated patients [31]. Long-term follow-up of CYCLOPS study has shown that pulse cyclophosphamide is associated with a higher relapse risk than daily oral cyclophosphamide. However, this is not associated with increased mortality or long-term morbidity [32].

Once the disease is into remission (usually within 3–6 months), azathioprine is as effective as cyclophosphamide and more effective than mycophenolate/mofetil to maintain remission [29, 33]. Methotrexate has also been shown to be equivalent to azathioprine, but it should not be used in patients with renal impairment [1]. A recent randomized trial has demonstrated a superiority of rituximab versus azathioprine in maintaining remission [34]. In this study, patients with newly diagnosed or relapsing granulomatosis with polyangiitis, microscopic polyangiitis, or renal-limited ANCA-associated vasculitis in complete remission after a cyclophosphamide–glucocorticoid regimen were randomly assigned to receive either 500 mg of rituximab on days 0 and 14 and at months 6, 12, and 18 after study entry or daily azathioprine until month 22. At month 28, major relapse had occurred in 17 (29%)

patients in the azathioprine group and in 3 (5%) patients in the rituximab group (hazard ratio for relapse 6.61, 95% CI 1.56–27.96, $p = 0.002$). The frequencies of severe adverse events were similar in the two groups [34].

How long to continue maintenance therapy is not known. A prospective randomized trial—that has compared two different durations of maintenance immunosuppressive therapy for the prevention of relapse in AAV—has shown that prolonged remission maintenance therapy with azathioprine/prednisolone beyond 24 months after diagnosis reduces relapse risk out to 48 months and improves renal survival in AAV [35]. On the contrary, a post hoc analysis of combined trial data has suggested that stopping azathioprine maintenance therapy does not lead to a significant increase in relapse rate and AZA maintenance for more than 18 months after diagnosis does not significantly influence relapse-free survival. ANCA specificity had more effect on relapse-free survival than duration of maintenance therapy and should be used to tailor therapy individually [36].

Patients with generalized vasculitis and renal involvement with a serum creatinine higher than 500 μmol/l (5.7 mg/dl) should be treated with a course of plasma exchange (seven sessions in 2 weeks) in addition to prednisone and oral cyclophosphamide [30]. In a randomized controlled trial, plasma exchange (PLEX) was shown to be more effective than methylprednisolone pulses (IV MeP) in terms of renal function recovery [30]. However, although short-term results with PLEX were encouraging, the long-term benefits remain unclear since, after a median of almost 4 years follow-up, there was no evidence of a net difference between PLEX and IV MeP in clinical outcomes [37].

Rituximab, a chimeric monoclonal antibody to CD20, is as effective as cyclophosphamide in inducing remission in AAV and should be preferred to cyclophosphamide in younger patients in order to preserve fertility [38, 39]. Rituximab was superior to cyclophosphamide in patients enrolled in the RAVE (Rituximab in ANCA-Associated Vasculitis) randomized controlled trial because of a severe flare and, therefore, these patients should be treated accordingly [38].

Worth of note, a *post hoc* analysis of this clinical trial data has demonstrated that patients with PR3-AAV were more than twice as likely to achieve complete remission at 6 months if treated with RTX rather than with cyclophosphamide/azathioprine. In addition, among patients with PR3-AAV who had relapsing disease at baseline, the risk of disease flare in RTX-treated patients was lower, not only at 6 months, but also at 12 and 18 months, despite the fact that patients randomized to RTX were not retreated preemptively with a maintenance regimen [40].

Rituximab has also some efficacy in refractory cases and may be used in patients who do not respond to standard treatment [41].

Preliminary results from small pilot studies indicate that mycophenolate mofetil is effective for induction and maintenance of remission in microscopic polyangiitis with mild-to-moderate renal involvement [42].

Accumulating evidence from animal models and clinical observations indicate that activation of the complement system—and the alternative pathway in particular—is crucial for the development of AAV, and that the complement activation product C5a has a central role. Recently, in a phase 2 randomized controlled trial,

C5a receptor inhibition with avacopan was effective in replacing high-dose glucocorticoids in treating vasculitis [43].

Prophylaxis and monitoring for many conditions, including *Pneumocystis jiroveci* infection, fungal and other opportunistic infections, osteoporosis should be considered in all patients [28].

A significant percentage of patients will remain with some degree of chronic renal impairment in terms of either reduced GFR or proteinuria or both. In this setting, antiproteinuric treatment with angiotensin-converting enzyme (ACE) inhibitors and/or angiotensin II receptor blockers (ARBs) is warranted in order to prevent or delay ESRD [1]. All the patients should be monitored closely in order to identify renal flares. Urinary sediment is fundamental for an early diagnosis of a renal flare and for differential diagnosis between proteinuria due to chronic damage from proteinuria due to active disease [1, 11].

Proteinuria due to renal scarring should not be treated as an active disease with corticosteroids and immunosuppressants. In doubtful cases, a repeat kidney biopsy should be performed if not contraindicated [1, 11].

11.8 End-Stage Renal Disease

Despite significant improvement in patient outcomes over the past decades, AAV still results in end-stage renal disease in a quarter of patients over 5 years [44, 45]. Renal replacement therapy (RRT) is required at diagnosis in a significant number of GPA and MPA patients who present with rapidly progressive renal insufficiency. Immunosuppressive treatment fails to obtain renal function recovery in one third of these patients and they need to continue RRT definitively [46]. Moreover, progressive renal insufficiency can develop in patients with less severe renal dysfunction at diagnosis because of the evolution of the histological lesions into glomerular, tubular, and vascular sclerosis. The occurrence of new renal relapses, together with arterial hypertension, atherosclerosis, and/or diabetes, contributes to the progressive deterioration of renal function. Hemodialysis and peritoneal dialysis are the treatment for acute and chronic forms of renal insufficiency. Renal transplantation is the best option for the treatment of AAV patients with irreversible ESRD.

11.9 Patients Requiring Acute Renal Replacement Therapy at Diagnosis

It is reported that from 29% to 55% of AAV patients are dialysis dependent at diagnosis [47, 48]. In our cohort of 92 AAV patients, 32% required dialysis at presentation or within the first week after diagnosis [11]. EUVAS investigators reported on the outcome of 41 AAV patients diagnosed between 2005 and 2010 and requiring RRT at presentation. Patients were treated with plasma exchange, corticosteroids, and intravenous cyclophosphamide. Three months later, 7.3% of patients had died on dialysis, 29.3% remained dialysis dependent, and 63.4% were dialysis independent. At 1-year follow-up, 13 (35%) patients remained dialysis dependent and 24 (65%) had independent renal function [46]. The Glomerular Disease Collaborative Network described 155 AAV patients diagnosed between 1985 and 2011, 87% of whom required dialysis at diagnosis. Four months after starting therapy, 35% of dialysis-dependent patients had not recovered renal function and 14% had died. At 12 months, four additional dialysis patients died and three new patients entered dialysis [49]. These data suggest that aggressive immunosuppressive treatment is unable to restore renal function in around one third of patients, while it can also cause potentially lethal adverse effects. For these reasons, it is a challenge for clinicians to decide which patients may benefit from treatment. To face this question, De Lind van Wijngaarden et al. [49] investigated the clinical and histological variables that determine the chances of dialysis independence, or death in 69 AAV dialysis-dependent patients. After 1 year of immunosuppressive therapy plus either intravenous methylprednisolone or plasma exchange, 43% of patients were dialysis independent, 32% were dialysis dependent, and 25% had died. Intravenous methylprednisolone as adjunctive therapy in the presence of less than 18% normal glomeruli and severe tubular atrophy increased the chance of therapy-related death over that of dialysis independence. Plasma exchange as adjunctive therapy increases the chance of renal recovery over that of death even in the presence of severe histological features (less than 2% of normal glomeruli). Lee et al. [50] found that low chronicity index and glomerular filtration rate (GFR) >10 ml/min were significantly associated with treatment response at 4 months. Notwithstanding these results, in cyclophosphamide-treated group, it was impossible to identify a threshold able to differentiate patients for whom the risks of therapy outweighs the benefits. Considering the low probability of achieving dialysis independence after 4 months therapy, the authors suggest that therapy should be discontinued after 4 months in nonresponders.

11.10 Patients Requiring Chronic Renal Replacement Therapy

The incidence and outcome of AAV patients requiring chronic RRT are poorly investigated. The incidence of chronic ESRD was 14% in 302 AAV patients included in six EUVAS trials and followed for 7.1 years [51]. A population-based study including 201 new cases of AAV diagnosed between 1997 and 2009 in southern Sweden (98 positive for PR3-ANCA and 85 positive for MPO-ANCA) reported the development of ESRD in 20% during a follow-up of around 5 years. Patients with MPO-ANCA were more likely to develop ESRD (38%) than those with PR3-ANCA (5%) [52].

Between 2002 and 2011, 425 AAV patients (166 MPA, 259 GPA) started chronic dialysis and were registered in the REIN (Renal Epidemiology and Information Network) registry accounting for 0.7% of all incident dialysis patients. The median age at initiation of dialysis was 70 years (range 7–93). Of the patients, 94% were treated with hemodialysis through central venous catheter in 66% of cases [53]. Peritoneal dialysis was less frequently employed in this cohort as in other studies [69, 71]. After a median follow-up of 23 months, 41% of patients died (61%

GPA and 39% MPA). The median survival time was 5.35 years (5.6 years for GPA, 4.7 years for MPA) and survival rates at 1 and 5 years were 85% and 53%, respectively [53]. Similar results have been reported in other studies [54]. Survival of AAV patients was not statistically different from that of non-AAV dialysis patients [53, 54]. Recently, Hruskova et al. [55] reported on 2511 (1.2%) patients with AAV (1755 GPA and 756 MPA) of the 207,855 who initiated RRT between 1993 and 2012 identified in 12 renal European registries. The 10-year probability patient survival in AAV on RRT after day 91 was 32.5% in comparison to 35.8% for patients with primitive glomerulonephritis, 17% for those with diabetes mellitus, and 30.2% for nondiabetes patients. Using Cox regression model and after adjusting for time period and country, patient survival on RRT after day 91 did not differ between AAV and matched nondiabetes patients, while it was lower than that of glomerulonephritis and higher than diabetes controls.

The main causes of death in dialysis patients were cardiovascular diseases (20–30%), followed by infections (10–23%) and malignancies (5–8%) [53–55]. Infections as cause of death was more frequent in AAV patients than in controls in some [53, 55] but not in all studies [54]. An important issue is the type and the duration of immunosuppressive therapy in patients on chronic RRT. Knowledge of the risk and the severity of relapses during dialysis is of paramount importance for the therapeutic management of patients on RRT. Lionaki et al. [56] reported that the AAV relapse rates were significantly lower on chronic dialysis (0.08 episodes/patient year) compared with the rate of the same patients before ESRD (0.20 episodes/patient/year) or with patients with preserved renal function (0.16 episodes). This was particularly true for patients with PR3-ANCA. However, it is not clear if the reduced rate of recurrences is due to the immunosuppressive treatment or a progressive quiescence of the disease during dialysis as reported for other autoimmune diseases attributed to an immunodeficiency status induced by uremia. Of note, infections were almost twice as frequent among patients with ESRD on maintenance immunosuppressants and were an important cause of death. Considering that, a minority of patients recover renal function after 3 months of dialysis, while infections are an important cause of mortality, international guidelines suggest to discontinue cyclophosphamide after 3 months in patients without extrarenal manifestation of AAV [57].

11.11 Renal Transplant

From 14% to 22% of AAV patients on chronic dialysis receive a renal transplant [53, 54]. Data from the United States Renal Data Service reported that among primitive and secondary glomerulonephritis on RRT, patients with vasculitis had the lowest rate of kidney transplantation (3.1 events for 100 patients years), and the highest rate of death that was more than double that of renal transplant (13.2 events for 100 patients years) [58]. Kidney transplantation was performed in 558 (22.2%) AAV patients included in 12 renal European registries. Patient and graft survival at 10 years were 74.8% and 63.7%, respectively. Using separate Cox regression models and after adjustments for time period and country, patients with AAV had mortality not different from the matched control group of primary glomerulonephritis and favorable transplant survival than each of the matched control groups [55]. In other studies including a lower number of patients, 10-year patient survival ranged between 65% and 87% and graft survival between 64% and 84% [59, 60]. Tang et al. [54] compared the outcome of 46 MPA and 47 GPA patients with that of 8193 non-AAV patients. The 10 years patient survival was significantly lower in MPA (68%) than in GPA (85%), and in non-AAV (92%), however, MPA patients were significantly older than GPA patients. The 10 years graft survival was 50% in MPA, 62% in GPA, and 70% in controls. After adjusting for a number of variables, MPA transplant patients had a risk of graft failure 1.87 times higher than that of controls. The MPA risk tended to be worse than that of GPA; instead, no differences were observed between GPA and controls. Despite some differences in the results of the various studies, transplantation is the therapeutic option able to assure the best survival and quality of life of ESRD patients as compared with dialysis regimens and with a graft survival not different from that of transplant in most renal pathologies. No difference in the causes of graft failure and death between AAV and non-AAV patients was reported by Marco et al. [59]. The only factor that has been reported to be associated with death post-transplant was transplant performed before 12 months of AAV remission.

A revision of the literature regarding the risk of AAV recurrence on renal graft was recently performed by Marco et al. [59]. This pooled analysis, that included 428 patients, found that recurrence of AAV occurred in 47 patients, which corresponds to a relapse rate of 11%. Recurrences occurred from 0.5 to 109 months after transplantation with an average time from transplantation to recurrence of 31 months [61]. The ANCA pattern, the duration of the original disease, the duration of dialysis, treatment with cyclosporine, and the source of donors did not influence the risk of recurrence [60], nor were clinical parameters very useful in predicting the risk of recurrence of AAV [60]. Single-center studies did not demonstrate the importance of persistent positive ANCA tests in predicting relapses after transplantation. Instead, the pooled analysis of Marco et al. reported that 17% of ANCA-positive patients at time of transplant had a recurrence in comparison to 5% of those ANCA-negative [59]. Relapses were more frequent in GPA than in MPA. The relapse rate after renal transplant has been reported to be lower than that observed before and during dialysis [60, 61]. Around 60% of recurrences involved the graft alone or in association with other organs, whereas the other 40% were primarily extrarenal [60]. Microscopic hematuria and proteinuria are the heralding signs for renal recurrences of AAV. These are generally associated with or followed by the deterioration of graft function [60]. The histologic picture is very similar to that observed in the native kidney and is characterized by focal or diffuse pauci-immune extracapillary necrotizing glomerulonephritis. In a recent study from the Dutch Transplant in Vasculitis (DUTRAVAS), the histological class of the 10 graft biopsies of renal AAV relapses were focal in 5 cases, crescentic in 1, and mixed in 4 [62]. Methylprednisolone pulses combined with cyclophosphamide and plasmapheresis while reducing the basal immunosuppression is the treatment of recurrence of AAV in renal transplant [63]. Recently, rituximab has been used with success to treat recurrences in renal transplant also [62]. The impact of recurrence on graft survival is not well defined. An Australian registry reported a graft loss of only 7.7% at 10 years due to recurrence of AAV in transplant patients [64]. In other studies, graft loss occurred in around one third of patients who had clinical recurrence of AAV [63, 64].

In conclusion, because clinical remission of AAV for less than 1 year at time of renal transplant is associated with a high mortality rate, AAV candidates for renal transplantation should be in a stable clinical remission at the time of transplantation. Prolonged immunosuppression may also expose patients to the risk of life-threatening infections after transplantation; thus, it is important that transplantation should be delayed after starting dialysis in patients who have received a prolonged or intense period of immunosuppression. We suggest checking for ANCA every 6–12 months, bearing in mind that negative results do not rule out completely the possibility of AAV relapse. As an increase in urine protein/creatinine ratio and/or the onset of hematuria and of erythrocyte casts in the urine sediment may herald a relapse of AAV, we suggest to monitor urinalysis every month during the first year after transplantation and every 3 months during the follow-up. The final diagnosis may require graft biopsy. Treatment of relapses is mainly based on methylprednisolone pulses, cyclophosphamide, and plasmapheresis or rituximab. Despite the unpredictable potential for recurrence, transplantation is the best option for AAV.

References

1. Sinico RA, Di Toma L, Radice A. Renal involvement in anti-neutrophil cytoplasmic autoantibody associated vasculitis. Autoimmun Rev. 2013;12:477–82.
2. Sinico RA, Di Toma L, Maggiore U, et al. Renal involvement in Churg–Strauss syndrome. Am J Kidney Dis. 2006;47(5):770–9.
3. Little MA, Pusey CD. Rapidly progressive glomerulonephritis: current and evolving treatment strategies. J Nephrol. 2004;17(Suppl. 8):10–9.
4. Mukhtyar C, Flossmann O, Hellmich B, et al. Outcomes from studies of antineutrophil cytoplasm antibody associated vasculitis: a systematic review by the European League Against Rheumatism systemic vasculitis task force. Ann Rheum Dis. 2008;67(7):1004–10.
5. Rutgers A, Sanders JS, Stegeman CA, Kallenberg CG. Pauci-immune necrotizing glomerulonephritis. Rheum Dis Clin N Am. 2010;36(3):559–72.
6. Chang SY, Keogh KA, Lewis JE, et al. IgG4-positive plasma cells in granulomatosis with polyangiitis (Wegener's): a clinicopathologic and immunohistochemical study on 43 granulomatosis with polyangiitis and 20 control cases. Hum Pathol. 2013;44:2432–7.
7. Danlos FX, Rossi GM, Blockmans D, et al. Antineutrophil cytoplasmic antibody-associated vasculitides and IgG4-related disease: a new overlap syndrome. Autoimmun Rev. 2017;16(10):1036–43.
8. Berden AE, Ferrario F, Hagen EC, et al. Histopathologic classification of ANCA-associated glomerulonephritis. J Am Soc Nephrol. 2010;21(10):1628–36.
9. Chang DY, Wu LH, Liu G, Chen M, Kallenberg CG, Zhao MH. Re-evaluation of the histopathologic classification of ANCA-associated glomerulonephritis: a study of 121 patients in a single center. Nephrol Dial Transplant. 2012;27:2343–9.
10. Muso E, Endo T, Itabashi M, et al. Evaluation of the newly proposed simplified histological classification in Japanese cohorts of myeloperoxidase-anti-neutrophil cytoplasmic antibody associated glomerulonephritis in comparison with other Asian and European cohorts. Clin Exp Nephrol. 2013;17(5):659–62.

11. Moroni G, Binda V, Leoni A, et al. Predictors of renal survival in ANCA associated vasculitis. Validation of a histopathological classification schema and review of the literature. Clin Exp Rheumatol. 2015;33(2 Suppl 89):S56–63.
12. Tanna A, Guarino L, Tam FW, et al. Long-term outcome of anti-neutrophil cytoplasm antibody-associated glomerulonephritis: evaluation of the international histological classification and other prognostic factors. Nephrol Dial Transplant. 2015;30:1185–92.
13. Hilhorst M, Wilde B, van Paassen P, et al. Improved outcome in anti-neutrophil cytoplasmic antibody (ANCA)-associated glomerulonephritis: a 30-year follow-up study. Nephrol Dial Transplant. 2013;28:373–9.
14. Ford SL, Polkinghorne KR, Longano A, et al. Histopathologic and clinical predictors of kidney outcomes in ANCA-associated vasculitis. Am J Kidney Dis. 2014;63:227–35.
15. Quintana LF, Peréz NS, De Sousa E, et al. ANCA serotype and histopathological classification for the prediction of renal outcome in ANCA-associated glomerulonephritis. Nephrol Dial Transplant. 2014;29:1764–9.
16. Bjørneklett R, Sriskandarajah S, Bostad L. Prognostic value of histologic classification of ANCA-associated glomerulonephritis. Clin J Am Soc Nephrol. 2016;11(12):2159–67.
17. Hauer HA, Bajema IM, Van Houwelingen HC, et al. Determinants of outcome in ANCA-associated glomerulonephritis: a prospective clinico-histopathological analysis of 96 patients. Kidney Int. 2002;62(5):1732–42.
18. Neumann I, Regele H, Kain R, Birck R, Meisl FT. Glomerular immune deposits are associated with increased proteinuria in patients with ANCA-associated crescentic nephritis. Nephrol Dial Transplant. 2003;18(3):524–31.
19. Haas M, Eustace JA. Immune complex deposits in ANCA-associated crescentic glomerulonephritis: a study of 126 cases. Kidney Int. 2004;65(6):2145–52.
20. de Lind van Wijngaarden RA, Hauer HA, et al. Clinical and histologic determinants of renal outcome in ANCA-associated vasculitis: a prospective analysis of 100 patients with severe renal involvement. J Am Soc Nephrol. 2006;17(8):2264–74.
21. Hogan SL, Falk RJ, Chin H, et al. Predictors of relapse and treatment resistance in anti-neutrophil cytoplasmic antibody-associated small-vessel vasculitis. Ann Intern Med. 2005;143(9):621–31.
22. Sinico RA, Bottero P. Churg–Strauss angiitis. Best Pract Res Clin Rheumatol. 2009;23(3):355–66.
23. Sinico RA, Radice A. Antineutrophil cytoplasmic antibodies (ANCA) testing: detection methods and clinical application. Clin Exp Rheumatol. 2014;32(3 Suppl 82):S112–7.
24. Sinico RA, Di Toma L, Maggiore U, et al. Prevalence and clinical significance of antineutrophil cytoplasmic antibodies in Churg–Strauss syndrome. Arthritis Rheum. 2005;52:2926–35.
25. Sable-Fourtassou R, Cohen P, Mahr A, et al. Antineutrophil cytoplasmic antibodies and the Churg–Strauss syndrome. Ann Intern Med. 2005;143:632–8.
26. Cottin V, Bel E, Bottero P, et al. Revisiting the systemic vasculitis in eosinophilic granulomatosis with polyangiitis (Churg-Strauss): a study of 157 patients by the Groupe d'Etudes et de Recherche sur les Maladies Orphelines Pulmonaires and the European Respiratory Society Taskforce on eosinophilic granulomatosis with polyangiitis (Churg-Strauss). Autoimmun Rev. 2017;16(1):1–9.
27. Guillevin L, Cohen P, Gayraud M, Lhote F, Jarrousse B, Casassus P. Churg–Strauss syndrome. Clinical study and long-term follow-up of 96 patients. Medicine. 1999;78:26–37.
28. Carruthers D, Sherlock J. Evidence-based management of ANCA vasculitis. Best Pract Res Clin Rheumatol. 2009;23(3):367–78.
29. Jayne D, Rasmussen N, Andrassy K, et al. A randomized trial of maintenance therapy for vasculitis associated with antineutrophil cytoplasmic autoantibodies. N Engl J Med. 2003;349(1):36–44.
30. Jayne DR, Gaskin G, Rasmussen N, et al. Randomized trial of plasma exchange or high-dosage methylprednisolone as adjunctive therapy for severe renal vasculitis. J Am Soc Nephrol. 2007;18(7):2180–8.

31. de Groot K, Harper L, Jayne DR, et al. Pulse versus daily oral cyclophosphamide for induction of remission in antineutrophil cytoplasmic antibody-associated vasculitis: a randomized trial. Ann Intern Med. 2009;150(10):670–80.
32. Harper L, Morgan MD, Walsh M, et al. EUVAS investigators. Pulse versus daily oral cyclophosphamide for induction of remission in ANCA-associated vasculitis: long-term follow-up. Ann Rheum Dis. 2012;71(6):955–60.
33. Hiemstra TF, Walsh M, Mahr A, et al. Mycophenolate mofetil vs azathioprine for remission maintenance in antineutrophil cytoplasmic antibody-associated vasculitis: a randomized controlled trial. JAMA. 2010;304(21):2381–8.
34. Guillevin L, Pagnoux C, Karras A, et al. French Vasculitis Study Group. Rituximab versus azathioprine for maintenance in ANCA-associated vasculitis. N Engl J Med. 2014;371(19):1771–80.
35. Karras A, Pagnoux C, Haubitz M, et al. European Vasculitis Society. Randomised controlled trial of prolonged treatment in the remission phase of ANCA-associated vasculitis. Ann Rheum Dis. 2017;76(10):1662–8.
36. de Joode AAE, Sanders JSF, Puéchal X, et al. Long term azathioprine maintenance therapy in ANCA-associated vasculitis: combined results of long-term follow-up data. Rheumatology (Oxford). 2017;56(11):1894–901.
37. Walsh M, Casian A, Flossmann O, et al. European Vasculitis Study Group (EUVAS). Long-term follow-up of patients with severe ANCA-associated vasculitis comparing plasma exchange to intravenous methylprednisolone treatment is unclear. Kidney Int. 2013;84(2):397–402.
38. Stone JH, Merkel PA, Spiera R, et al. Rituximab versus cyclophosphamide for ANCA-associated vasculitis. N Engl J Med. 2010;363(3):221–32.
39. Jones RB, Tervaert JW, Hauser T, et al. Rituximab versus cyclophosphamide in ANCA-associated renal vasculitis. N Engl J Med. 2010;363(3):211–20.
40. Unizony S, Villarreal M, Miloslavsky EM, et al. RAVE-ITN Research Group. Clinical outcomes of treatment of anti-neutrophil cytoplasmic antibody (ANCA)-associated vasculitis based on ANCA type. Ann Rheum Dis. 2016;75(6):1166–9.
41. Jones RB, Ferraro AJ, Chaudhry AN, et al. A multicenter survey of rituximab therapy for refractory antineutrophil cytoplasmic antibody-associated vasculitis. Arthritis Rheum. 2009;60(7):2156–68.
42. Silva F, Specks U, Kalra S, et al. Mycophenolate mofetil for induction and maintenance of remission in microscopic polyangiitis with mild to moderate renal involvement—a prospective, open-label pilot trial. Clin J Am Soc Nephrol. 2010;5(3):445–53.
43. Jayne DRW, Bruchfeld AN, Harper L, et al. Randomized trial of C5a receptor inhibitor avacopan in ANCA-associated vasculitis. J Am Soc Nephrol. 2017;28(9):2756–67.
44. Booth AD, Almond MK, Burns A, et al. Outcome of ANCA-associated renal vasculitis: a 5-year retrospective study. Am J Kidney Dis. 2003;41:776–84.
45. de Lind van Wijngaarden RA, Hauer HA, Wolterbeek R, et al. Clinical and histologic determinants of renal outcome in ANCA-associated vasculitis: a prospective analysis of 100 patients with severe renal involvement. J Am Soc Nephrol. 2006;17:2264–74.
46. Pepper RJ, Chanouzas D, Tarzi R, European Vasculitis Study (EUVAS) investigators, et al. Intravenous cyclophosphamide and plasmapheresis in dialysis-dependent ANCA-associated vasculitis. Clin J Am Soc Nephrol. 2013;8:219–24.
47. Slot MC, Tervaert JW, Franssen CF, et al. Renal survival and prognostic factors in patients with PR3-ANCA associated vasculitis with renal involvement. Kidney Int. 2003;63:670–7.
48. Little MA, Nazar L, Farrington K. Outcome in glomerulonephritis due to systemic small vessel vasculitis: effect of functional status and non-vasculitic co-morbidity. Nephrol Dial Transplant. 2004;19:356–64.
49. de Lind van Wijngaarden RA, Hauer HA, Wolterbeek R, EUVAS, et al. Chances of renal recovery for dialysis-dependent ANCA-associated glomerulonephritis. J Am Soc Nephrol. 2007;18:2189–97.
50. Lee T, Gasim A, Derebail VK, et al. Predictors of treatment outcomes in ANCA-associated vasculitis with severe kidney failure. Clin J Am Soc Nephrol. 2014;9:905–13.

51. Robson J, Doll H, Suppiah R, et al. Damage in the ANCA-associated vasculitides: long-term data from the European vasculitis study group (EUVAS) therapeutic trials. Ann Rheum Dis. 2015;74:177–84.
52. Mohammad AJ, Segelmark M. A population-based study showing better renal prognosis for proteinase 3 antineutrophil cytoplasmic antibody (ANCA)-associated nephritis versus myeloperoxidase ANCA-associated nephritis. J Rheumatol. 2014;41:1366–73.
53. Romeu M, Couchoud C, Delarozière JC, et al. Survival of patients with ANCA-associated vasculitis on chronic dialysis: data from the French REIN registry from 2002 to 2011. QJM. 2014;107:545–55.
54. Tang W, Bose B, McDonald SP, et al. The outcomes of patients with ESRD and ANCA-associated vasculitis in Australia and New Zealand. Clin J Am Soc Nephrol. 2013;8:773–80.
55. Hruskova Z, Stel VS, Jayne D, et al. Characteristics and outcomes of granulomatosis with polyangiitis (Wegener) and microscopic polyangiitis requiring renal replacement therapy: results from the European Renal Association-European Dialysis and Transplant Association Registry. Am J Kidney Dis. 2015;66:613–20.
56. Lionaki S, Hogan SL, Jennette CE, et al. The clinical course of ANCA small-vessel vasculitis on chronic dialysis. Kidney Int. 2009;76:644–51.
57. Rovin BH, Caster DJ, Cattran DC, et al. Management and treatment of glomerular diseases (part 2): conclusions from a Kidney Disease: Improving Global Outcomes (KDIGO) Controversies Conference. Kidney Int. 2019;95(2):281–95.
58. O'Shaughnessy MM, Liu S, Montez-Rath ME, et al. Kidney transplantation outcomes across GN subtypes in the United States. J Am Soc Nephrol. 2017;28:632–44.
59. Marco H, Mirapeix E, Arcos E, Catalan Study Group of Glomerular Diseases (GLOMCAT), et al. Long-term outcome of antineutrophil cytoplasmic antibody-associated small vessel vasculitis after renal transplantation. Clin Transpl. 2013;27:338–47.
60. Moroni G, Torri A, Gallelli B, et al. The long-term prognosis of renal transplant in patients with systemic vasculitis. Am J Transplant. 2007;7:2133–9.
61. Nachman PH, Segelmark M, Westman K, et al. Recurrent ANCA-associated small vessel vasculitis after transplantation: a pooled analysis. Kidney Int. 1999;56:1544–50.
62. Göçeroğlu A, Rahmattulla C, Berden AE, et al. The Dutch transplantation in vasculitis (DUTRAVAS) study: outcome of renal transplantation in antineutrophil cytoplasmic antibody-associated glomerulonephritis. Transplantation. 2016;100:916–24.
63. Ponticelli C, Moroni G, Glassock RJ. Recurrence of secondary glomerular disease after renal transplantation. Clin J Am Soc Nephrol. 2011;6:1214–21.
64. Briganti EM, Russ GR, McNeil JJ, Atkins RC, Chadban SJ. Risk of renal allograft loss from recurrent glomerulonephritis. N Engl J Med. 2002;347:103–9.

Peripheral Nervous System Involvement 12

Michael P. Collins and P. James B. Dyck

Abbreviations

AAV	ANCA-associated vasculitides
ACR	American College of Rheumatology
AIF	Allograft inflammatory factor
ANA	Antinuclear antibody
ANCA	Anti-neutrophil cytoplasmic antibody
AZA	Azathioprine
CHCC	Chapel Hill Consensus Conference
CIDP	Chronic inflammatory demyelinating polyneuropathy
CMV	Cytomegalovirus
CS	Corticosteroids
CTD	Connective tissue disease
CTL	Cytotoxic T lymphocyte
CYC	Cyclophosphamide
DCVAS	Diagnostic and Classification Criteria in Vasculitis Study
DIF	Direct immunofluorescence
EGPA	Eosinophilic granulomatosis with polyangiitis
EMG	Electromyography
ESR	Erythrocyte sedimentation rate

M. P. Collins (✉)
Medical College of Wisconsin, Milwaukee, WI, USA
e-mail: mcollins@mcw.edu

P. J. B. Dyck
Mayo Clinic, Rochester, MN, USA
e-mail: dyck.pjames@mayo.edu

R. A. Sinico, L. Guillevin (eds.), *Anti-Neutrophil Cytoplasmic Antibody (ANCA) Associated Vasculitis*, Rare Diseases of the Immune System,
https://doi.org/10.1007/978-3-030-02239-6_12

EULAR	European League Against Rheumatism
FVSG	French Vasculitis Study Group
GCA	Giant cell arteritis
GPA	Granulomatosis with polyangiitis
HNPP	Hereditary neuropathy with liability to pressure palsies
ICOS	Inducible costimulator
IHC	Immunohistochemical
IVIg	Intravenous immunoglobulins
MMF	Mycophenolate mofetil
MMP	Matrix metalloproteinase
MPA	Microscopic polyangiitis
MPO	Myeloperoxidase
MTX	Methotrexate
NCS	Nerve conduction studies
NSVN	Nonsystemic vasculitic neuropathy
PAN	Polyarteritis nodosa
PE	Plasma exchange
PR3	Proteinase 3
RCT	Randomized controlled trial
RF	Rheumatoid factor
SVN	Systemic vasculitic neuropathy
VEGF	Vascular endothelial growth factor
VN	Vasculitic neuropathy
VZV	Varicella zoster virus

12.1 Introduction

The vasculitides are a clinically, pathogenically, and etiologically diverse group of disorders, which share the pathologic signature of inflammatory damage to blood vessel walls, resulting in inflammatory and ischemic injury to the affected tissues [1]. They can develop from direct infections of the vessel wall, but in most cases, the process involves autoimmune mechanisms. While immune-mediated vasculitides can be triggered by identifiable factors, such as drugs, infections, cancers, connective tissue diseases (CTDs), other medical conditions, or environmental toxins, the underlying cause is often unknown. Some vasculitides are mild and self-limited; others produce multi-organ failure and death. Multiple combinations of organ systems can be affected, resulting in a wide variety of clinical manifestations. Specific clinical features depend on the location and size of the involved vessels, severity and tempo of the inflammatory process, underlying etiology, and comorbid conditions.

Systemic vasculitides that involve small-to-medium-sized vessels commonly affect epineurial vessels in the vasa nervorum resulting in peripheral neuropathies [2, 3]. In contrast, vasculitides with primarily large vessel involvement tend to spare epineurial vessels. For example, neuropathies occur in 60–75% of patients with polyarteritis nodosa (PAN), eosinophilic granulomatosis with polyangiitis (EGPA), and cryoglobulinemic vasculitis and up to 40–50% of those with microscopic polyangiitis (MPA) and rheumatoid vasculitis. On the other hand, neuropathies are rare in large-vessel vasculitides, such as giant cell arteritis (GCA). Peripheral nerve vasculitis is usually just one of many clinical manifestations of a systemic disease, but vasculitis can be restricted to individual organs, tissues, or body regions [4]. These localized vasculitides have been reported for almost all organs, including the PNS.

The studies of Kernohan and Woltman (1938), Boyd (1940), and Lovshin and Kernohan (1948) focused attention on PNS involvement in PAN [5–7]. These investigators observed that vasculitic neuropathy (VN) may herald the systemic disease, spontaneously regress, and present not only as a multifocal neuropathy ("mononeuritis multiplex") but also in a distal, symmetric fashion. Kernohan and Woltman were the first to report a case of PAN restricted to the PNS. Single-organ vasculitis of the PNS was established as a distinct entity by Kissel et al. in 1985 and Dyck et al. in 1987 [8, 9]. Dyck coined the term nonsystemic vasculitic neuropathy (NSVN). In the last four decades, numerous series of patients with systemic vasculitic neuropathy (SVN) and NSVN have been reported, better defining the clinical and pathological spectrum of these disorders [10–42]. Single-organ PNS vasculitis is still referred to as NSVN, but various forms of clinically isolated peripheral nerve vasculitis are now recognized and can be considered NSVN variants [43]. A Peripheral Nerve Society guideline group published consensus recommendations on the classification, diagnosis, and treatment of NSVN in 2010 [44].

12.2 Nomenclature, Classification, and Epidemiology

Numerous classifications for the vasculitides have been proposed since the 1950s contingent on advances in our understanding of the etiology, mechanisms, clinical features, laboratory findings, and pathological alterations of these disorders. Most have distinguished primary vasculitides, which lack an identified cause, from secondary vasculitides, resulting from a known cause or predisposing condition. The most widely used classification criteria for the primary systemic vasculitides are those published by the American College of Rheumatology (ACR) in 1990 for PAN, Churg-Strauss syndrome, Wegener's granulomatosis, hypersensitivity vasculitis, Henoch-Schönlein purpura, GCA, and Takayasu arteritis [45]. While useful for *classifying* already diagnosed patients for clinical studies, these criteria were not appropriate for *diagnosis* because they did not distinguish vasculitic from non-vasculitic conditions. In 1994, the Chapel Hill Consensus Conference (CHCC) defined ten vasculitides based on size and pathology of involved vessels—GCA, Takayasu arteritis, PAN, Kawasaki disease, microscopic polyangiitis (MPA), Wegener's granulomatosis, Churg-Strauss syndrome, Henoch-Schönlein purpura, essential cryoglobulinemic vasculitis, and cutaneous leukocytoclastic angiitis [46]. To address some of the failings of the 1994 CHCC and ACR criteria, vasculitis experts developed a new consensus methodology for classification of Wegener's granulomatosis, Churg-Strauss syndrome, MPA, and PAN in 2007 that, for the first time, incorporated anti-cytoplasmic antibodies (ANCAs) [47]. In vasculitis, ANCAs are usually directed against proteinase 3 (PR3) or myeloperoxidase (MPO).

The 2012 Revised International CHCC (CHCC2012) convened for the purpose of improving nomenclature for previously defined vasculitides and adding vasculitides not included in CHCC1994 [1]. Eponyms were eliminated for most disorders. In this system, the first level of categorization is size of predominantly involved vessels. Large vessels are the aorta, vena cavae, and their major branches; medium vessels comprise the main visceral arteries and veins and their initial branches; and small vessels consist of the intraparenchymal vessels. The "large-vessel vasculitides" are GCA and Takayasu arteritis, but they sometimes also affect small-to-medium-sized vessels. "Medium-vessel vasculitides" are PAN and Kawasaki disease. They affect small- and medium-sized arteries but not the microvasculature. ANCAs exclude PAN. "Small-vessel vasculitides" primarily affect small arteries, arterioles, capillaries, and venules, but medium-sized vessels are also sometimes involved. The small-vessel vasculitides are, in turn, divided into those associated with sparse versus prominent vascular wall deposits of immunoglobulin and complement. The "pauci-immune" disorders are the ANCA-associated vasculitides (AAVs), i.e., Wegener's granulomatosis, Churg-Strauss syndrome, and MPA, with Wegener's granulomatosis renamed granulomatosis with polyangiitis (GPA) and Churg-Straus syndrome renamed EGPA. The "immune complex small-vessel vasculitides" exhibit "moderate-to-marked" immune deposits in small vessels. They include anti-glomerular basement disease (Goodpasture syndrome), cryoglobulinemic vasculitis, IgA vasculitis (Henoch-Schönlein purpura), and hypocomplementemic urticarial vasculitis. The "variable-vessel vasculitides" are Behçet disease and Cogan syndrome. They affect vessels of all sizes and types non-preferentially. "Single-organ vasculitis" affects vessels of any type in a single organ/tissue with no signs of an underlying systemic vasculitis. NSVN should be included in this group. The many secondary causes of vasculitis are incorporated into "vasculitis associated with systemic disease" (e.g., rheumatoid arthritis and lupus) and "vasculitis associated with a probable etiology" (e.g., hepatitis B-associated PAN and hepatitis C-associated cryoglobulinemic vasculitis).

The Diagnostic and Classification Criteria in Vasculitis Study (DCVAS) is a multinational, observational study designed to develop and validate new diagnostic and classification criteria for the primary systemic vasculitides, which will be applicable to both clinical practice and clinical trials [48]. More than 6800 patients were recruited from 2011 to 2017. Provisional classification criteria have been presented at national and international meetings but will require further testing before endorsement by the ACR and European League Against Rheumatism (EULAR).

For the primary small-to-medium-vessel vasculitides most routinely associated with neuropathy—MPA, PAN, EGPA, and GPA—annual incidence rate is ~10–20 cases/million [49]. No study has determined the incidence or prevalence of any form of VN, but the *relative* frequency of these disorders can be derived from investigations ascertaining patients with VN based, in part, on nerve biopsy findings [8, 9, 14, 17, 20, 22, 23, 26–28, 30, 33, 37, 38, 40, 50–57]. These frequencies (Table 12.1) differ from those of the corresponding systemic vasculitides because of the variable

Table 12.1 Prevalence of vasculitis types in vasculitic neuropathy

Series	NSVN	PAN[a]/ MPA[b]	RV	EGPA	UCTD	GPA	SLE	Cancer	pSS	EMC/ HCV	Other
Kissel [8]	7	3	0	0	5	0	1	0	0	0	0
Harati [17]	21	2	2	0	4	0	0	3	0	0	Scl-1
Dyck [9]	20	32	2	4	0	1	1	3	0	0	Scl-1, HIV-1
Said [26]	25	24	26	6	6	0	1	1	2	0	Scl-1. HIV-3, Sarcoid-1, GCA-1, PM-1
Panegyres [23]	7	0	5	3	0	1	0	0	1	0	MGUS-1
Hawke & McCombe [20, 50]	2	11	7	3	8	1	3	1	1	0	0
Midroni [51]	4	3	8	3	10	0	2	0	1	0	HV-1
Nicolai [22]	2	2	1	4	7	0	0	0	0	3	HIV-1
Singhal [28]	7	6	0	2	4	1	4	0	0	0	0
Ohkoshi [52]	1	6	1	3	0	0	2	0	0	0	0
Cartier [53]	6	21	1	0	11	0	1	2	0	0	
Collins [14]	11	6	8	0	0	2	1	2	0	0	MGUS-3, VZV-1, HV-2
Sanchez [27]	5	12	0	3	0	2	2	1	0	0	Sarcoid-1
Vital & Vital [37, 38]	37	28	9	17	0	4	1	0	3	6	Skin/nerve-5, HIV-4, Sarcoid-2, Eos-2, EBV-1
Gorson [56]	8	1	1	3	0	0	0	3	3	1	DM-1, GCA-1
Mathew [40]	11	27	12	22	6	14	4	4	0	4	IgAV-1, meningococcemia-1
Oka [54]	8	13	3	6	0	0	1	0	3	0	0
Zivkovic [55]	12	4	6	0	1	2	4	4	1	2	Scl-2, Sarcoid-1, MCTD-1
Bennett [30]	22	10	3	3	2	3	0	2	2	2	HIV-2, Scl-1, GVHD-1
Agadi [33]	21	1	1	4	0	0	0	0	0	0	0
Zhang [57]	3	4	3	2	0	0	0	0	1	0	Behcet-1

(continued)

Table 12.1 (continued)

Series	NSVN	PAN[a]/ MPA[b]	RV	EGPA	UCTD	GPA	SLE	Cancer	pSS	EMC/ HCV	Other
Total (percent) *n* = 873	**240** (27.5)	**216** (24.7)	**99** (11.3)	**88** (10.0)	**60** (6.9)	**31** (3.6)	**28** (3.2)	**24** (2.7)	**21** (2.4)	**18** (2.1)	**All 48** (5.5) HIV 11 Scl 6 MGUS 5 Sarcoid 5 Nerve/skin 5 HV 3 Eos 2 GCA 2 Behcet 1 DM 1 EBV 1 GVHD 1 IgAV 1 MCTD 1 Meningococcemia 1 PM 1 VZV 1

DM dermatomyositis, *EBV* Epstein-Barr virus, *EGPA* eosinophilic granulomatosis with polyangiitis, *EMC* essential mixed cryoglobulinemia, *Eos* hypereosinophilia without lung involvement, *GCA* giant cell arteritis, *GPA* granulomatosis with polyangiitis, *GVHD* chronic graft versus host disease, *HCV* hepatitis C virus, *HIV* human immunodeficiency virus, *HV* hypersensitivity vasculitis, *IgAV* IgA vasculitis (Henoch-Schönlein Purpura), *MCTD* mixed connective tissue disease, *MGUS* monoclonal gammopathy of undetermined significance, *MPA* microscopic polyarteritis, *NSVN* = nonsystemic vasculitic neuropathy, *PAN* polyarteritis nodosa, *PM* polymyositis, *pSS* primary Sjogren's syndrome, *RV* rheumatoid vasculitis, *sarcoid* sarcoidosis, *Scl* scleroderma, *SLE* systemic lupus erythematosus, *UCTD* undifferentiated connective tissue disease, *VZV* varicella zoster virus

[a]Includes cases of hepatitis B-associated PAN

[b]MPA combined with PAN because these disorders were not distinguished in vasculitic neuropathy series prior to 1997

prevalence of neuropathy in these conditions and the existence of NSVN. In these studies, the most common VNs are NSVN (27.5%) and those associated with MPA/PAN (25%), rheumatoid vasculitis (11%), and EGPA (10%).

The primary systemic vasculitides most likely to produce a neuropathy are PAN, EGPA, and MPA [58–60]. Of the secondary systemic vasculitides, nerves are most commonly affected in hepatitis B-associated PAN, hepatitis C-related cryoglobulinemic vasculitis, and rheumatoid vasculitis [2, 3, 58, 61]. Conversely, neuropathies are uncommon in GCA and rare in Behçet disease and the non-cryoglobulinemic immune complex vasculitides. Pathologically proven VN has not been reported in Kawasaki disease, Takayasu arteritis, anti-glomerular basement membrane disease, and Cogan syndrome [44]. On the basis of these and other observations, the 2010 Peripheral Nerve Society guideline group derived a consensus classification for vasculitides associated with neuropathy that categorized VNs into the primary systemic vasculitides, secondary systemic vasculitides, and localized vasculitides [44]. In 2017, we updated this classification, adapting the CHCC2012 nomenclature and including a new formulation of the single-organ VNs (Box 12.1) [43].

Box 12.1: Classification of Vasculitides Associated with Neuropathy (Reproduced with Permission from [43])

Primary systemic vasculitides

- Predominantly small-vessel vasculitis
  - Anti-neutrophil cytoplasmic antibody (ANCA)-associated vasculitis
    - Microscopic polyangiitis
    - Eosinophilic granulomatosis with polyangiitis (Churg-Strauss)
    - Granulomatosis with polyangiitis (Wegener's)
  - Immune complex small-vessel vasculitis
    - Cryoglobulinemic vasculitis
    - IgG vasculitis (Henoch-Schönlein purpura)
    - Hypocomplementemic urticarial vasculitis
- Predominantly medium-vessel vasculitic
  - Polyarteritis nodosa
- Predominantly large-vessel vasculitis
  - Giant cell arteritis
- Variable-vessel vasculitis
  - Behçet's disease

Vasculitis associated with systemic disease

- Connective tissue diseases
  - Rheumatoid arthritis
  - Systemic lupus erythematosus
  - Primary Sjogren's syndrome
  - Systemic sclerosis
  - Mixed connective tissue disease
  - Dermatomyositis

Sarcoidosis
Inflammatory bowel disease

Vasculitis associated with probable etiology

Infection (such as hepatitis B virus, hepatitis C virus, HIV, cytomegalovirus, leprosy, Lyme disease, human T-cell-lymphotropic virus-I, parvovirus B19)
Drugs
Malignancy
Vaccinations

Single-organ vasculitis of the PNS (nonsystemic vasculitic neuropathy)

Includes but is not limited to following subtypes:
- Wartenberg migratory sensory neuropathy (non-mechanical cases)
- Postsurgical inflammatory neuropathy
- Diabetic radiculoplexus neuropathy
  - Predominantly lumbosacral
  - Predominantly thoracic (diabetic thoracic radiculopathy or radiculoneuropathy)
  - Predominantly cervical
- Neuralgic amyotrophy (probably)
- Nonsystemic skin/nerve vasculitis
  - Cutaneous polyarteritis nodosa
  - Other

While most neurologists recognize NSVN as a distinct entity, non-neurologists often classify it as a variant of MPA or PAN [4]. However, arguing against MPA, NSVN is not pauci-immune and has no association with ANCAs [44]. Excluding PAN, nerve biopsies in patients with NSVN routinely show microvascular involvement [3]. Clinically, in patients carefully selected for absence of systemic features and conditions predisposing to systemic vasculitis, the likelihood of spread to organs other than regional skin or muscle is very low, assuming immunosuppressive treatment is instituted [15]. Patients with NSVN frequently relapse as treatment is tapered, but unlike the SVNs, relapses are almost always restricted to the PNS. Furthermore, the PNS is resistant to ischemia and should not be preferentially susceptible to a systemic ischemic process [51]. There is also the "proof of principle" argument provided by numerous examples of localized vasculitis involving other organs [4].

VNs can also be divided into two groups based on the size of predominantly involved vessels: nerve large arteriole vasculitis and nerve microvasculitis [62]. All vessels in peripheral nerves are, by definition, "small vessels." Microvessels are venules, capillaries, and small arterioles (diameters <40 μm). Larger arterioles have diameters up to 100 μm. Arterial vessels with diameters >100 μm are small arteries. While all endoneurial and perineurial vessels are microscopic, most

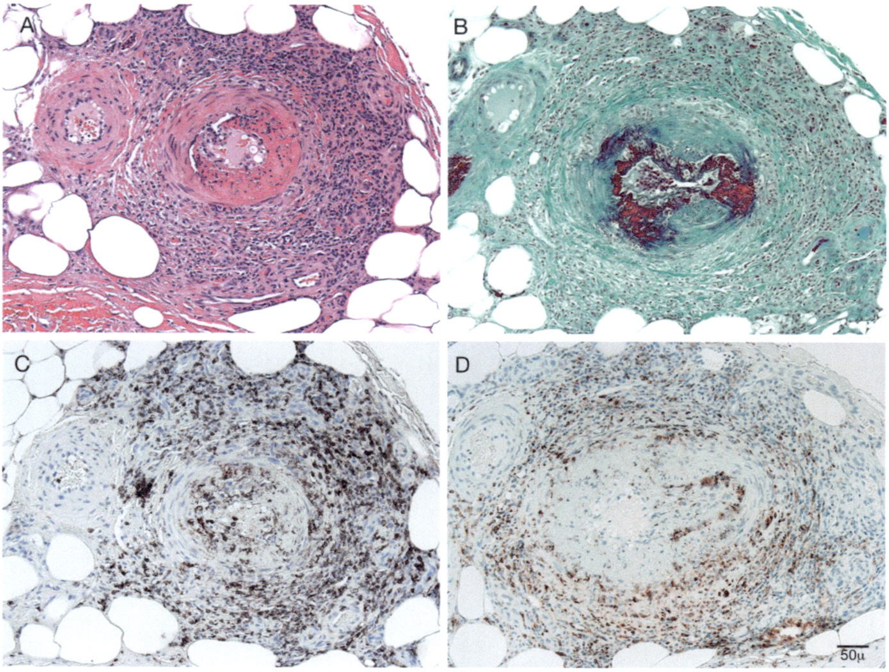

Fig. 12.1 Serial paraffin cross sections of nerve showing large inflammatory collection involving a large arteriole exhibiting sectoral fibrinoid necrosis in **a** (H&E) and **b** (Masson's trichrome). Vessel wall inflammation highlighted with pan-leukocyte marker CD45 in **c** and macrophage marker CD68 in **d**. Taken together, the findings are diagnostic of nerve large arteriole necrotizing vasculitis

epineurial vessels are larger in size (50–300 μm) [51]. The nerve large arteriole vasculitides demonstrate primary involvement of small arteries and large arterioles combined with variable involvement of smaller vessels (Fig. 12.1). They include most of the SVNs. Nerve microvasculitis is restricted to microvessels and can occur in NSVN, Sjogren's syndrome, some virus-associated vasculitic neuropathies (e.g., HIV), diabetic radiculoplexus neuropathy, and non-diabetic radiculoplexus neuropathy (clinical variant of NSVN) (Fig. 12.2). Of note, NSVN can also affect large arterioles and small arteries and is thus not, strictly speaking, a pure microvasculitis. It tends to involve smaller vessels (<100 μm) but is not limited to microvessels [31, 32].

12.3 Clinical Presentation of Vasculitic Neuropathy

The clinical presentation of PNS vasculitis depends on the distribution of affected nerves, disease severity, and spectrum of systemic involvement. Signs and symptoms of multi-organ dysfunction are indicative of a systemic vasculitis or underlying CTD. Combining information from numerous series of patients with SVN, skin is

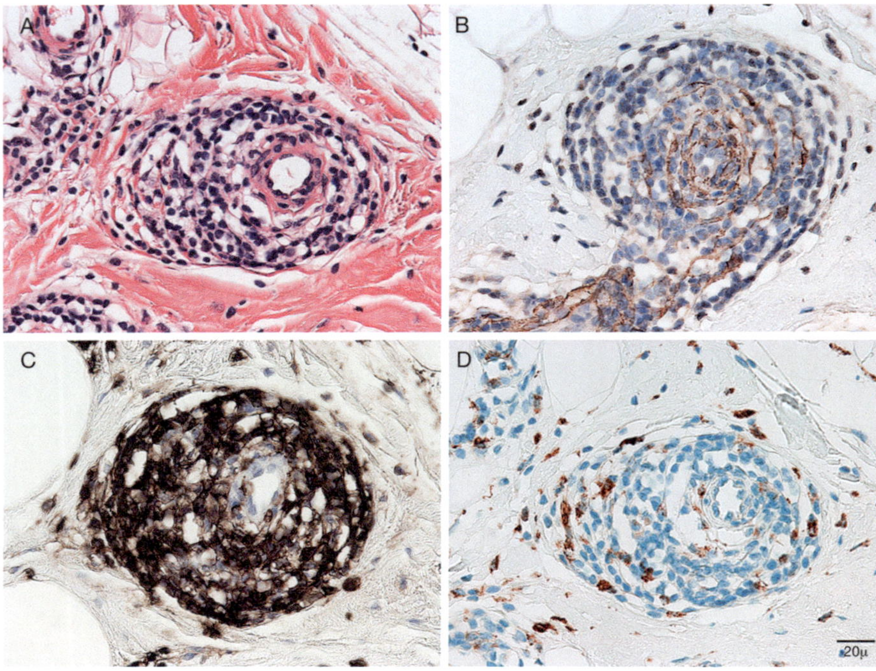

Fig. 12.2 Serial paraffin cross sections of a microvessel showing lymphocytic-predominant inflammation and only rare macrophages in vessel wall in **a** (H&E), **c** (CD45), and **d** (CD68). Human smooth muscle actin stain in **b** shows separation and fragmentation of smooth muscle layers of the vessel wall. Taken together, these findings are diagnostic of nerve microvasculitis

affected in 1/3 of patients, while renal, GI tract, lung (excluding EGPA), and heart involvement occurs in <15% [10, 12, 18–21, 24–26, 29, 63–67]. Consistent with this data, analysis of 506 patients with GPA or MPA who participated in clinical trials conducted by European Vasculitis Study Group revealed that SVNs were associated with skin, mucous membrane, and ENT manifestations but not renal, cardiac, pulmonary, or GI involvement [68]. An assessment of 955 patients with AAV included in the DCVAS revealed that SVN was significantly associated with skin, musculoskeletal, and cardiovascular involvement and with the absence of renal, eye, and GI involvement [69]. Prevalence of SVN was also higher in GPA and EGPA lacking in pulmonary involvement. In summary, SVN tends to occur in association with cutaneous, musculoskeletal, and ENT manifestations and independent of more life-threatening internal organ involvement. SVNs are accompanied by fevers and other constitutional symptoms in 60–65% of patients [7, 8, 10, 11, 14, 22, 24, 28–31, 66, 67, 70, 71]. By definition, NSVN is not accompanied by clinical evidence of extra-neurologic involvement, but constitutional symptoms occur in almost 30% of patients and fevers in 10–15% [43]. In patients with SVN, neuropathic symptoms are one of the presenting features in 70% of cases; in the other 30%, systemic symptoms precede the neuropathy by weeks to months [5, 7, 11, 12, 18, 20, 21, 24, 25, 39, 72–74].

VN has a characteristic clinical picture whether occurring alone or as one feature of a systemic vasculitis. Studies have shown that NSVN is clinically similar to SVN except for reduced severity and more indolent progression [16, 19, 20, 30, 31]. VN can develop at any age but most commonly occurs in the 6th–8th decades. The mean age at onset of SVN ranges from 53 to 67 years in various series if not restricted to EGPA, which tends to develop at a younger age [11, 14, 19, 20, 26, 30, 41]. For NSVN, the mean age at diagnosis is 60 years [43]. In the primary SVNs, men are more frequently affected than women in PAN, MPA, and rheumatoid vasculitis, but there is no association with gender for GPA and EGPA [75]. In NSVN, both genders are equally affected [43]. Most patients follow a stepwise or relapsing course, but the disease steadily progresses in 40% [9, 14, 30]. Some 5–10% of patients with NSVN and up to 35–40% of those with an SVN present with acute, rapidly progressive deficits and are diagnosed within 1 month, but most patients progress subacutely over several months [8, 16, 20, 25, 30, 34, 36, 41, 42, 65]. Still others follow an indolent course over multiple years prior to diagnosis, highlighting the need to maintain vigilance for NSVN in patients with long-standing neuropathies [76]. Median delay from symptom onset to diagnosis has ranged from 2 to 8 months in most series [14–16, 20, 30, 31].

Three patterns of clinical involvement in NSVN and SVN have been identified: multifocal neuropathy (also referred to as multiple mononeuropathy), asymmetric polyneuropathy (also referred to as overlapping or confluent multifocal neuropathy), and distal symmetric polyneuropathy (Fig. 12.3). Most distinctive is a *multifocal neuropathy,* wherein patients develop pain, weakness, and/or sensory loss in the distribution of a single peripheral nerve, followed by stepwise involvement of other nerves. Although distinctive, this pattern is not pathognomonic for vasculitis. An asymmetric polyneuropathy restricted to the lower limbs with proximal involvement can be labeled a lumbosacral radiculoplexus neuropathy. The distribution most difficult to recognize as vasculitic is a distal, symmetric polyneuropathy. The reported frequencies of these three phenotypes are highly variable due to a lack of standardized definitions. For example, in a 2003 Ohio State series of patients with NSVN where no asymmetry was ignored, asymmetric polyneuropathy was the most common pattern (85%) followed by multifocal neuropathy (13%) and distal symmetric polyneuropathy (2%) [15], but combined data from all series and case reports of NSVN yield a different distribution (45% asymmetric polyneuropathy, 33% multifocal neuropathy, and 23% symmetric polyneuropathy) [43], as do pooled data from many studies of SVN (48% multifocal neuropathy, 32% asymmetric polyneuropathy, and 20% symmetric polyneuropathy) [8, 10, 19–22, 28, 29, 33, 36, 51, 55, 65, 77]. In vasculitis, symmetric polyneuropathies are necessarily overlapping multifocal neuropathies at the microscopic level, suggesting that clinical findings in VN should always be at least slightly asymmetric or multifocal.

To address this problem, we recently proposed new definitions for these patterns [43]. We defined multifocal neuropathy as a peripheral neuropathy that affects two or more noncontiguous, individual, named, somatic, sensory, motor or sensorimotor peripheral or cranial nerves simultaneously or sequentially. Conversely, a distal symmetric polyneuropathy was defined as a length-dependent neuropathy that

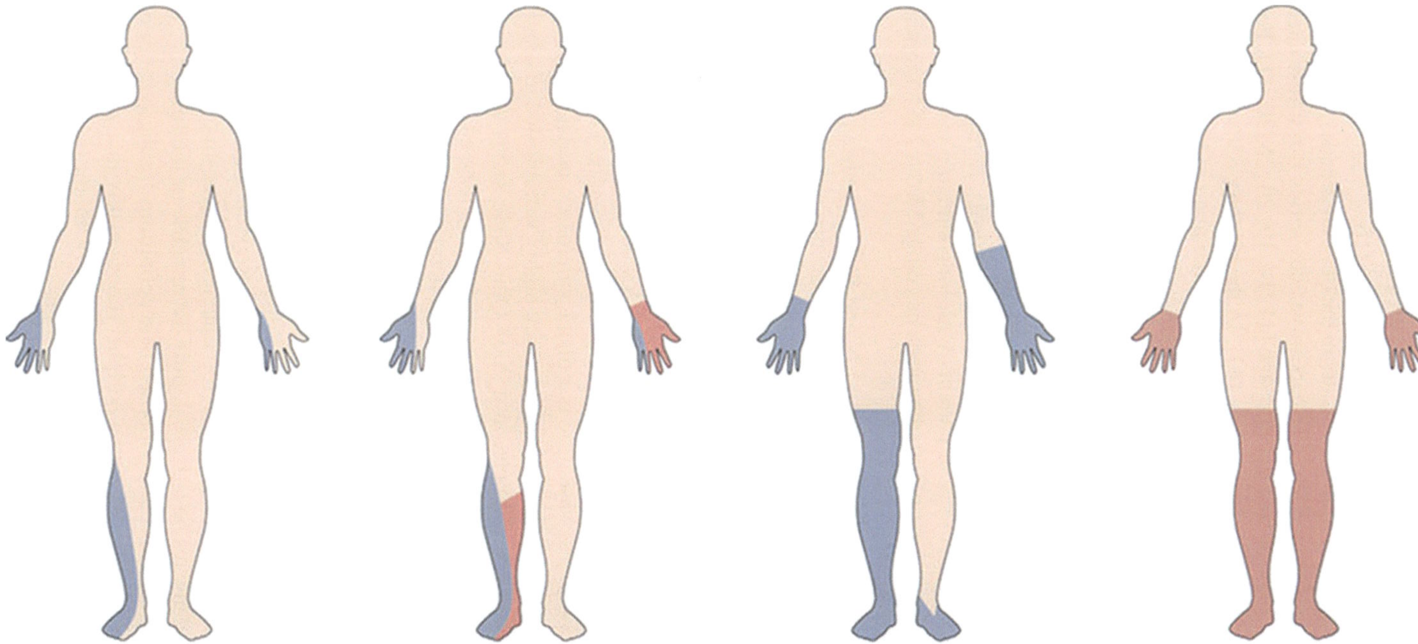

Fig. 12.3 Anatomical patterns of neuropathy. In the multifocal neuropathy and early overlapping multifocal neuropathy figures, the two colors differentiate between distributions of different cutaneous nerves. In the late overlapping multifocal neuropathy and distal symmetric polyneuropathy figures, the single color depicts involvement by multiple overlapping cutaneous nerves. Reproduced with permission from [45]

affects multiple somatic nerves diffusely and symmetrically, commencing distally and spreading proximally with continued distal predominance. We defined an early overlapping multifocal neuropathy as a multifocal neuropathy in which contiguous cranial or individual peripheral nerves distal to the plexuses are involved. In a late overlapping multifocal neuropathy, there is more extensive involvement of contiguous nerves, to the extent that individual mononeuropathies are no longer distinguishable and the anatomical pattern loses its multifocal features. The neuropathy then appears as a diffuse process, mimicking a distal symmetric polyneuropathy, but can be identified by residual asymmetries. A late overlapping multifocal neuropathy is identical to an asymmetric polyneuropathy.

Certain nerves have a propensity for vasculitic involvement, but at presentation, the most commonly affected nerves are a diffuse, overlapping mixture of lower limb nerves derived from the lumbosacral plexus [14, 15, 35]. The tendency of VN to affect certain nerves has generally been attributed to poor collateral vascular supply, but variability in vascular topography, antigen expression, and adhesion molecules might also play a role [78]. The most frequently affected nerve is the common peroneal or peroneal division of the distal sciatic nerve. In the arms, the ulnar nerve is most commonly involved. Combined data from several studies indicate that the prevalence of individual distal motor nerve involvement is as follows: common peroneal 93% of patients, tibial 61%, ulnar 48%, median 43%, and radial 20% [9, 12, 14, 18, 25, 30, 33, 39, 65, 79, 80]. Data on proximal nerve involvement are more limited, variable, and confounded by superimposed myopathies. Cranial neuropathies occur in 5–10% of patients with SNV and NSVN [25, 39, 43, 57, 60, 68, 80, 81].

PNS vasculitis affects mixed or purely sensory peripheral nerves rather than anterior horn cells or sensory/autonomic ganglia [82]. As such, most patients develop both sensory and motor deficits, but 10–15% have purely or predominantly sensory signs and symptoms due to cutaneous nerve involvement (more common in NSVN than SVN) [7, 11, 13, 14, 18, 21, 30, 31, 36, 43, 64, 67, 70]. Sensory dysfunction usually involves all modalities, but exceptional patients have small fiber-predominant neuropathies [30]. Pure motor presentations are rare [34]. Vasculitic neuropathy is generally considered to be a painful neuropathy, but based on our review of the literature, 25% of patients with SVN and NSVN have no pain.

Summarizing, patients with [1] no asymmetries, [2] pure motor involvement, or [3] entirely proximal findings are unlikely to have a VN.

12.4 Clinical Features of Vasculitic Neuropathy in PAN and AAV

The clinical features of the AAVs—GPA, MPA, and EGPA—are detailed in Chapters 8–10. The clinical manifestations of the VNs—both nonsystemic and systemic—are described in Section 3. In this section, we summarize the non-ANCA-associated primary systemic vasculitis most closely associated with SNV, PAN, and contrast this condition from the AAVs, followed by up-to-date analyzes of the prevalence of VN in these vasculitides.

12.4.1 Polyarteritis Nodosa

PAN is a systemic vasculitis that affects small- and medium-sized arteries [58, 83]. It is sometimes triggered by hepatitis B, hepatitis C, or HIV infection, but in the 2012 Revised International CHCC Nomenclature of Vasculitides, infection-related vasculitides were recast as "vasculitis associated with a probable etiology" [1]. PAN has traditionally represented the most common small-to-medium-vessel systemic vasculitis and most common cause of SVN. However, its incidence was reduced by the 1994 and 2012 CHCC nomenclature, which mandated that any pathologically proven microvessel involvement excluded the diagnosis, making MPA the more prevalent disease in most studies [84]. It is also excluded by lung vasculitis, glomerulonephritis, cryoglobulins, or ANCAs [1, 58, 83].

PAN usually develops between the ages of 40 and 70 years [58, 83, 85, 86]. The onset is subacute, characterized by constitutional symptoms emerging over weeks to months. Fevers and weight loss occur in 60–70% of patients. Symptoms referable to specific organ involvement soon follow. The most commonly affected tissues are the PNS, skin (55–60%), joints (50%), kidneys (40–50%), muscles (25–50%), GI tract (30%), and testes (2–29%) [2]. Lungs and spleen are rarely involved. Angiography shows microaneursyms in renal, hepatic, and mesenteric arteries in 2/3 of patients and nonspecific occlusive changes in 98% [87]. About 30% of patients relapse [58]. Death most commonly ensues from mesenteric vasculitis.

There are no diagnostic criteria for PAN, but the 2007 European Medicines Agency classification criteria allow for a PAN designation in patients having histology compatible with CHCC PAN (no microvascular involvement or granulomas) or typical angiographic features of PAN but no ANCAs, surrogate clinical markers of upper/lower airway granulomatous disease, surrogate markers of glomerulonephritis, or eosinophilic lung disease [47].

Based on a review of over 1000 patients in 13 old series (prior to 1994), neuropathies occur in 60% of patients with PAN [88]. In the only large post-CHCC study of 348 patients with PAN, neuropathies occurred in 74% of patients, including 85% of those with hepatitis B-related PAN and 68% of those with non-viral PAN [58]. In five much smaller series since 1994, neuropathies developed in 52% of patients [89–93]. None of the post-CHCC studies presented data on cranial nerve involvement.

12.4.2 Microscopic Polyangiitis

MPA is a "microscopic" form of PAN that primarily affects arterioles, capillaries, and venules [59, 72, 94]. In contrast to GPA and EGPA, there are no granulomas. Unlike the immune complex vasculitides, immune deposits are inconspicuous. Clinically, MPA is similar to PAN, but distinguishing features include rapidly progressive glomerulonephritis in ~80% of patients, occasional pulmonary involvement (20% with alveolar hemorrhage), ANCAs, and the absence of visceral aneurysms. MPO-ANCAs are positive in 71–88% of patients and PR3-ANCAs in another 5–9% [95].

Peripheral neuropathy was consistently identified in 20% of patients with MPA in the 1980s nephrology literature [96–100]. However, in 19 series since the 1994 CHCC, the prevalence of neuropathy in MPA has been highly variable (7–58%), indicative of implicit biases [39, 59, 68, 69, 72, 89, 101–113]. The 7% incidence in one retrospective study was likely an underestimate due to insensitivity of the screening process [68]. Combined data from these 20 studies yield an overall prevalence of 30%. In all of these cohorts, the percentage of patients with renal involvement was high (57–100%). In these studies, neuropathies were more commonly identified in patients lacking in renal involvement. This observation is consistent with the inverse relationship between PNS and renal involvement in MPA revealed in the DCVAS analysis cited above [69]. Possible reasons for this relationship include a true pathogenic interaction, varying attention to neuropathy between nephrology and non-nephrology centers, and misclassification. The prevalence of neuropathy in childhood-onset MPA is much lower (3%) [114–116]. Cranial neuropathies occur in 8% of patients with MPA [39, 68, 107].

12.4.3 Eosinophilic Granulomatosis with Polyangiitis

EGPA is another AAV, but ANCAs only occur in 30–40% of patients (usually MPO-ANCAs) [60, 73, 117, 118]. Its salient histopathologic alterations are (1) eosinophilic tissue infiltration, (2) extravascular granulomas, and (3) small-vessel vasculitis [118]. The Lanham diagnostic criteria require (1) asthma, (2) eosinophilia (>1500/mm^3), and (3) vasculitis involving two or more non-pulmonary sites [118]. Clinical features distinguishing EGPA from PAN are (1) asthma (100% of patients), (2) pulmonary infiltrates (50–75%), (3) allergic rhinosinusitis (60–80%), (4) glomerulonephritis (15–30%), and (5) congestive heart failure (25%) [2]. In adults, neuropathies occur in 65% of patients [60, 66, 69, 73, 104, 118–122], contrasting with only 35% of children [123–125]. Cranial neuropathies develop in about 5% of patients [18, 39, 60, 66, 107, 126, 127].

In 2017, a European task force proposed a revised nomenclature for EGPA and a new entity referred to as eosinophilic asthma with systemic manifestations (HASM), designed to restrict the diagnosis of EGPA to patients with clinical or pathological evidence of systemic vasculitis [128]. Under this proposal, EGPA is defined as hypereosinophilic asthma accompanied by biopsy-proven vasculitis, biopsy-revealed leukocytoclastic capillaritis or eosinophilic infiltration of arterial wall, alveolar hemorrhage, palpable purpura, myocardial infarction due to coronary arteritis, clinical surrogates of glomerulonephritis, multifocal neuropathy, or ANCAs occurring with any systemic manifestations. The incidence of neuropathy in EGPA will undoubtedly increase with this new definition.

12.4.4 Granulomatosis with Polyangiitis

GPA is defined by the pathological triad of granulomatous inflammation, necrosis, and vasculitis predominating in the respiratory tracts and kidneys [129–131].

Vasculitis affects the microvasculature and small-to-medium-sized arteries and veins. In patients with active, generalized disease, ANCAs directed against PR3 occur in 77–81% of patients, while MPO-ANCAs are found in 9–12% [95]. ANCA positivity decreases to 40–60% in those with inactive or limited disease.

In numerous studies and literature reviews dating back to 1975, the prevalence of neuropathy in GPA has consistently ranged from 15% to 20% [69, 80, 81, 103, 107, 108, 112, 129, 131, 132], except for a higher prevalence in Germany, where 40% of GPA patients develop neuropathy [130]. Hence, patients with GPA or PR3-related AAV are less likely to develop a SVN than those with EGPA, MPA, or MPO-related AAV. Neuropathies are rare (2%) in childhood-onset GPA [133–135]. Cranial neuropathies, often multiple and most commonly involving nerves II, VI, or VII, occur in ~10% of patients, but they usually result from contiguous extension of nasal or paranasal granulomas rather than vasculitis [25, 68, 80, 81].

12.5 Nerve Pathology

Nerve biopsies in patients with SVN and NSVN reveal changes indicative of an axonal neuropathy because axons are more vulnerable to ischemia than Schwann cells [26, 51]. Affected fascicles usually exhibit decreased myelinated nerve fiber density, prominent Wallerian-like degeneration, and regenerating axonal clusters [14, 20, 26, 31, 51] (Fig. 12.4). Axon loss tends to be centrofascicular in proximal watershed areas (e.g., sciatic nerve bifurcation in distal thigh) but becomes multifocal in distal parts of the nerve due to intermingling of descending fibers (Fig. 12.4) [82, 136, 137]. Segmental demyelination/remyelination is also sometimes increased, but tends to cluster on individual teased fibers and consecutive internodes, consistent with secondary demyelination induced by axonal atrophy [138]. Some studies have reported preferential involvement of larger myelinated nerve fibers [139], while others have not [31]. In fulminant vasculitis, Schwann cells, fibroblasts, and all other cellular elements are lost.

Nerve large arteriole or systemic PNS vasculitis primarily affects epineurial vessels with diameters of 50–300 μm [9, 20, 26, 31, 37, 51]. NSVN tends to involve smaller vessels (<100 μm) within this range but is not limited to the microvasculature [31, 32]. All endoneurial and perineurial vessels are microscopic (<40 μm); these vessels are only infrequently affected in vasculitis [51]. Active vasculitic lesions are characterized by epineurial T-cells and macrophages surrounding and invading vessel walls, producing fibrinoid necrosis and other signs of vascular damage (Fig. 12.1). Cellular infiltrates are perivascular and predominate in the epineurium. They consist primarily of T-cells and macrophages, with T-cells generally outnumbering macrophages by a factor of 2–3 [18, 31, 140–144]. B-cells are uncommon (2–6% of cells), and natural killer cells and polymorphonuclear leukocytes rare. Epineurial T-cells are almost always CD4+ or CD8+ with varying CD4+/CD8+ ratios. No immunohistochemical (IHC) studies of plasma, dendritic, or T-regulatory cells have appeared. Direct immunofluorescence (DIF) shows immune deposits of IgM, fibrinogen, C3, or complement terminal membrane attack complex (C5b9) in

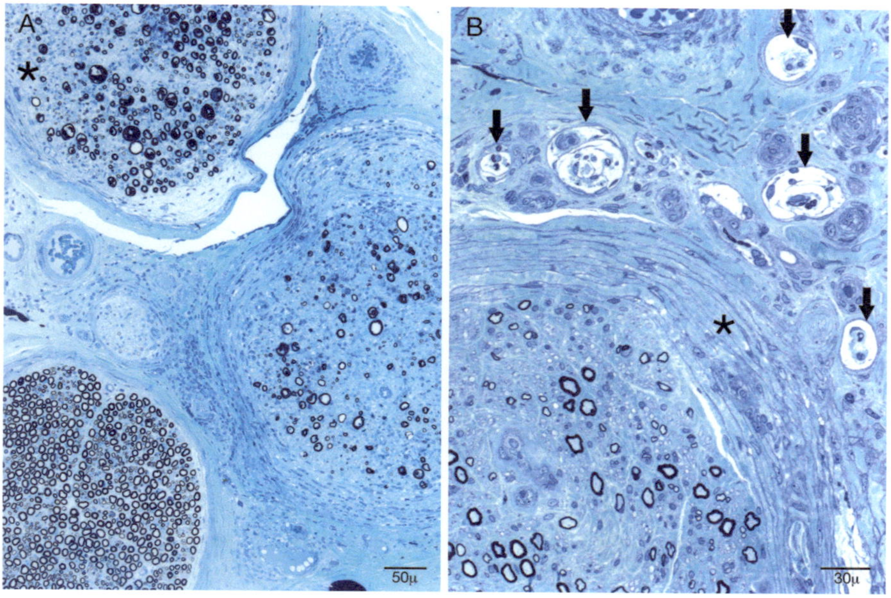

Fig. 12.4 Typical findings of ischemic injury of nerve. Two epoxy cross sections of nerve stained with methylene blue. In **a**, there is multifocal fiber loss. The lower fascicle has a normal density and size distribution of myelinated nerve fibers. The upper fascicle (asterisk) has a mildly reduced density and many actively degenerating fibers. The middle fascicle has thickened perineurium and marked reduction in fiber density. Three microvessels surrounding the middle fascicle are surrounded by mononuclear inflammatory cells (perivascular inflammation). In **b**, there are multiple microfascicles (arrows), sometimes containing small myelinated nerve fibers, surrounding a parent fascicle at the bottom left with thickened perineurium (asterisk) and reduced density of myelinated fibers

epineurial vessel walls in 55–80% of patients (Fig. 12.5) [16, 20, 140, 145]. C3d epineurial vascular deposits were more common in NSVN than MPA-associated SVN in one study [146].

The final common pathway of tissue damage is regional ischemia due to occlusion of the involved epineurial or nutrient vessels. Peripheral nerves have a rich anastomotic vascular supply composed of two integrated but distinct systems [147]. This rich blood supply, coupled with the ability of the nerve to tolerate anaerobic conditions, enables the PNS to resist the effects of chronic ischemia [148]. Only with extensive involvement of the vasa nervorum does ischemia induce axonal degeneration. In experimental models of small vessel occlusion, the central regions of large fascicles in proximal nerves degenerate most consistently [136]. Autopsy studies of peripheral nerves in patients with SVN (MPA and rheumatoid vasculitis) have shown that vasculitis is distributed in the epineurium throughout the proximal and distal segments of nerves, but myelinated fiber loss and Wallerian-like degeneration begin in the middle nerve segments, corresponding to the distal upper arm and distal thigh [82, 137]. Likewise, the ischemic pattern of centrofascicular degeneration occurs only in proximal and middle nerve segments, while diffuse nerve

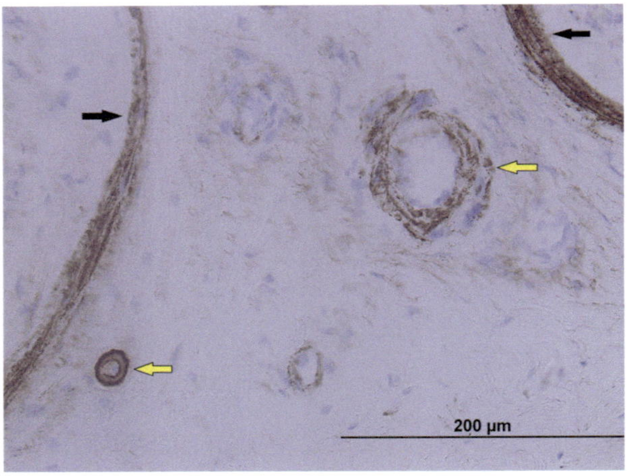

Fig. 12.5 High-power frozen section of nerve immunostained for C5b9 (complement membrane attack complex) showing deposits of C5b9 in the perineuria of two adjacent fascicles (black arrows), a normal finding, and in the vessel walls of an epineurial capillary and large arteriole (yellow arrows) in a patient with vasculitic neuropathy

loss predominates distally. In teased nerve fiber examinations, myelin wrinkling and mild demyelination/remyelination predominate in proximal sections, contrasting with axonal degeneration in distal sections. The spinal cord, dorsal root and sympathetic ganglia, and ventral/dorsal roots are spared. Systemic vasculitis thus tends to affect the PNS diffusely but produces maximal damage in a border zone vulnerable to ischemia in the proximal/middle portions of the extremities.

12.6 Pathogenesis of Vasculitic Neuropathy

While ANCAs appear important to the pathogenesis of AAV, they are unlikely to mediate VNs. For example, nerve biopsies in patients with SVN and NSVN only rarely reveal neutrophils, the chief effector cells in AAV [18, 31, 140]. In addition, while biopsies in most tissues in patients with AAV are "pauci-immune" (i.e., few immunoglobulins and complement deposits in involved tissues), vascular immune deposits are common in nerve biopsies of patients with VN [145]. Moreover, in EGPA—the AAV most closely associated with neuropathy—most patients with neuropathy are ANCA-negative [61]. Finally, in the most common VN—NSVN—ANCAs are rarely present [44].

The available evidence suggests that NSVN and most SVNs are mediated primarily by T-cell mechanisms (cytokine-mediated inflammation, macrophage activation, and/or direct T-cell cytotoxicity). First, a DNA microarray analysis of nerve biopsies in patients with VN revealed many genes involved in T-cell and macrophage responses to be differentially upregulated [149]. Second, an analysis of mRNA expression in nerve biopsies of patients with SVN revealed a Th1 cytokine profile and upregulation of chemokines and chemokine receptors involved in the migration and activation of T-cells and macrophages [150]. Third, nerve biopsies in patients with NSVN and SVN consistently demonstrate a predominance of CD4+ or CD8+ T-cells and macrophages in the epineurium, with many of the T-cells expressing markers of cytotoxic T lymphocytes (CTLs) [31, 140, 141, 151]. Fourth, antigen-presenting cells (macrophages and—to a lesser extent—T-cells, Schwann cells, endothelial cells, and perineurial cells) are increased in the epineurium and endoneurium [140, 143, 152]. Fifth, co-stimulatory molecule CD86, which interacts with CD28 on naïve T-cells, is upregulated on endothelial cells in NSVN [152]. Sixth, co-stimulatory molecule ICOS (inducible costimulator), which is expressed preferentially by effector memory T-cells, is upregulated on epineurial T-cells, while ICOS-ligand is upregulated on epineurial macrophages, suggesting that macrophages act as antigen-presenting cells to re-stimulate activated T-cells [54]. Seventh, CD58—an adhesion/co-stimulatory molecule that interacts with CD2 on T-cells—is upregulated on Schwann cells and endothelial cells [152]. Eighth, allograft inflammatory factor (AIF)-1 expression is upregulated in T-cells, macrophages, and vascular smooth muscle cells in patients with VNs. AIF-1 promotes macrophage and T-cell activation, proliferation, and migration [153].

These and other observations support a pathogenic model wherein disease-specific, autoreactive T-cells are recruited to the PNS; recognize self-glycolipid or peptide antigens presented by macrophages, Schwann cells, and/or endothelial cells; undergo activation; and then mature into CTLs or Th1 helper cells that stimulate inflammation and activate other leukocytes, thereby damaging targeted epineurial vessels. However, arguing against this model, one analysis of T-cell receptor Vβ gene utilization in epineurial infiltrates in sural nerve biopsies of five NSVN patients demonstrated no evidence of clonally expanded populations of T-cells, suggesting that polyclonal T-cells had been recruited nonspecifically to the PNS during the course of the inflammatory response, and in another investigation of patients with both NSVN and SVN, apoptosis was restricted to perivascular mononuclear cells, implicating apoptosis in recovery from rather than mediation of vascular injury [151, 154]. These studies imply that T-cells might have a nonspecific or regulatory rather than pathogenic role in VN.

Humoral mechanisms probably also contribute to the pathogenesis of VN. As noted above, epineurial vessel walls often contain deposits of immunoglobulin and complement [145]. Compellingly, an analysis of differential gene expression in patients with VN revealed immunoglobulin genes to be maximally upregulated, indicative of B-cell selection and antigen recognition [149]. A C1q gene was also upregulated, suggesting concomitant activation of the classical complement pathway. Therefore, immune complex deposition or in situ formation with subsequent activation of complement and recruitment of phagocytes might constitute another mechanism of vascular damage in VN.

A recent histopathological study offered further support for humoral mechanisms in VN and suggested that NSVN and MPA might be mediated by distinct pathways [146]. In this investigation, sural nerve biopsies from 24 patients with NSVN and 37 with MPA-associated neuropathy (MPAN) were examined. IHC stains for C3d revealed significantly more frequent epineurial vascular deposits in NSVN than MPAN. On the other hand, electron microscopy showed attachment of neutrophils to endothelial cells of epineurial small vessels more frequently in MPAN than NSVN, and IHC stains demonstrated MPO-positive neutrophils adhering to the endothelial cells of epineurial vessels more often in MPAN than

NSVN. The authors concluded that attachment of neutrophils to endothelial cells might be an early lesion in MPAN but not NSVN, consistent with the frequent occurrence of ANCAs in MPA but not NSVN. Complement participated in the pathogenesis of vasculitis of both neuropathies but was a more salient feature of NSVN. This study had several methodological flaws, including the failure to control for duration of vasculitis, therapy, and duration of the surgical procedure.

Many other inflammatory mediators are upregulated or over-produced in nerve specimens from patients with SVN and NSVN, including pro-inflammatory cytokines [142, 150, 155, 156]; nitric oxide [141, 150]; cyclooxygenase-2 [141, 157]; matrix metalloproteinase (MMP)-1, 2 and 9 [141, 150, 158–160]; receptor for advanced glycation end-products [161]; nuclear factor κβ [156, 161, 162]; various cellular adhesion molecules [152, 156, 163, 164]; oxidative and hypoxic stress-induced proteins [54, 150, 161]; components of the plasminogen activator system [150]; and neutrophil extracellular traps [165].

12.7 Differential Diagnosis

The differential diagnosis of VN includes numerous non-vasculitic etiologies of a sensory-motor or sensory asymmetric/multifocal neuropathy. The full list is extensive and was recently reviewed [43]. Among the more common or important conditions to consider are hereditary neuropathy with liability to pressure palsies (HNPP), non-HNPP-related multiple nerve entrapments, multiple compressive radiculopathies, Lewis–Sumner syndrome or multifocal chronic inflammatory demyelinating polyneuropathy (CIDP), sarcoidosis, sensory neuronopathy (paraneoplastic or Sjögren syndrome-related), leprosy, Lyme disease, HIV infection (with secondary cytomegalovirus (CMV) infection, varicella-zoster virus (VZV) infection, or diffuse infiltrative lymphocytosis syndrome), amyloidosis, porphyria, neoplastic cell infiltration, other paraneoplastic neuropathies, chronic graft-versus-host disease, and motor neuron disease with sensory involvement. Electrodiagnostic testing permits differentiation of the demyelinating features of Lewis–Sumner syndrome, HNPP, and leprosy from the axonal pattern of VN.

The differential diagnosis for a rapidly progressive, symmetric, axonal, sensory-motor presentation of VN includes but is not limited to the acute inflammatory demyelinating and acute motor-sensory axonal variants of Guillain–Barré syndrome; critical illness neuropathy; acute alcohol-nutritional deficiency neuropathies; other causes of severe polynutritional deficiency, such as inadequate dietary intake, repeated vomiting after gastric reduction surgery, other GI disorders, beriberi, and emesis gravidarum; acute exposures to certain drugs or toxins; the acute painful diabetic neuropathy; and high-grade neoplastic infiltrative neuropathies.

For patients diagnosed with definite or clinically probable VN, the differential diagnosis includes all conditions associated with PNS vasculitis (Box 12.1). Determination of the type of VN depends on evaluation of the clinical presentation, laboratory findings, and nerve pathology.

Pathologically, almost all vasculitides have the potential to involve vessels in a size range atypical for that disease [51]. Because of this overlap, identification of the

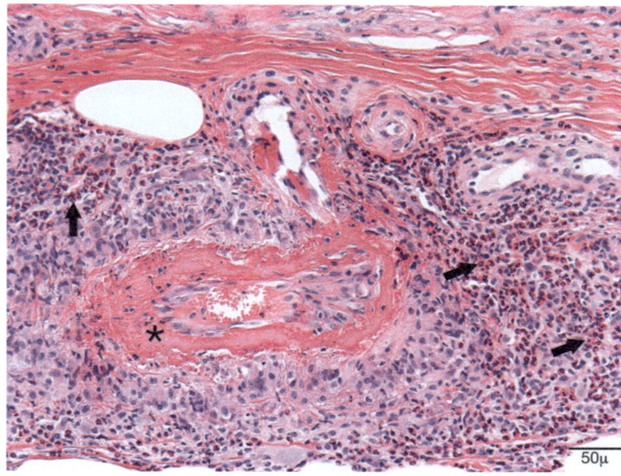

Fig. 12.6 Paraffin section of nerve showing definite necrotizing vasculitis, featuring fibrinoid necrosis of the vessel wall (asterisk) and frequent eosinophils (arrows). The robust eosinophilic infiltration suggests that this vasculitis is due to eosinophilic granulomatosis with polyangiitis (EGPA)

caliber and type of affected vessels does not indicate a specific disorder but can be used to refine the differential diagnosis. Similarly, the cellular composition of the vasculitic infiltrates does not reliably distinguish between the vasculitides [51]. PAN is a necrotizing vasculitis involving small- to medium-sized arteries [166]. Granulomas and eosinophilic infiltrates are rare. Considering the CHCC restriction of PAN to small-to-medium-sized arteries, microvascular or venular involvement excludes PAN [1]. MPA is also a necrotizing vasculitis that affects arterioles, capillaries, and venules primarily [167]. In contrast to GPA and EGPA, there are no granulomas, and unlike NSVN or the immune-complex small-vessel vasculitides, few immune deposits are seen. The three salient histopathological alterations of EGPA are eosinophilic tissue infiltration, extravascular granulomas, and small-vessel necrotizing vasculitis (Fig. 12.6) [1, 118]. In six series reporting nerve biopsy findings in EGPA, necrotizing vasculitis was observed in 30%, eosinophilic infiltrates in 35–40%, and granulomas in 5% [18, 38, 63–65, 70]. CD4+/CD8+ T-cells are the predominant cellular constituent in the vascular aggregates. GPA is defined by the pathological triad of granulomatous inflammation, necrosis, and vasculitis [168]. Vasculitis affects the microvasculature and small-to-medium-sized arteries and veins. Open lung biopsies are the most reliable method of diagnosis, yielding vasculitis, necrosis, and granulomas in 90% of specimens [169]. Information on nerve pathology is sparse [170]. NSVN exhibits nonspecific, non-granulomatous changes reminiscent of PAN, MPA, or the microvasculitides, albeit with frequent vascular immune deposits [43].

12.8 Diagnosis of Vasculitic Neuropathy

The important first step in diagnosis is to recognize the clinical pattern as one compatible with a VN. This process requires characterization of the neuropathy's tempo (acute, subacute, chronic), clinical course (steadily or stepwise progressive, stable, improving), functional involvement (sensory-motor, pure sensory, pure motor), anatomic pattern (distal symmetric, distal and proximal symmetric, asymmetric, multifocal), and inferred pathology (axonal, demyelinating). Painful, stepwise progressive, distal-predominant, asymmetric/multifocal, axonal, sensory-motor neuropathies are particularly concerning for vasculitis, even with a clinical course of several years. Conversely, pure motor or indolently progressive, distal, symmetric polyneuropathies are rarely vasculitic.

12.8.1 Electrodiagnostic Evaluation

Electromyography (EMG) and nerve conduction studies (NCS) help to determine the distribution of nerve involvement (focal, multifocal, or length-dependent), identify the involved functional modalities (sensory and/or motor), infer the probable nerve pathology (axon loss versus demyelination), and select an appropriate nerve to biopsy [55, 171]. Electrodiagnostic findings in VN usually reflect the underlying pathology of multifocal axonal damage to motor and sensory fibers. NCS demonstrate low-amplitude or absent compound sensory nerve and muscle action potentials with normal or mildly reduced conduction velocities, indicative of axon loss. H reflexes and F waves are often impersistent with normal or mildly prolonged latencies. Needle EMG demonstrates active denervation (fibrillation potentials) in 70% of patients, decreased recruitment in clinically weak muscles, and motor unit potential remodeling consistent with chronic reinnervation in those with sufficiently long-standing disease or pre-existing neurogenic disorders [44]. Short-duration motor unit potentials, suggestive of a concomitant myopathy, occur in 10–15% of patients with SVN [10, 23, 29, 30], but not in those with NSVN [15, 23, 30]. Pre-existing neuropathies, entrapments, and radiculopathies need to be kept in mind when interpreting the data.

Findings of axon loss in an asymmetric or multifocal pattern are supportive of a VN [55]. Conversely, symmetric findings reduce the likelihood of vasculitis. In motor and sensory NCS, an inter-side amplitude asymmetry of ≥50% is generally taken as significant, but evidence suggests that the cutoff should be lower for the ulnar motor nerve (25–30%) and higher for the peroneal motor and sural sensory nerves (at least 60%) [172–174]. Other NCS findings suggestive of an asymmetric/multifocal process are a significant amplitude differences between nerves of similar length in one limb and significantly lower amplitudes in upper limb nerves than lower limb nerves unexplained by entrapments. In a multifocal neuropathy, needle EMG usually reveals active and/or chronic partial denervation in a non-length-dependent distribution, e.g., conspicuous inter-side differences in denervation between homologous muscles, greater denervation in proximal than distal muscles, disproportionate involvement of a single nerve in one limb, and greater denervation in upper limb than lower limb muscles [172].

"Pseudo" conduction blocks are identified in ~10% of patients with VN. They occur when motor NCS are performed shortly after an ischemic insult to the nerve [9, 15, 30, 32, 34, 36, 41]. In this situation, the amplitude/area of the compound muscle action potential drops with proximal stimulation because Wallerian-like degeneration has not yet developed in the distal stump of the damaged nerve, which, therefore, continues to conduct action potentials, contrasting with failure of conduction across the non-functional, ischemic nerve fibers. Following axonal degeneration, which develops over the next week, conduction failure occurs with both proximal and distal stimulation and the apparent "conduction block" disappears. Sensory nerve action potentials also decline in amplitude and often disappear over 7–10 days after the ischemic event. True demyelinating but generally transient partial motor conduction blocks are more rarely seen [175], but significantly reduced conduction velocities or other findings indicative of demyelination, such as abnormal temporal dispersion or persistent conduction block, are rare and should prompt consideration of an alternative diagnosis, such as Lewis–Sumner syndrome.

12.8.2 Laboratory Evaluation

Laboratory evaluation of a patient with a suspected VN is designed to assess for (1) extra-neurologic organ dysfunction, (2) measures of systemic inflammation, and (3) specific causes of a multifocal neuropathy or vasculitis. In the Peripheral Nerve Society guideline on NSVN, consensus was reached on laboratory tests to be considered when evaluating a patient with an unexplained, progressive neuropathy suspicious for vasculitis [44]. Routinely obtained laboratory tests include complete blood count, metabolic panel, urinalysis, erythrocyte sedimentation rate (ESR), C-reactive protein (CRP), antinuclear antibodies (ANA), ANCAs, rheumatoid factor (RF), angiotensin-converting enzyme, serum protein immunofixation electrophoresis, glucose tolerance testing and/or glycosylated hemoglobin, cryoglobulins, complement, hepatitis B surface antigen, hepatitis C antibodies, and chest X-ray. Testing for other inflammatory, genetic, or infectious disorders (e.g., HIV, PB19, CMV, VZV, Lyme disease, porphyria, and transthyretin amyloidosis) should be considered in select cases. As malignancies underlie only 2–3% of reported cases of VN (Table 12.1), cancer screening should be performed only if indicated by other clinical features, laboratory findings, or risk factors. Laboratory studies predictive of biopsy-confirmed VN include elevated ESR, CRP, RF, β2-microglobulin, MPO-ANCAs, plasma vascular endothelial growth factor (VEGF), and neurofilament light chain levels [44, 176]. Based on direct comparisons of cohorts of patients with NSVN and SVN, the best laboratory predictors of an underlying systemic vasculitis in a patient presenting with VN are ANCAs and ESR $\geq$ 100 mm/h [44].

In NSVN, a mildly to moderately elevated ESR occurs in 50% of patients, but extreme elevation is concerning for a systemic condition [43]. Other laboratory markers of inflammation or immune system activation (e.g., ANA, RF, anemia, leukocytosis, and hypocomplementemia) are abnormal in less than 25% of patients [43]. ANCAs are rare and, if present, exclude the diagnosis [44]. In patients with SVN, laboratory abnormalities are more common. In PAN, laboratory studies reveal highly elevated ESR in more than 85% of patients and leukocytosis, anemia, and thrombocytosis in 60–70%. ANAs, RFs, and reduced circulating complement occur less commonly (15–30%) [2, 58]. ANCAs are absent. In MPA, the incidence of increased ESR, anemia, leukocytosis, ANAs, and RFs is similar to that in PAN, but hypocomplementemia is rare. ANCAs are positive in 85–90% of MPA patients, mostly MPO-ANCAs. In EGPA, elevated ESR, leukocytosis, and anemia occur in 80–90% of patients, but ANAs, cryoglobulins, and complement are usually normal or negative. IgE levels are elevated in 75% of patients and RFs in 40–50%. ANCAs occur in 30–40%, usually MPO-ANCAs. Laboratory findings in GPA include markedly elevated ESR in 80–85% of patients, anemia in ~75%, thrombocytosis in ~55%, leukocytosis in 35%, RFs in 50–60%, and ANAs in 25%. PR3-ANCAs occur in 90% of patients with active disease.

CSF analysis is not usually helpful. Pleocytosis is uncommon (5–10% of patients), and mild-to-moderate protein elevation occurs in 30–35% of patients with both NSVN and SVN [9–11, 14, 15, 20, 22, 23, 30, 31, 34]. Lumbar puncture should be considered in patients with (1) proximal signs and symptoms suggestive of root involvement; (2) electrodiagnostic evidence of demyelinating or mixed axonal/demyelinating features; or (3) clinically suspected sarcoidosis, cancer, or meningeal infection [44].

12.8.3 Pathological Diagnostic Criteria

The gold standard for diagnosis of VN is nerve biopsy evidence of *definite vasculitis.* In 2010, the Peripheral Nerve Society guideline group published consensus criteria for *pathologically definite VN* [44]. The group's consensus was that vascular wall inflammation must be accompanied by active or chronic vascular damage to qualify as definite vasculitis (Fig. 12.1). Microvasculitis, defined as inflammation of microvessels *without vascular damage*, was deemed nonspecific, as it can occur in many non-vasculitic neuropathies [37, 177–179]. The Peripheral Nerve Society guideline group's definition was subsequently adapted by the Brighton Collaboration Vasculitic Peripheral Neuropathy Working Group in 2017 [180].

Nerve biopsies that fail to satisfy criteria for definite vasculitis sometimes meet less specific criteria for *pathologically probable VN.* The Peripheral Nerve Society guideline group formulated such criteria after reviewing the evidence on pathological findings associated with definite VN [44]. Their consensus was that a diagnosis of pathologically probable VN required predominantly axonal alterations together with either (1) perivascular inflammation and pathological signs of vascular damage or (2) perivascular or vascular inflammation accompanied by one of five pathological predictors of VN (vascular deposits of complement, IgM or fibrinogen detectable with DIF; hemosiderin deposits detectable with Perls' stain; asymmetric nerve fiber loss or degeneration; prominent active axonal degeneration; and myofiber necrosis, regeneration, or infarcts in concomitant peroneus brevis muscle biopsy) (Figs. 12.4, 12.5, 12.7) [44].

Subsequent to the formulation of the Peripheral Nerve Society criteria, a case–control study showed that vessel-bound T-cells and CD68+ macrophages were significantly more prevalent in skin biopsies from 17 patients with untreated NSVN than those from 10 patients with non-inflammatory axonal neuropathies and nine

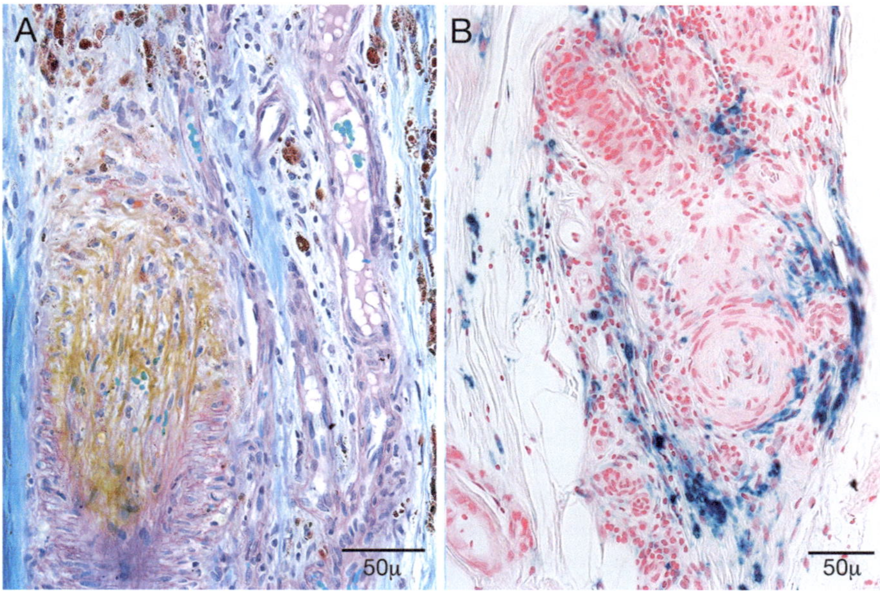

Fig. 12.7 Longitudinal paraffin sections from vasculitic nerves showing prior bleeding due to vessel wall damage and leakage in necrotizing vasculitis. In **a** (LFB/PAS), there are frequent macrophages laden with dark brown balls of mature hemosiderin (upper and right sectors), contrasting with earlier appearing, light brown hemosiderin or biliverdin (left center) in the occluded vessel lumen having a more dispersed appearance and not arranged in balls. In **b** (Turnbull Blue), blue-staining, hemosiderin-laden macrophages surround an inflamed blood vessel

healthy controls [181]. Based on this finding, the Brighton Collaboration case definition of VN included "perivascular mononuclear inflammation in skin biopsy obtained concurrently with nerve biopsy" as a sixth criterion to support a diagnosis of pathologically probable VN [180]. The association between increased cutaneous perivascular T-cells/macrophages and biopsy-confirmed VN was recently extended to six patients with SVN [144]. Focal perineurial damage/thickening, injury neuroma with microfasciculation, endoneurial hemorrhage, and epineurial neovascularization are also utilized as supportive features by some workers, but their specificity for vasculitis is not fully established (Fig. 12.4) [37, 44, 182].

12.8.4 Clinical Diagnostic Criteria

Evidence of *pathologically definite VN* in a nerve biopsy permits a diagnosis of *clinically definite VN*, irrespective of clinical phenotype. Without such evidence, patients can still be diagnosed with *clinically probable VN* if their clinicopathological profile matches that of a typical biopsy-proven case of VN, but to facilitate this diagnosis, a case definition is required. The Peripheral Nerve Society guideline group on NSVN designed such a case definition after reviewing the evidence on clinical and laboratory predictors of definite VN and analyzing uncontrolled NSVN/SVN series to determine the typical phenotype of a VN [44]. Features with high sensitivity for VN were electrodiagnostically revealed axonal neuropathy, distal predominance, electrodiagnostic evidence of asymmetric/multifocal process, clinically asymmetric/multifocal neuropathy, pain, fibrillation potentials in at least one muscle by EMG, and clinical course characterized by at least one acute attack. Conversely, factors with very low sensitivity were electrodiagnostic evidence of a demyelinating neuropathy, pure motor involvement, upper limb predominance, CSF pleocytosis, and CSF protein level >110 mg/dl.

The Brighton Collaboration case definition of VN was developed in 2015 and published in 2017 as a practical tool to help non-specialists identify patients with VN [180]. Although intended for use in epidemiological studies of adverse effects of vaccination, the definition was also applicable to vaccination-unrelated cases. It was adapted from the Peripheral Nerve Society criteria. The Brighton definition included three levels of diagnostic certainty (Boxes 12.2 and 12.3). The highest level required definite vasculitis in a nerve biopsy. The lowest level permitted a diagnosis of clinically probable VN based on history and examination alone. The intermediate level of certainty required biopsy evidence of definite vasculitis in another organ or nerve biopsy showing pathologically probable VN.

Box 12.2: Brighton Collaboration Case Definition of Vasculitic Neuropathy (Reproduced with Permission from [180])

Level 1 definition (gold standard)

Biopsy of peripheral nerve meets criteria for pathologically definite vasculitis

Level 2 definition

Clinical features are suggestive of vasculitic neuropathy (Box 12.3); and Histopathological support for the existence of vasculitis:

- Biopsy of peripheral nerve meets criteria for pathologically probable vasculitis; or
- Diagnosis of systemic vasculitis confirmed by biopsy; or
- Biopsy of skin or muscle meets criteria for pathologically definite vasculitis

Level 3 definition (minimum acceptable evidence)

- Biopsy of peripheral nerve or muscle not done or does not meet criteria for definite or probable vasculitis; and
- Clinical features are suggestive of vasculitic neuropathy (Box 12.3)

Box 12.3: Clinical Features Suggestive of Vasculitic Neuropathy (Brighton Collaboration) (Reproduced with Permission from [180])

1. Evidence of peripheral neuropathy
   (a) Electrodiagnostic evidence of an axonal neuropathy; or
   (b) Clinical examinations signs indicative of a peripheral neuropathy;
   AND
2. Clinical presentation typical of a vasculitic neuropathy
   (a) Sensory-motor or sensory (*not pure motor*); and
   (b) Multifocal[a] or asymmetric pattern,[b] not attributable to compression of peripheral nerves or nerve roots[c]; AND
   (c) Either:
      - Additional clinical features:
         - Lower limb predominant; and
         - Painful; and
         - One or more acute attacks,[d] or variable speed of progression, or improvement of motor or sensory deficit

      OR
      - Biopsy of nerve shows pathologically probable vasculitis

[a] "Multifocal" requires discrete involvement of multiple, individual, non-confluent peripheral nerves.

[b] "Asymmetric pattern" encompasses focal or multifocal neuropathies and all other neuropathies exhibiting significant inter-side differences or non-length-dependent features. Asymmetry and compression/entrapment may be demonstrated by history, examination, EMG/NCS, or imaging.

[c] If there are specific clinical features to suggest any of the following rare alternative diagnoses, which may cause asymmetric/multifocal neuropathy through a mechanism other than vasculitis, then further investigations may be necessary to distinguish these from VN: hereditary neuropathy, neoplastic cell infiltration in peripheral nerve, non-vasculitic paraneoplastic neuropathies, amyloidosis, sarcoidosis, Lewis–Sumner syndrome (multifocal CIDP), idiopathic brachial plexus neuropathy (neuralgic amyotrophy), chronic graft-versus-host disease, motor neuron disease with sensory involvement, neuroborreliosis (Lyme disease), leprosy.

[d] Onset to maximum severity within 1 month followed by spontaneous stabilization.

12.8.5 Nerve Biopsy

Considering the broad differential diagnosis of a multifocal/asymmetric neuropathy, serious risks of long-term immunosuppressive therapy, and absence of specific biomarkers for NSVN, most patients with clinically suspected VN should undergo nerve biopsy. One possible exception is a patient with an established diagnosis of systemic vasculitis who develops a multifocal neuropathy. Given the 20% prevalence of distal symmetric polyneuropathy in reported patients with VN, nerve biopsy should be considered in all patients with progressive axonal neuropathies, irrespective of symmetry, with the caveat that nerve biopsy in patients with an idiopathic, chronic, symmetric polyneuropathy yields definite vasculitis in only ~3% [13, 183, 184]. This low yield must be weighed against the risks of nerve biopsy, such as permanent sensory loss, chronic pain, delayed wound healing, and wound infection.

When performed, an accessible, clinically affected sensory nerve should be selected for biopsy. The most commonly biopsied nerves are the sural and superficial peroneal nerves, but other sensory nerves can be biopsied if clinically indicated, e.g., saphenous, intermediate femoral cutaneous, lateral antebrachial cutaneous, dorsal ulnar, and superficial radial nerves. Although nerve biopsy is more often diagnostic than muscle biopsy, especially in NSVN, one meta-analysis showed that muscle biopsy increased the yield for definite vasculitis by 15% in patients with a final diagnosis of VN [185]. However, in the only study in which a proximal muscle was biopsied (quadriceps), yield was not increased, suggesting that this conclusion pertains only to distal muscles [30]. Superficial peroneal nerve biopsy is always combined with peroneus brevis muscle biopsy through the same incision. Sural nerve biopsies can be combined with anterior tibialis, gastrocnemius, or soleus muscle biopsies. Others advocate fascicular biopsies of mixed proximal nerves in patients with abnormal MRIs of a proximal nerve or plexus [186].

In the absence of an independent gold standard, the true sensitivity of nerve or nerve/muscle biopsy for SVN or NSVN cannot be determined, but in patients for whom nerve biopsy does not provide proof of VN, clinically probable VN can still be diagnosed by recourse to the Peripheral Nerve Society or Brighton Collaboration case definitions. Assuming these clinically probable cases truly have VN, estimated sensitivities can be derived. On the basis of data from multiple studies, the estimated sensitivity of a finding of definite vasculitis in sural nerve biopsy alone is 50–55%, while that for combined SPN/PBM or sural nerve/distal leg muscle biopsy is about 60% [2].

12.8.6 Radiographic Evaluation

There is no established radiographic technique for diagnosing or monitoring VN. MRI guidance prior to targeted fascicular biopsies of proximal nerves and plexuses is routinely performed at the Mayo Clinic, but a comparison of its diagnostic accuracy in VN to that of distal lower limb cutaneous nerve biopsies has not been reported [186]. No series dedicated to peripheral nerve MRI findings in patients with pathologically proven VN has been published. There is a similar paucity of evidence on the use of PET scans to evaluate PNS disease activity in patients with SVN or NSVN, but a single case report suggested that it might have a role in identifying foci of extra-neurological involvement in patients presenting with clinically isolated VN [187].

Peripheral nerve ultrasonography has been investigated in VN. One study used ultrasonography to evaluate clinically involved tibial nerves in the ankles of eight patients with SVN. Compared to those in healthy controls, tibial nerves in patients with SVN had significantly larger mean cross-sectional areas [188]. In another study of 14 patients with SVN, ultrasound of 31 clinically involved nerves revealed focal enlargements in 22 [189]. Mean cross-sectional areas of the tibial, peroneal and—to a lesser extent—median and ulnar nerves were larger than those in healthy controls. In a third study, the sural, superficial peroneal, tibial, and peroneal nerves were assessed ultrasonically in six patients with biopsy-proven VN (four with NSVN), six with CIDP, five with non-immune neuropathies, and 26 healthy controls [190]. In patients with VN, the cross-sectional area of the sural nerve was significantly greater than that in healthy and disease controls, and the longitudinal diameter of the superficial peroneal nerve was greater than that in healthy controls. A fourth study, which compared ultrasonography of bilateral brachial plexus, median, ulnar, tibial, peroneal, and sural nerves in 16 patients with VN (11 SVN, 5 NSVN) to 16 controls with non-inflammatory axonal neuropathies, showed that multifocal nerve enlargements in proximal arm nerves were 94% sensitive and 88% specific for VN (Fig. 12.8) [191]. Hence, focal nerve enlargements might have a role in directing nerve biopsies and monitoring disease activity in VN, but further study is necessary.

12.9 Treatment

As previously noted, VN produces axon loss. Clinical recovery is thus dependent on the slow process of axonal regeneration. By inference, even if immunomodulatory therapy is successful in controlling the vasculitis, recovery of sensory and motor function will occur gradually over many months and may be incomplete in severely affected nerves. Hence, the short-term goal of therapy is to stabilize (not reverse) pre-existing neurologic deficits and prevent the development of new PNS lesions. During the initial weeks of therapy, caution must be exercised to avoid overtreatment if the patient is stable but unimproved. The long-term goal of therapy is, of course, to improve neurologic deficits, understanding that complete recovery from a severe axonal neuropathy is uncommon.

VN that develops in the setting of a systemic AAV is generally treated according to evidence-based guidelines for those diseases [192, 193]. However, in almost all treatment trials of systemic vasculitis, neuropathy outcome measures were nonexistent or unreliable, and to assume that the best treatment for life-threatening forms of systemic vasculitis, such as those affecting the kidneys or heart, are necessarily optimal for SVN would be incorrect. Nonetheless, data revealed or implied in these studies suggest that VNs do typically improve in concert with the nonneurologic manifestations [44, 127].

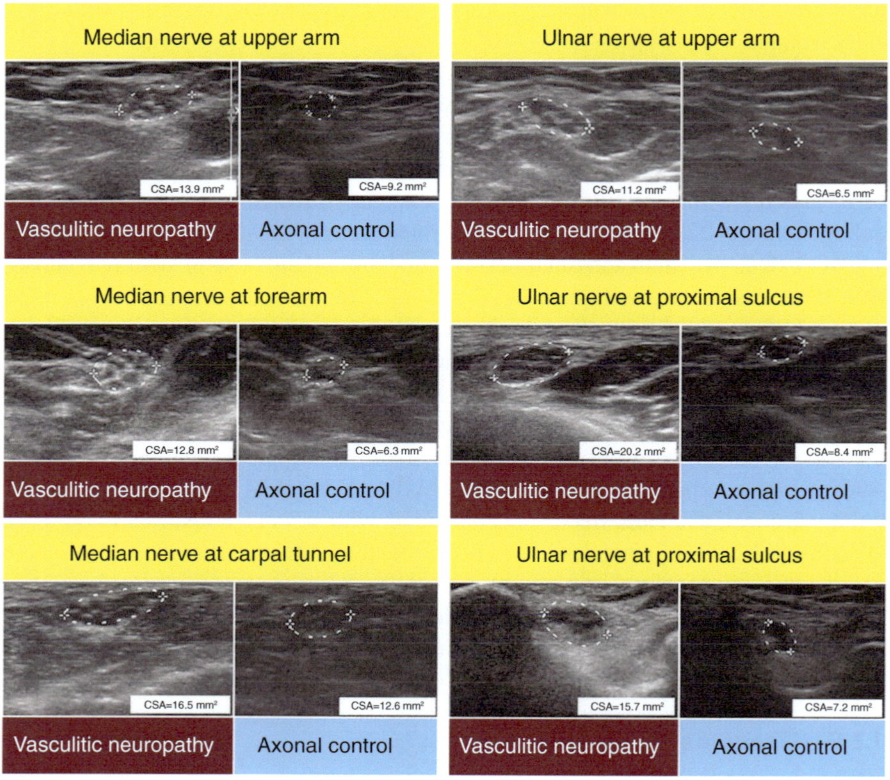

Fig. 12.8 Nerve sonography findings in patient with vasculitic neuropathy and non-inflammatory axonal disease control showing median and ulnar nerve enlargement (cross-sectional area >9 mm^2) at multiple sites outside common sites of nerve compression in patient with vasculitic neuropathy (left panels) but only in median nerve at carpal tunnel in non-inflammatory axonal disease control (right panels). Reproduced with permission from [191]

Extensive evidence on treatment of the primary small-to-medium-vessel systemic vasculitides was reviewed in the Peripheral Nerve Society guideline published in 2010 [44]. The introduction of corticosteroids (CS) and cyclophosphamide (CYC) in the 1950s transformed the survival rate of patients with PAN and GPA from only 10–15% at 1 year to 85–90% at 5 years. The serious adverse effects of long-term exposure to oral CYC have, since the 1990s, been reduced by lowering the cumulative dose of CYC via a pulse induction regime or by substituting potentially less toxic immunosuppressive agents for induction (e.g., methotrexate (MTX) or mycophenolate mofetil (MMF)) and/or maintenance (e.g., MTX or azathioprine (AZA)) of remission, albeit at the expense of higher relapse rates [194–198].

The current approach to the AAVs is to initiate induction therapy for 3–6 months to arrest the inflammatory process, followed by long-term immunosuppression with a maintenance drug [192, 193]. Maintenance therapy is generally continued for

18–24 months, but one large retrospective cohort survey and one randomized controlled trial (RCT) showed that longer duration maintenance therapy with AZA or MTX for >36 months or 48 months significantly reduced relapses [199, 200]. Since publication of the Peripheral Nerve Society guideline, evidence from three RCTs has shown that rituximab is at least as effective as CYC for induction of remission and more effective than AZA for maintenance of remission in the AAVs [201–203]. Hence, rituximab is now an option for both induction and maintenance therapy of AAV and may be preferred to CYC in PR3-associated AAV, relapsing patients, and those with fertility, compliance, and malignancy issues [192]. None of the RCTs of rituximab in AAV analyzed neuropathic endpoints, but eight retrospective series detailing the use of rituximab in treatment-refractory AAV provided data on neuropathies [61]. Almost 90% of neuropathies improved in these studies.

Relevant to patients with SVN are trials conducted by the French Vasculitis Study Group (FVSG) in patients with skin/nerve-predominant vasculitides. One prospective study of 124 patients with PAN or MPA and no poor-prognostic factors (renal, GI, cardiac, or CNS involvement) was conducted between 1993 and 2005 [204]. Vasculitis affected skin in 79% of patients and nerve in 66% of patients. Additional manifestations were uncommon (5–30% of patients). All patients initially received prednisone 1.0 mg/kg/day. Prednisone induced remission in 79% of patients, but the disease could not be controlled with CS alone in 45%, and 40% received second-line agents. Five-year survival was 92%. Long-term follow-up of this cohort was reported in 2014: CS monotherapy induced remission in 82% of patients, but 53% relapsed [205]. Throughout follow-up, 47% of patients required treatment with a second agent. Five-year survival was still 93%, but 78% of patients had chronic sequelae, including 49% with neuropathy. The investigators concluded that CS monotherapy commonly resulted in relapses and long-term sequelae.

In a subsequent study, the FVSG analyzed 118 patients from the same cohort in combination with 75 patients with EGPA who had no poor-prognostic factors and received similar treatment in order to identify patient characteristics associated with the need for immunosuppressive agents [206]. CS induced remission in 87% of patients, but add-on therapy was required in 45%, of which 60% developed chronic neuropathy. The only factor associated with the need for add-on therapy was multifocal neuropathy, suggesting that patients with multifocal neuropathy were more likely to fail CS monotherapy.

These observations prompted performance of a randomized, double-blind, placebo-controlled trial of AZA for 12 months added to CS for induction and maintenance of remission in patients with PAN, MPA, and EGPA lacking in poor prognostic factors [207]. In the 95 randomized patients, vasculitis predominated in the PNS (65%), skin (53%), and ENT domain (42%). Unfortunately, there were no significant differences favoring AZA in remission rate, relapse risk, or CS exposure.

This evidence suggests that patients with neuropathy-predominant SVN treated with CS monotherapy frequently relapse and develop chronic neuropathic sequelae, with the implication that combination therapy (CS and a second immunosuppressive agent) at baseline might improve long-term outcomes, but an alternative to AZA should be evaluated.

Treatment-resistant or refractory disease is defined as unchanged or increased disease activity after 4–6 weeks of CYC/CS therapy or improved but persistent disease activity after 8 weeks of therapy [208]. The Peripheral Nerve Society guideline group on NSVN reviewed 16 studies addressing treatment of refractory disease in patients with small-to-medium-vessel primary systemic vasculitis [44]. One study was class I and the rest were uncontrolled studies of 10 or more patients. The class I study was a double-blind RCT of IVIg in refractory GPA or MPA. Patients were randomized to IVIg 0.4 g/kg/day for 5 days versus placebo added to unchanged doses of immunosuppressive drugs [209]. Significantly more patients responded to IVIg (82%) than placebo (35%). Five of seven patients with neuropathy remitted. Hence, add-on therapy with IVIg is effective in improving disease activity in patients with refractory AAV. The agents investigated in the uncontrolled studies were IVIg, MMF, rituximab, anti-human thymocyte globulin, 15-deoxyspergualin, infliximab, and alemtuzumab. The group concluded that rituximab and IVIg were the most promising agents for refractory patients with SVN.

Three controlled studies of IVIg in newly diagnosed patients with small-to-medium-vessel SVN have been reported. Two prospective cohort surveys enrolled patients with EGPA [127, 210]. Neuropathy-related disability was measured with the modified Rankin scale. One study analyzed the addition of repeated cycles of IVIg and plasma exchange (PE) every 1–2 months for 1 year to CS in all patients and CYC in those with severe disease [127]. There were no significant differences in mortality or relapse rate, but IVIg/PE significantly improved the modified Rankin scale and Vasculitis Damage Index. In the second study, IVIg every 1–2 months for 1 year was added to CS or CYC/CS, yielding similar results plus significantly reduced relapses [210]. A blinded, placebo-controlled trial of IVIg 2 g/kg over 5 days in 23 patients with EGPA who were in remission by laboratory indices but had "residual" neuropathy-related weakness and numbness showed significantly improved strengths at 2 weeks as assessed by a manual muscle testing sum score, with the caveat that strengths in patients with chronic axon-loss neuropathies do not usually improve over 2-week intervals [211]. These studies suggest but do not prove that IVIg may be effective in patients with newly diagnosed and refractory EGPA-related SVN.

12.9.1 Evaluation of Outcome

A major difficulty in treating patients with VN is the absence of a simple way to monitor disease activity and remission, e.g., by recourse to a laboratory study or radiographic procedure. Subjective responses are important to consider, but improvements in pain, fatigue, and malaise more often reflect improvements in mood and sense of well-being than PNS function. Objective monitoring is crucial and depends on assessment of such measures as manual muscle testing-quantified weakness, sensory loss, maximized compound muscle and sensory nerve action potential amplitudes, needle EMG findings (fibrillation potentials),

ESR/CRP if elevated, ANCA titers (in AAV-related SVN), neuropathy impairment scores, and disability scales (e.g., Overall Neuropathy Limitations Scale) [212, 213].

While there is still no validated biomarker of SVN or NSVN, two candidates have emerged. One small study showed that plasma VEGF levels were significantly higher in five patients with VN (4 SVN and 1 NSVN) than in 18 control patients with Guillain–Barré syndrome, CIDP, or ALS [214]. In three patients with SVN, VEGF levels improved following successful therapy. Hence, plasma VEGF may be a reliable marker for the diagnosis and monitoring of SVN and NSVN, but larger trials are required. More recently, Bischof and colleagues showed that serum neurofilament light chain levels were significantly elevated in 10 patients with VN (8 SVN, 2 NSVN) compared to 10 patients with systemic vasculitis but no neuropathy, 30 healthy individuals, and three patients with non-vasculitic neuropathy (sensitivity 82% and specificity 100%) [176]. Levels were not increased in the two patients with NSVN. In SVN patients, the levels normalized in remission. This evidence suggests that serum neurofilament light chain level may be a useful biomarker in the diagnosis and management of SVN, but the finding should be confirmed.

Treatment of VN usually continues for more than 1 year. During this time, the clinician needs to frequently re-assess motor, sensory, and functional findings to ensure that the patient is not developing new deficits. Surveillance electrodiagnostic studies are usually unnecessary but can be helpful in equivocal situations. In patients with no other evidence of active vasculitis, worsening pain is not an indication to intensify immunosuppression unless concomitant neurologic deficits emerge. New motor or sensory deficits that arise during treatment are an indication to escalate therapy or change to a new agent. Stable deficits do not necessarily signify treatment failure, as recovery is a slow process.

12.9.2 Symptom Management

Supportive care of the patient with VN includes pain management, rehabilitation, counseling, and education. Immunosuppressive therapy is often effective in reducing neuropathic pain, but for many patients, pain control is still a high-priority issue, mandating the use of tricyclic antidepressants, gabapentin, pregabalin, serotonin-norepinephrine reuptake inhibitors, tramadol, topical lidocaine, topical capsaicin, and—in carefully selected patients—scheduled narcotics [215]. Second-line agents with unproven efficacy that can be tried in patients refractory to the first-line drugs include carbamazepine, oxcarbazepine, divalproex sodium, lamotrigine, topiramate, and mexilitine. In general, continued pain in the absence of progressive neurologic deficits is not an indication to continue high-dose CS.

Clinical research on rehabilitation interventions in VN is lacking. Rehabilitation issues can usually be addressed only after the patient's pain is reduced, neurologic status stabilized, and non-neurologic complications controlled. Physical therapy

Table 12.2 Neurologic outcomes in survivors of nonsystemic and systemic vasculitic neuropathies

Final disability [14–16, 18, 20, 21, 34, 41, 42, 127]	NSVN	SVN
No or essentially no symptoms	16/119 (13%)	16/102 (16%)
Mild symptoms, no restrictions	49/119 (41%)	36/102 (35%)
Mildly to moderately impaired, ambulatory without assistance	33/119 (28%)	32/102 (31%)
Ambulatory with assistance, dependent in some ADLs	17/119 (14%)	15/102 (15%)
Non-ambulatory	4/119 (3%)	3/102 (3%)

ADLs activities of daily living, *NSVN* nonsystemic vasculitic neuropathy, *SVN* systemic vasculitic neuropathies

is designed to improve strength, maintain range of motion, prevent contractures, limit osteoporosis, and minimize or prevent CS-induced myopathy. Occupational therapy is tailored to maximize function, especially for activities of daily living, sometimes facilitated by bracing of joints. Walking aids or even a manual or power wheelchair may be required to maintain mobility. Speech therapy is of lesser importance in VN.

The value of counseling and psychological support for patients with VN cannot be overemphasized. Because of chronic pain, physical limitations, exposure to CS, prolonged recovery, other disease-related morbidity, loss of gainful employment, and uncertain prognosis, patients with SVN are at high risk for developing depression and anxiety. Physicians need to educate patients about the chronic nature of their disease, including the fact that improvement may not occur for weeks to months after therapy has begun. Patients should be closely monitored for the emergence of depression, which if identified, should trigger pharmacologic support and psychiatric referral.

12.10 Outcome

For treated VN, the final outcome in long-term survivors is fairly good, but up to 60% report chronic pain [15]. No study has compared final disability in patients with NSVN and SVN, but data compiled from several series reveal similar outcomes (Table 12.2) [14–16, 18, 20, 21, 34, 41, 42, 127]. The favorable recovery seen in most patients with VN suggests that neurologic deficits do not exclusively result from ischemia-induced axon loss. True demyelinating or functional conduction blocks likely also contribute, supported by the observation that many patients show improved motor function (especially in proximal muscles) during the first 1–2 months of therapy, prior to the expected effects of axonal regeneration.

References

1. Jennette JC, Falk RJ, Bacon PA, et al. 2012 revised international Chapel Hill consensus conference nomenclature of vasculitides. Arthritis Rheum. 2013;65(1):1–11.
2. Collins MP, Arnold WD, Kissel JT. The neuropathies of vasculitis. Neurol Clin. 2013;31(2):557–95.
3. Gwathmey KG, Burns TM, Collins MP, Dyck PJ. Vasculitic neuropathies. Lancet Neurol. 2014;13(1):67–82.
4. Hernandez-Rodriguez J, Hoffman GS. Updating single-organ vasculitis. Curr Opin Rheumatol. 2012;24(1):38–45.
5. Boyd LJ. Periarteritis Nodosa. Neuromyositic manifestations. Bulletin NY Med Coll nd Flower Hospital. 1940;3(4):272–9.
6. Kernohan JW, Woltman HW. Periarteritis nodosa. A clinicopathologic study with special refereence to the nervous system. Arch Neurol Psychiatr. 1938;39:655–86.
7. Lovshin LL, Kernohan JW. Peripheral neuritis in periarteritis nodosa; a clinicopathologic study. Arch Intern Med (Chic). 1948;82(4):321–38.
8. Kissel JT, Slivka AP, Warmolts JR, Mendell JR. The clinical spectrum of necrotizing angiopathy of the peripheral nervous system. Ann Neurol. 1985;18(2):251–7.
9. Dyck PJ, Benstead TJ, Conn DL, Stevens JC, Windebank AJ, Low PA. Nonsystemic vasculitic neuropathy. Brain. 1987;110(Pt 4):843–53.
10. Bouche P, Leger JM, Travers MA, Cathala HP, Castaigne P. Peripheral neuropathy in systemic vasculitis: clinical and electrophysiologic study of 22 patients. Neurology. 1986;36(12):1598–602.
11. Castaigne P, Brunet P, Hauw JJ, Leger JM, Gherardi R, Guillevin L. Peripheral nervous system and panarteritis nodosa. Review of 27 cases. Rev Neurol (Paris). 1984;140(5):343–52.
12. Chang RW, Bell CL, Hallett M. Clinical characteristics and prognosis of vasculitic mononeuropathy multiplex. Arch Neurol. 1984;41(6):618–21.
13. Chia L, Fernandez A, Lacroix C, Adams D, Plante V, Said G. Contribution of nerve biopsy findings to the diagnosis of disabling neuropathy in the elderly. A retrospective review of 100 consecutive patients. Brain. 1996;119(Pt 4):1091–8.
14. Collins MP, Mendell JR, Periquet MI, et al. Superficial peroneal nerve/peroneus brevis muscle biopsy in vasculitic neuropathy. Neurology. 2000;55(5):636–43.
15. Collins MP, Periquet MI, Mendell JR, Sahenk Z, Nagaraja HN, Kissel JT. Nonsystemic vasculitic neuropathy: insights from a clinical cohort. Neurology. 2003;61(5):623–30.
16. Davies L, Spies JM, Pollard JD, McLeod JG. Vasculitis confined to peripheral nerves. Brain. 1996;119(Pt 5):1441–8.
17. Harati Y, Niakan E. The clinical spectrum of inflammatory-angiopathic neuropathy. J Neurol Neurosurg Psychiatry. 1986;49(11):1313–6.
18. Hattori N, Ichimura M, Nagamatsu M, et al. Clinicopathological features of Churg-Strauss syndrome-associated neuropathy. Brain. 1999;122(Pt 3):427–39.
19. Hattori N, Mori K, Misu K, Koike H, Ichimura M, Sobue G. Mortality and morbidity in peripheral neuropathy associated Churg-Strauss syndrome and microscopic polyangiitis. J Rheumatol. 2002;29(7):1408–14.
20. Hawke SH, Davies L, Pamphlett R, Guo YP, Pollard JD, McLeod JG. Vasculitic neuropathy. A clinical and pathological study. Brain. 1991;114(Pt 5):2175–90.
21. Moore PM, Fauci AS. Neurologic manifestations of systemic vasculitis. A retrospective and prospective study of the clinicopathologic features and responses to therapy in 25 patients. Am J Med. 1981;71(4):517–24.
22. Nicolai A, Bonetti B, Lazzarino LG, Ferrari S, Monaco S, Rizzuto N. Peripheral nerve vasculitis: a clinico-pathological study. Clin Neuropathol. 1995;14(3):137–41.
23. Panegyres PK, Blumbergs PC, Leong AS, Bourne AJ. Vasculitis of peripheral nerve and skeletal muscle: clinicopathological correlation and immunopathic mechanisms. J Neurol Sci. 1990;100(1-2):193–202.

24. Puechal X, Said G, Hilliquin P, Coste J, et al. Peripheral neuropathy with necrotizing vasculitis in rheumatoid arthritis. A clinicopathologic and prognostic study of thirty-two patients. Arthritis Rheum. 1995;38(11):1618–29.
25. de Groot K, Schmidt DK, Arlt AC, Gross WL, Reinhold-Keller E. Standardized neurologic evaluations of 128 patients with Wegener granulomatosis. Arch Neurol. 2001;58(8):1215–21.
26. Said G, Lacroix-Ciaudo C, Fujimura H, Blas C, Faux N. The peripheral neuropathy of necrotizing arteritis: a clinicopathological study. Ann Neurol. 1988;23(5):461–5.
27. Sanchez J, Coll-Canti J, Ariza A, Olive A, Cuixart A, Teixido J. Neuropathy due to necrotizing vasculitis: a study of the clinical anatomy, neurophysiological characteristics, and clinical course of the disorder in 27 patients. Rev Neurol. 2001;33(11):1033–6.
28. Singhal BS, Khadilkar SV, Gursahani RD, Surya N. Vasculitic neuropathy: profile of twenty patients. J Assoc Physicians India. 1995;43(7):459–61.
29. Wees SJ, Sunwoo IN, Oh SJ. Sural nerve biopsy in systemic necrotizing vasculitis. Am J Med. 1981;71(4):525–32.
30. Bennett DL, Groves M, Blake J, et al. The use of nerve and muscle biopsy in the diagnosis of vasculitis: a 5 year retrospective study. J Neurol Neurosurg Psychiatry. 2008;79(12):1376–81.
31. Sugiura M, Koike H, Iijima M, et al. Clinicopathologic features of nonsystemic vasculitic neuropathy and microscopic polyangiitis-associated neuropathy: a comparative study. J Neurol Sci. 2006;241(1-2):31–7.
32. Kararizou E, Davaki P, Karandreas N, Davou R, Vassilopoulos D. Nonsystemic vasculitic neuropathy: a clinicopathological study of 22 cases. J Rheumatol. 2005;32(5):853–8.
33. Agadi JB, Raghav G, Mahadevan A, Shankar SK. Usefulness of superficial peroneal nerve/peroneus brevis muscle biopsy in the diagnosis of vasculitic neuropathy. J Clin Neurosci. 2012;19(10):1392–6.
34. Uceyler N, Geng A, Reiners K, Toyka KV, Sommer C. Non-systemic vasculitic neuropathy: single-center follow-up of 60 patients. J Neurol. 2015;262(9):2092–100.
35. Dyck PJ, Norell JE, Dyck PJ. Non-diabetic lumbosacral radiculoplexus neuropathy: natural history, outcome and comparison with the diabetic variety. Brain. 2001;124(Pt 6):1197–207.
36. Seo JH, Ryan HF, Claussen GC, Thomas TD, Oh SJ. Sensory neuropathy in vasculitis: a clinical, pathologic, and electrophysiologic study. Neurology. 2004;63(5):874–8.
37. Vital C, Vital A, Canron MH, et al. Combined nerve and muscle biopsy in the diagnosis of vasculitic neuropathy. A 16-year retrospective study of 202 cases. J Peripher Nerv Syst. 2006;11(1):20–9.
38. Vital A, Vital C, Viallard JF, Ragnaud JM, Canron MH, Lagueny A. Neuro-muscular biopsy in Churg-Strauss syndrome: 24 cases. J Neuropathol Exp Neurol. 2006;65(2):187–92.
39. Cattaneo L, Chierici E, Pavone L, et al. Peripheral neuropathy in Wegener's granulomatosis, Churg-Strauss syndrome and microscopic polyangiitis. J Neurol Neurosurg Psychiatry. 2007;78(10):1119–23.
40. Mathew L, Talbot K, Love S, Puvanarajah S, Donaghy M. Treatment of vasculitic peripheral neuropathy: a retrospective analysis of outcome. QJM. 2007;100(1):41–51.
41. Wolf J, Schmitt V, Palm F, Grau AJ, Bergner R. Peripheral neuropathy as initial manifestation of primary systemic vasculitides. J Neurol. 2013;260(4):1061–70.
42. Hirahara T, Yamashita S, Misumi Y, et al. Gait disturbance due to foot drop is refractory to treatment in nonsystemic vasculitic neuropathy. Eur Neurol. 2014;71(3-4):180–6.
43. Collins MP, Hadden RD. The nonsystemic vasculitic neuropathies. Nat Rev Neurol. 2017;13(5):302–16.
44. Collins MP, Dyck PJ, Gronseth GS, et al. Peripheral nerve society guideline on the classification, diagnosis, investigation, and immunosuppressive therapy of non-systemic vasculitic neuropathy: executive summary. J Peripher Nerv Syst. 2010;15(3):176–84.
45. Fries JF, Hunder GG, Bloch DA, et al. The American College of Rheumatology 1990 criteria for the classification of vasculitis. Summary. Arthritis Rheum. 1990;33(8):1135–6.

46. Jennette JC, Falk RJ, Andrassy K, et al. Nomenclature of systemic vasculitides. Proposal of an international consensus conference. Arthritis Rheum. 1994;37(2):187–92.
47. Watts R, Lane S, Hanslik T, et al. Development and validation of a consensus methodology for the classification of the ANCA-associated vasculitides and polyarteritis nodosa for epidemiological studies. Ann Rheum Dis. 2007;66(2):222–7.
48. Luqmani RA, Suppiah R, Grayson PC, Merkel PA, Watts R. Nomenclature and classification of vasculitis - update on the ACR/EULAR diagnosis and classification of vasculitis study (DCVAS). Clin Exp Immunol. 2011;164(Suppl 1):11–3.
49. Watts RA, Mahr A, Mohammad AJ, Gatenby P, Basu N, Flores-Suarez LF. Classification, epidemiology and clinical subgrouping of antineutrophil cytoplasmic antibody (ANCA)-associated vasculitis. Nephrol Dial Transplant. 2015;30(Suppl 1):i14–22.
50. McCombe PA, McLeod JG, Pollard JD, Guo YP, Ingall TJ. Peripheral sensorimotor and autonomic neuropathy associated with systemic lupus erythematosus. Clinical, pathological and immunological features. Brain. 1987;110(Pt 2):533–49.
51. Midroni G, Bilbao JM. Biopsy diagnosis of peripheral neuropathy. Boston: Butterworth-Heinemann; 1995.
52. Ohkoshi N, Mizusawa H, Oguni E, Shoji S. Sural nerve biopsy in vasculitic neuropathies: morphometric analysis of the caliber of involved vessels. J Med. 1996;27(3-4):153–70.
53. Cartier L, Garcia M, Penaherrera P, Vergara C. Multiple mononeuropathy and vasculitis. Rev Med Chil. 1999;127(2):189–96.
54. Oka N, Kawasaki T, Mizutani K, Sugiyama H, Akiguchi I. Hypoxia-inducible factor 1alpha may be a marker for vasculitic neuropathy. Neuropathology. 2007;27(6):509–15.
55. Zivkovic SA, Ascherman D, Lacomis D. Vasculitic neuropathy–electrodiagnostic findings and association with malignancies. Acta Neurol Scand. 2007;115(6):432–6.
56. Gorson KC. Therapy for vasculitic neuropathies. Curr Treat Options Neurol. 2006;8(2): 105–17.
57. Zhang Y, Sun A, Zhang B, Zhong Y, Dong R, Fan D. The clinical electrophysiology and pathological characteristics of 15 cases of vasculitic neuropathy. Zhonghua Nei Ke Za Zhi. 2014;53(5):384–9.
58. Pagnoux C, Seror R, Henegar C, et al. Clinical features and outcomes in 348 patients with polyarteritis nodosa: a systematic retrospective study of patients diagnosed between 1963 and 2005 and entered into the French Vasculitis study group database. Arthritis Rheum. 2010;62(2):616–26.
59. Guillevin L, Durand-Gasselin B, Cevallos R, et al. Microscopic polyangiitis: clinical and laboratory findings in eighty-five patients. Arthritis Rheum. 1999;42(3):421–30.
60. Comarmond C, Pagnoux C, Khellaf M, et al. Eosinophilic granulomatosis with polyangiitis (Churg-Strauss): clinical characteristics and long-term followup of the 383 patients enrolled in the French Vasculitis study group cohort. Arthritis Rheum. 2013;65(1):270–81.
61. Collins MP. The vasculitic neuropathies: an update. Curr Opin Neurol. 2012;25(5):573–85.
62. Dyck PJB, Engelstad J, Dyck PJ. Microvasculitis. In: Dyck PJ, Thomas PK, editors. Peripheral neuropathy. 4th ed. Philadelphia: Elsevier Saunders; 2005. p. 2405–14.
63. Shimoi T, Shojima K, Murota A, Takizawa Y, Maruyama J, Setoguchi K. Clinical and pathological features of Churg Strauss syndrome among a Japanese population: a case series of 18 patients. Asian Pac J Allergy Immunol. 2012;30(1):61–70.
64. Kararizou E, Davaki P, Spengos K, Karandreas N, Dimitracopoulos A, Vassilopoulos D. Churg-Strauss syndrome complicated by neuropathy: a clinicopathological study of nine cases. Clin Neuropathol. 2011;30(1):11–7.
65. Oka N, Kawasaki T, Matsui M, Shigematsu K, Unuma T, Sugiyama H. Two subtypes of Churg-Strauss syndrome with neuropathy: the roles of eosinophils and ANCA. Mod Rheumatol. 2011;21(3):290–5.
66. Cho HJ, Yune S, Seok JM, et al. Clinical characteristics and treatment response of peripheral neuropathy in the presence of eosinophilic granulomatosis with polyangiitis (churg-strauss syndrome): experience at a single tertiary center. J Clin Neurol. 2017;13(1):77–83.

67. Santos-Pinheiro F, Li Y. Eosinophilic granulomatosis with polyangiitis (Churg-Strauss syndrome) presenting with polyneuropathy--a case series. J Clin Neuromuscul Dis. 2015;16(3):125–30.
68. Suppiah R, Hadden RD, Batra R, et al. Peripheral neuropathy in ANCA-associated vasculitis: outcomes from the European Vasculitis study group trials. Rheumatology (Oxford). 2011;50(12):2214–22.
69. Collins MP, Bischof A, Jaeger VK, et al. Prevalence and associations of peripheral neuropathy at disease-onset in ANCA-associated vasculitides: data from the DCVAS study. J Peripher Nerv Syst. 2018;23:315–6.
70. Giusti Del Giardino L, Cavallaro T, Anzola GP, Lombardi C, Ferrari S. Neuropathy in eosinophilic granulomatosis with polyangiitis: a comparison study of 24 cases with or without prior leukotriene antagonist exposure. Eur Ann Allergy Clin Immunol. 2014;46(6):201–9.
71. Lozeron P, Lacroix C, Michon M, et al. Vasculitis neuropathy mimicking lower limb monoradiculopathy: a study and follow-up of 8 cases. Intern Emerg Med. 2013;8(7):601–9.
72. Schirmer JH, Wright MN, Vonthein R, et al. Clinical presentation and long-term outcome of 144 patients with microscopic polyangiitis in a monocentric German cohort. Rheumatology (Oxford). 2016;55(1):71–9.
73. Moosig F, Bremer JP, Hellmich B, et al. A vasculitis Centre based management strategy leads to improved outcome in eosinophilic granulomatosis and polyangiitis (Churg-Strauss, EGPA): monocentric experiences in 150 patients. Ann Rheum Dis. 2013;72(6):1011–7.
74. Grayson PC, Cuthbertson D, Carette S, et al. New features of disease after diagnosis in 6 forms of systemic vasculitis. J Rheumatol. 2013;40(11):1905–12.
75. Gonzalez-Gay MA, Garcia-Porrua C. Epidemiology of the vasculitides. Rheum Dis Clin N Am. 2001;27(4):729–49.
76. Cassereau J, Baguenier-Desormeaux C, Letournel F, et al. Necrotizing vasculitis revealed in a case of multiple mononeuropathy after a 14-year course of spontaneous remissions and relapses. Clin Neurol Neurosurg. 2012;114(3):290–3.
77. Ford RG, Siekert RG. Central nervous system manifestations of periarteritis nodosa. Neurology. 1965;15:114–22.
78. Hoffman GS, Calabrese LH. Vasculitis: determinants of disease patterns. Nat Rev Rheumatol. 2014;10(8):454–62.
79. Said G, Lacroix C. Primary and secondary vasculitic neuropathy. J Neurol. 2005;252(6): 633–41.
80. Nishino H, Rubino FA, DeRemee RA, Swanson JW, Parisi JE. Neurological involvement in Wegener's granulomatosis: an analysis of 324 consecutive patients at the Mayo Clinic. Ann Neurol. 1993;33(1):4–9.
81. Anderson JM, Jamieson DG, Jefferson JM. Non-healing granuloma and the nervous system. Q J Med. 1975;44(174):309–23.
82. Morozumi S, Koike H, Tomita M, et al. Spatial distribution of nerve fiber pathology and vasculitis in microscopic polyangiitis-associated neuropathy. J Neuropathol Exp Neurol. 2011;70(5):340–8.
83. Forbess L, Bannykh S. Polyarteritis nodosa. Rheum Dis Clin N Am. 2015;41(1):33–46. vii
84. Watts RA, Jolliffe VA, Carruthers DM, Lockwood M, Scott DG. Effect of classification on the incidence of polyarteritis nodosa and microscopic polyangiitis. Arthritis Rheum. 1996;39(7):1208–12.
85. Lightfoot RW Jr, Michel BA, Bloch DA, et al. The American College of Rheumatology 1990 criteria for the classification of polyarteritis nodosa. Arthritis Rheum. 1990;33(8): 1088–93.
86. Hernandez-Rodriguez J, Alba MA, Prieto-Gonzalez S, Cid MC. Diagnosis and classification of polyarteritis nodosa. J Autoimmun. 2014;48-49:84–9.
87. Stanson AW, Friese JL, Johnson CM, et al. Polyarteritis nodosa: spectrum of angiographic findings. Radiographics. 2001;21(1):151–9.
88. Collins MP, Kissel JT. Neuropathies with systemic Vasculitis. In: Dyck PJ, Thomas PK, editors. Peripheral neuropathy. 4th ed. Philadelphia: Elsevier Saunders; 2005. p. 2335–404.

89. Kirkland GS, Savige J, Wilson D, Heale W, Sinclair RA, Hope RN. Classical polyarteritis nodosa and microscopic polyarteritis with medium vessel involvement--a comparison of the clinical and laboratory features. Clin Nephrol. 1997;47(3):176–80.
90. Selga D, Mohammad A, Sturfelt G, Segelmark M. Polyarteritis nodosa when applying the Chapel Hill nomenclature--a descriptive study on ten patients. Rheumatology (Oxford). 2006;45(10):1276–81.
91. Alibaz-Oner F, Koster MJ, Crowson CS, et al. Clinical Spectrum of medium-sized vessel Vasculitis. Arthritis Care Res (Hoboken). 2017;69(6):884–91.
92. Kint N, De Haes P, Blockmans D. Comparison between classical polyarteritis nodosa and single organ vasculitis of medium-sized vessels: a retrospective study of 25 patients and review of the literature. Acta Clin Belg. 2016;71(1):26–31.
93. Sharma A, Pinto B, Dhooria A, et al. Polyarteritis nodosa in North India: clinical manifestations and outcomes. Int J Rheum Dis. 2017;20(3):390–7.
94. Greco A, De Virgilio A, Rizzo MI, et al. Microscopic polyangiitis: advances in diagnostic and therapeutic approaches. Autoimmun Rev. 2015;14(9):837–44.
95. Bossuyt X, Cohen Tervaert JW, Arimura Y, et al. Position paper: revised 2017 international consensus on testing of ANCAs in granulomatosis with polyangiitis and microscopic polyangiitis. Nat Rev Rheumatol. 2017;13(11):683–92.
96. Fuiano G, Cameron JS, Raftery M, Hartley BH, Williams DG, Ogg CS. Improved prognosis of renal microscopic polyarteritis in recent years. Nephrol Dial Transplant. 1988;3(4):383–91.
97. Serra A, Cameron JS, Turner DR, et al. Vasculitis affecting the kidney: presentation, histopathology and long-term outcome. Q J Med. 1984;53(210):181–207.
98. Savage CO, Winearls CG, Evans DJ, Rees AJ, Lockwood CM. Microscopic polyarteritis: presentation, pathology and prognosis. Q J Med. 1985;56(220):467–83.
99. Rodgers H, Guthrie JA, Brownjohn AM, Turney JH. Microscopic polyarteritis: clinical features and treatment. Postgrad Med J. 1989;65(766):515–8.
100. Adu D, Howie AJ, Scott DG, Bacon PA, McGonigle RJ, Micheal J. Polyarteritis and the kidney. Q J Med. 1987;62(239):221–37.
101. Itabashi M, Takei T, Morito T, et al. Estimation of BVAS in patients with microscopic polyangiitis in Japan. Clin Rheumatol. 2011;30(11):1499–505.
102. Oh JS, Lee CK, Kim YG, Nah SS, Moon HB, Yoo B. Clinical features and outcomes of microscopic polyangiitis in Korea. J Korean Med Sci. 2009;24(2):269–74.
103. Furuta S, Chaudhry AN, Hamano Y, et al. Comparison of phenotype and outcome in microscopic polyangiitis between Europe and Japan. J Rheumatol. 2014;41(2):325–33.
104. Solans-Laque R, Fraile G, Rodriguez-Carballeira M, et al. Clinical characteristics and outcome of Spanish patients with ANCA-associated vasculitides: impact of the vasculitis type, ANCA specificity, and treatment on mortality and morbidity. Medicine (Baltimore). 2017;96(8):e6083.
105. Miloslavsky EM, Lu N, Unizony S, et al. Myeloperoxidase-antineutrophil cytoplasmic antibody (ANCA)-positive and ANCA-negative patients with granulomatosis with polyangiitis (Wegener's): distinct patient subsets. Arthritis Rheumatol. 2016;68(12):2945–52.
106. Wu CS, Hsieh CJ, Peng YS, Chang TH, Wu ZY. Antineutrophil cytoplasmic antibody-associated vasculitis in Taiwan: a hospital-based study with reference to the population-based National Health Insurance database. J Microbiol Immunol Infect. 2015;48(5):477–82.
107. Zhang W, Zhou G, Shi Q, Zhang X, Zeng XF, Zhang FC. Clinical analysis of nervous system involvement in ANCA-associated systemic vasculitides. Clin Exp Rheumatol. 2009;27(1 Suppl 52):S65–9.
108. Lane SE, Watts RA, Shepstone L, Scott DG. Primary systemic vasculitis: clinical features and mortality. QJM. 2005;98(2):97–111.
109. Ahn JK, Hwang JW, Lee J, Jeon CH, Cha HS, Koh EM. Clinical features and outcome of microscopic polyangiitis under a new consensus algorithm of ANCA-associated vasculitides in Korea. Rheumatol Int. 2012;32(10):2979–86.
110. Wang L, Li J, Qian M, et al. Clinical features of microscopic polyangiitis associated with peripheral neuropathy. Zhonghua Yi Xue Za Zhi. 2015;95(27):2190–3.

111. Shuai ZW, Lv YF, Zhang MM, Hu ZY. Clinical analysis of patients with myeloperoxidase anti-neutrophil cytoplasmic antibody-associated vasculitis. Genet Mol Res. 2015;14(2):5296–303.
112. Cisternas M, Soto L, Jacobelli S, et al. Clinical features of Wegener granulomatosis and microscopic polyangiitis in Chilean patients. Rev Med Chil. 2005;133(3):273–8.
113. Unizony S, Villarreal M, Miloslavsky EM, et al. Clinical outcomes of treatment of anti-neutrophil cytoplasmic antibody (ANCA)-associated vasculitis based on ANCA type. Ann Rheum Dis. 2016;75(6):1166–9.
114. Peco-Antic A, Bonaci-Nikolic B, Basta-Jovanovic G, et al. Childhood microscopic polyangiitis associated with MPO-ANCA. Pediatr Nephrol. 2006;21(1):46–53.
115. Yu F, Huang JP, Zou WZ, Zhao MH. The clinical features of anti-neutrophil cytoplasmic antibody-associated systemic vasculitis in Chinese children. Pediatr Nephrol. 2006;21(4):497–502.
116. Basu B, Mahapatra TK, Mondal N. Favourable renal survival in paediatric microscopic polyangiitis: efficacy of a novel treatment algorithm. Nephrol Dial Transplant. 2015;30(Suppl 1):i113–8.
117. Mouthon L, Dunogue B, Guillevin L. Diagnosis and classification of eosinophilic granulomatosis with polyangiitis (formerly named Churg-Strauss syndrome). J Autoimmun. 2014;48-49:99–103.
118. Lanham JG, Elkon KB, Pusey CD, Hughes GR. Systemic vasculitis with asthma and eosinophilia: a clinical approach to the Churg-Strauss syndrome. Medicine (Baltimore). 1984;63(2):65–81.
119. Keogh KA, Specks U. Churg-Strauss syndrome: clinical presentation, antineutrophil cytoplasmic antibodies, and leukotriene receptor antagonists. Am J Med. 2003;115(4):284–90.
120. Sinico RA, Di Toma L, Maggiore U, et al. Prevalence and clinical significance of antineutrophil cytoplasmic antibodies in Churg-Strauss syndrome. Arthritis Rheum. 2005;52(9):2926–35.
121. Durel CA, Berthiller J, Caboni S, Jayne D, Ninet J, Hot A. Long-term followup of a multicenter cohort of 101 patients with eosinophilic granulomatosis with polyangiitis (Churg-Strauss). Arthritis Care Res (Hoboken). 2016;68(3):374–87.
122. Uchiyama M, Mitsuhashi Y, Yamazaki M, Tsuboi R. Elderly cases of Churg-Strauss syndrome: case report and review of Japanese cases. J Dermatol. 2012;39(1):76–9.
123. Gendelman S, Zeft A, Spalding SJ. Childhood-onset eosinophilic granulomatosis with polyangiitis (formerly Churg-Strauss syndrome): a contemporary single-center cohort. J Rheumatol. 2013;40(6):929–35.
124. Zwerina J, Eger G, Englbrecht M, Manger B, Schett G. Churg-Strauss syndrome in childhood: a systematic literature review and clinical comparison with adult patients. Semin Arthritis Rheum. 2009;39(2):108–15.
125. Eleftheriou D, Gale H, Pilkington C, Fenton M, Sebire NJ, Brogan PA. Eosinophilic granulomatosis with polyangiitis in childhood: retrospective experience from a tertiary referral Centre in the UK. Rheumatology (Oxford). 2016;55(7):1263–72.
126. Wolf J, Bergner R, Mutallib S, Buggle F, Grau AJ. Neurologic complications of Churg-Strauss syndrome--a prospective monocentric study. Eur J Neurol. 2010;17(4):582–8.
127. Danieli MG, Cappelli M, Malcangi G, Logullo F, Salvi A, Danieli G. Long term effectiveness of intravenous immunoglobulin in Churg-Strauss syndrome. Ann Rheum Dis. 2004;63(12):1649–54.
128. Cottin V, Bel E, Bottero P, et al. Revisiting the systemic vasculitis in eosinophilic granulomatosis with polyangiitis (Churg-Strauss): a study of 157 patients by the Groupe d'Etudes et de Recherche sur les maladies Orphelines Pulmonaires and the European Respiratory Society taskforce on eosinophilic granulomatosis with polyangiitis (Churg-Strauss). Autoimmun Rev. 2017;16(1):1–9.
129. Hoffman GS, Kerr GS, Leavitt RY, Hallahan CW, Lebovics RS, Travis WD, et al. Wegener granulomatosis: an analysis of 158 patients. Ann Intern Med. 1992;116(6):488–98.

130. Holle JU, Gross WL, Latza U, et al. Improved outcome in 445 patients with Wegener's granulomatosis in a German vasculitis center over four decades. Arthritis Rheum. 2011;63(1):257–66.
131. Terrier B, Dechartres A, Deligny C, et al. Granulomatosis with polyangiitis according to geographic origin and ethnicity: clinical-biological presentation and outcome in a French population. Rheumatology (Oxford). 2017;56(3):445–50.
132. Sharma A, Naidu GS, Rathi M, et al. Clinical features and long-term outcomes of 105 granulomatosis with polyangiitis patients: a single center experience from North India. Int J Rheum Dis. 2017;21(1):278–84.
133. Cabral DA, Uribe AG, Benseler S, et al. Classification, presentation, and initial treatment of Wegener's granulomatosis in childhood. Arthritis Rheum. 2009;60(11):3413–24.
134. Iudici M, Puechal X, Pagnoux C, et al. Brief report: childhood-onset systemic necrotizing vasculitides: long-term data from the French vasculitis study group registry. Arthritis Rheumatol. 2015;67(7):1959–65.
135. Akikusa JD, Schneider R, Harvey EA, et al. Clinical features and outcome of pediatric Wegener's granulomatosis. Arthritis Rheum. 2007;57(5):837–44.
136. Nukada H, Dyck PJ. Microsphere embolization of nerve capillaries and fiber degeneration. Am J Pathol. 1984;115(2):275–87.
137. Dyck PJ, Conn DL, Okazaki H. Necrotizing angiopathic neuropathy. Three-dimensional morphology of fiber degeneration related to sites of occluded vessels. Mayo Clin Proc. 1972;47(7):461–75.
138. Dyck PJ, Johnson WJ, Lambert EH, O'Brien PC. Segmental demyelination secondary to axonal degeneration in uremic neuropathy. Mayo Clin Proc. 1971;46(6):400–31.
139. Fujimura H, Lacroix C, Said G. Vulnerability of nerve fibres to ischaemia. A quantitative light and electron microscope study. Brain. 1991;114(Pt 4):1929–42.
140. Kissel JT, Riethman JL, Omerza J, Rammohan KW, Mendell JR. Peripheral nerve vasculitis: immune characterization of the vascular lesions. Ann Neurol. 1989;25(3):291–7.
141. Satoi H, Oka N, Kawasaki T, Miyamoto K, Akiguchi I, Kimura J. Mechanisms of tissue injury in vasculitic neuropathies. Neurology. 1998;50(2):492–6.
142. Lindenlaub T, Sommer C. Cytokines in sural nerve biopsies from inflammatory and non-inflammatory neuropathies. Acta Neuropathol. 2003;105(6):593–602.
143. Khalili-Shirazi A, Gregson NA, Londei M, Summers L, Hughes RA. The distribution of CD1 molecules in inflammatory neuropathy. J Neurol Sci. 1998;158(2):154–63.
144. Uceyler N, Braunsdorf S, Kunze E, et al. Cellular infiltrates in skin and sural nerve of patients with polyneuropathies. Muscle Nerve. 2017;55(6):884–93.
145. Collins MP, Periquet-Collins I, Sahenk Z, Kissel JT. Direct immunofluoresence in vasculitic neuropathy: specificity of vascular immune deposits. Muscle Nerve. 2010;42(1):62–9.
146. Takahashi M, Koike H, Ikeda S, et al. Distinct pathogenesis in nonsystemic vasculitic neuropathy and microscopic polyangiitis. Neurol Neuroimmunol Neuroinflamm. 2017;4(6):e407.
147. Lundborg G. Structure and function of the intraneural microvessels as related to trauma, edema formation, and nerve function. J Bone Joint Surg Am. 1975;57(7):938–48.
148. Low PA, Lagerlund TD, McManis PG. Nerve blood flow and oxygen delivery in normal, diabetic, and ischemic neuropathy. Int Rev Neurobiol. 1989;31:355–438.
149. Kinter J, Broglio L, Steck AJ, et al. Gene expression profiling in nerve biopsy of vasculitic neuropathy. J Neuroimmunol. 2010;225(1–2):184–9.
150. Saadoun D, Bieche I, Maisonobe T, et al. Involvement of chemokines and type 1 cytokines in the pathogenesis of hepatitis C virus-associated mixed cryoglobulinemia vasculitis neuropathy. Arthritis Rheum. 2005;52(9):2917–25.
151. Heuss D, Probst-Cousin S, Kayser C, Neundorfer B. Cell death in vasculitic neuropathy. Muscle Nerve. 2000;23(7):999–1004.

152. Van Rhijn I, Van den Berg LH, Bosboom WM, Otten HG, Logtenberg T. Expression of accessory molecules for T-cell activation in peripheral nerve of patients with CIDP and vasculitic neuropathy. Brain. 2000;123(Pt 10):2020–9.
153. Broglio L, Erne B, Tolnay M, et al. Allograft inflammatory factor-1: a pathogenetic factor for vasculitic neuropathy. Muscle Nerve. 2008;38(4):1272–9.
154. Bosboom WM, Van den Berg LH, Mollee I, et al. Sural nerve T-cell receptor Vbeta gene utilization in chronic inflammatory demyelinating polyneuropathy and vasculitic neuropathy. Neurology. 2001;56(1):74–81.
155. Deprez M, Lubke U, Verlaet M, Debrus S, Delvenne P, Martin JJ. Detection of cytokines in human sural nerve biopsies: an immunohistochemical and molecular study. Acta Neuropathol. 2001;101(4):393–404.
156. Kawamura N, Dyck PJ, Schmeichel AM, Engelstad JK, Low PA, Dyck PJ. Inflammatory mediators in diabetic and non-diabetic lumbosacral radiculoplexus neuropathy. Acta Neuropathol. 2008;115(2):231–9.
157. Hu W, Mathey E, Hartung HP, Kieseier BC. Cyclo-oxygenases and prostaglandins in acute inflammatory demyelination of the peripheral nerve. Neurology. 2003;61(12):1774–9.
158. Gurer G, Erdem S, Kocaefe C, Ozguc M, Tan E. Expression of matrix metalloproteinases in vasculitic neuropathy. Rheumatol Int. 2004;24(5):255–9.
159. Leppert D, Hughes P, Huber S, et al. Matrix metalloproteinase upregulation in chronic inflammatory demyelinating polyneuropathy and nonsystemic vasculitic neuropathy. Neurology. 1999;53(1):62–70.
160. Renaud S, Erne B, Fuhr P, et al. Matrix metalloproteinases-9 and -2 in secondary vasculitic neuropathies. Acta Neuropathol. 2003;105(1):37–42.
161. Haslbeck KM, Bierhaus A, Erwin S, et al. Receptor for advanced glycation endproduct (RAGE)-mediated nuclear factor-kappaB activation in vasculitic neuropathy. Muscle Nerve. 2004;29(6):853–60.
162. Mazzeo A, Aguennouz M, Messina C, Vita G. Immunolocalization and activation of transcription factor nuclear factor kappa B in dysimmune neuropathies and familial amyloidotic polyneuropathy. Arch Neurol. 2004;61(7):1097–102.
163. Coll-Vinent B, Cebrian M, Cid MC, et al. Dynamic pattern of endothelial cell adhesion molecule expression in muscle and perineural vessels from patients with classic polyarteritis nodosa. Arthritis Rheum. 1998;41(3):435–44.
164. Schneider C, Wunderlich G, Bleistein J, et al. Lymphocyte antigens targetable by monoclonal antibodies in non-systemic vasculitic neuropathy. J Neurol Neurosurg Psychiatry. 2017;88(9):756–60.
165. Takeuchi H, Kawasaki T, Shigematsu K, Kawamura K, Oka N. Neutrophil extracellular traps in neuropathy with anti-neutrophil cytoplasmic autoantibody-associated microscopic polyangiitis. Clin Rheumatol. 2017;36(4):913–7.
166. Bonsib SM. Polyarteritis nodosa. Semin Diagn Pathol. 2001;18(1):14–23.
167. Jennette JC, Thomas DB, Falk RJ. Microscopic polyangiitis (microscopic polyarteritis). Semin Diagn Pathol. 2001;18(1):3–13.
168. Yi ES, Colby TV. Wegener's granulomatosis. Semin Diagn Pathol. 2001;18(1):34–46.
169. Travis WD, Hoffman GS, Leavitt RY, Pass HI, Fauci AS. Surgical pathology of the lung in Wegener's granulomatosis. Review of 87 open lung biopsies from 67 patients. Am J Surg Pathol. 1991;15(4):315–33.
170. Finkelman R, Munsat T, Mandell H, Adelman L, Logigian E. Neuromuscular manifestations of Wegener's granulomatosis: a case report. Neurology. 1993;43(3 Pt 1):617–8.
171. Lacomis D, Zivkovic SA. Approach to vasculitic neuropathies. J Clin Neuromuscul Dis. 2007;9(1):265–76.
172. Olney RK. AAEM minimonograph #38: neuropathies in connective tissue disease. Muscle Nerve. 1992;15(5):531–42.
173. Bromberg MB, Jaros L. Symmetry of normal motor and sensory nerve conduction measurements. Muscle Nerve. 1998;21(4):498–503.

174. Buschbacher RM, Kumbhare DA, Robinson LR. Buschbacher's manual of nerve conduction studies. 3rd ed. New York: Demos Medical; 2016.
175. Jamieson PW, Giuliani MJ, Martinez AJ. Necrotizing angiopathy presenting with multifocal conduction blocks. Neurology. 1991;41(3):442–4.
176. Bischof A, Manigold T, Barro C, et al. Serum neurofilament light chain: a biomarker of neuronal injury in vasculitic neuropathy. Ann Rheum Dis. 2017;77(7):1093–4.
177. Terrier B, Lacroix C, Guillevin L, et al. Diagnostic and prognostic relevance of neuromuscular biopsy in primary Sjogren's syndrome-related neuropathy. Arthritis Rheum. 2007;57(8):1520–9.
178. Vincent D, Dubas F, Hauw JJ, et al. Nerve and muscle microvasculitis: 50 cases. Rev Neurol (Paris). 1985;141(6-7):440–6.
179. Leger JM, Bouche P, Chaunu MP, et al. Peripheral neuropathies with neural vasculitis. Clinical and electrophysiological aspects of 33 cases. Presse Med. 1988;17(15): 733–7.
180. Hadden RDM, Collins MP, Zivkovic SA, et al. Vasculitic peripheral neuropathy: case definition and guidelines for collection, analysis, and presentation of immunisation safety data. Vaccine. 2017;35(11):1567–78.
181. Uceyler N, Devigili G, Toyka KV, Sommer C. Skin biopsy as an additional diagnostic tool in non-systemic vasculitic neuropathy. Acta Neuropathol. 2010;120(1):109–16.
182. Dyck PJ, Norell JE, Dyck PJ. Microvasculitis and ischemia in diabetic lumbosacral radiculoplexus neuropathy. Neurology. 1999;53(9):2113–21.
183. Schweikert K, Fuhr P, Probst A, Tolnay M, Renaud S, Steck AJ. Contribution of nerve biopsy to unclassified neuropathy. Eur Neurol. 2007;57(2):86–90.
184. Deprez M, de Groote CC, Gollogly L, Reznik M, Martin JJ. Clinical and neuropathological parameters affecting the diagnostic yield of nerve biopsy. Neuromuscul Disord. 2000;10(2):92–8.
185. Vrancken AF, Gathier CS, Cats EA, Notermans NC, Collins MP. The additional yield of combined nerve/muscle biopsy in vasculitic neuropathy. Eur J Neurol. 2011;18(1): 49–58.
186. Capek S, Amrami KK, Dyck PJ, Spinner RJ. Targeted fascicular biopsy of the sciatic nerve and its major branches: rationale and operative technique. Neurosurg Focus. 2015;39(3):E12.
187. Fujikawa S, Omoto M, Ogasawara J, Koga M, Kawai M, Kanda T. Systemic vasculitic neuropathy diagnosed by means of (18)F-FDG PET CT. Rinsho Shinkeigaku. 2016;56(2): 88–92.
188. Ito T, Kijima M, Watanabe T, Sakuta M, Nishiyama K. Ultrasonography of the tibial nerve in vasculitic neuropathy. Muscle Nerve. 2007;35(3):379–82.
189. Grimm A, Decard BF, Bischof A, Axer H. Ultrasound of the peripheral nerves in systemic vasculitic neuropathies. J Neurol Sci. 2014;347(1-2):44–9.
190. Uceyler N, Schafer KA, Mackenrodt D, Sommer C, Mullges W. High-resolution ultrasonography of the superficial peroneal motor and sural sensory nerves may be a non-invasive approach to the diagnosis of vasculitic neuropathy. Front Neurol. 2016;7:48.
191. Goedee HS, van der Pol L, van Asseldonk JH, Vrancken AF, Notermans NC, Visser LH, et al. Nerve sonography to detect peripheral nerve involvement in vasculitis syndromes. Neurol Clin Pract. 2016;6:1–11.
192. Yates M, Watts RA, Bajema IM, et al. EULAR/ERA-EDTA recommendations for the management of ANCA-associated vasculitis. Ann Rheum Dis. 2016;75(9):1583–94.
193. Ntatsaki E, Carruthers D, Chakravarty K, et al. BSR and BHPR guideline for the management of adults with ANCA-associated vasculitis. Rheumatology (Oxford). 2014;53(12): 2306–9.
194. Puechal X, Pagnoux C, Perrodeau E, et al. Long-term outcomes among participants in the WEGENT trial of remission-maintenance therapy for granulomatosis with polyangiitis (Wegener's) or microscopic polyangiitis. Arthritis Rheumatol. 2016;68:690–701.

195. Jones RB, Hiemstra TF, Ballarin J, et al. Mycophenolate mofetil versus cyclophosphamide for remission induction in ANCA-associated vasculitis: a randomised, non-inferiority trial. Ann Rheum Dis. 2019;78:399–405.
196. Walsh M, Faurschou M, Berden A, et al. Long-term follow-up of cyclophosphamide compared with azathioprine for initial maintenance therapy in ANCA-associated vasculitis. Clin J Am Soc Nephrol. 2014;9(9):1571–6.
197. Faurschou M, Westman K, Rasmussen N, et al. Brief report: long-term outcome of a randomized clinical trial comparing methotrexate to cyclophosphamide for remission induction in early systemic antineutrophil cytoplasmic antibody-associated vasculitis. Arthritis Rheum. 2012;64(10):3472–7.
198. Harper L, Morgan MD, Walsh M, et al. Pulse versus daily oral cyclophosphamide for induction of remission in ANCA-associated vasculitis: long-term follow-up. Ann Rheum Dis. 2012;71(6):955–60.
199. Springer J, Nutter B, Langford CA, Hoffman GS, Villa-Forte A. Granulomatosis with polyangiitis (Wegener's): impact of maintenance therapy duration. Medicine (Baltimore). 2014;93(2):82–90.
200. Karras A, Pagnoux C, Haubitz M, et al. Randomised controlled trial of prolonged treatment in the remission phase of ANCA-associated vasculitis. Ann Rheum Dis. 2017;76(10): 1662–8.
201. Stone JH, Merkel PA, Spiera R, et al. Rituximab versus cyclophosphamide for ANCA-associated vasculitis. N Engl J Med. 2010;363(3):221–32.
202. Jones RB, Tervaert JW, Hauser T, et al. Rituximab versus cyclophosphamide in ANCA-associated renal vasculitis. N Engl J Med. 2010;363(3):211–20.
203. Pagnoux C, Guillevin L. French Vasculitis study group, MAINRITSAN investigators. Rituximab or azathioprine maintenance in ANCA-associated vasculitis. N Engl J Med. 2015;372(4):386–7.
204. Ribi C, Cohen P, Pagnoux C, et al. Treatment of polyarteritis nodosa and microscopic polyangiitis without poor-prognosis factors: a prospective randomized study of one hundred twenty-four patients. Arthritis Rheum. 2010;62(4):1186–97.
205. Samson M, Puechal X, Devilliers H, et al. Long-term follow-up of a randomized trial on 118 patients with polyarteritis nodosa or microscopic polyangiitis without poor-prognosis factors. Autoimmun Rev. 2014;13(2):197–205.
206. Samson M, Puechal X, Devilliers H, et al. Mononeuritis multiplex predicts the need for immunosuppressive or immunomodulatory drugs for EGPA, PAN and MPA patients without poor-prognosis factors. Autoimmun Rev. 2014;13(9):945–53.
207. Puechal X, Pagnoux C, Baron G, et al. Adding azathioprine to remission-induction glucocorticoids for eosinophilic granulomatosis with polyangiitis (Churg-Strauss), microscopic polyangiitis, or polyarteritis nodosa without poor prognosis factors: a randomized, controlled trial. Arthritis Rheumatol. 2017;69(11):2175–86.
208. Hellmich B, Flossmann O, Gross WL, et al. EULAR recommendations for conducting clinical studies and/or clinical trials in systemic vasculitis: focus on anti-neutrophil cytoplasm antibody-associated vasculitis. Ann Rheum Dis. 2007;66(5):605–17.
209. Jayne DR, Chapel H, Adu D, et al. Intravenous immunoglobulin for ANCA-associated systemic vasculitis with persistent disease activity. QJM. 2000;93(7):433–9.
210. Danieli MG, Calcabrini L, Marchetti A, et al. Intravenous immunoglobulin treatment in autoimmune diseases. Recenti Prog Med. 2007;98(6):322–6.
211. Koike H, Akiyama K, Saito T, Sobue G. Research group for IVIg for EGPA/CSS in Japan. Intravenous immunoglobulin for chronic residual peripheral neuropathy in eosinophilic granulomatosis with polyangiitis (Churg-Strauss syndrome): a multicenter, double-blind trial. J Neurol. 2015;262(3):752–9.
212. Graham RC, Hughes RA. A modified peripheral neuropathy scale: the overall neuropathy limitations scale. J Neurol Neurosurg Psychiatry. 2006;77(8):973–6.

213. Hatemi G, Esatoglu SN, Yazici Y. Biomarkers in vasculitis. Curr Opin Rheumatol. 2018;30(1):30–5.
214. Sakai K, Komai K, Yanase D, Yamada M. Plasma VEGF as a marker for the diagnosis and treatment of vasculitic neuropathy. J Neurol Neurosurg Psychiatry. 2005;76(2):296.
215. Zilliox LA. Neuropathic pain. Continuum (Minneap Minn). 2017;23(2, Selected Topics in Outpatient Neurology):512–32.

Central Nervous System Involvement in ANCA-Associated Vasculitis

13

Hubert de Boysson

13.1 Introduction

Antineutrophil cytoplasmic antibodies (ANCA)-associated vasculitides (AAV) involve small- and medium-sized vessels and can affect the central nervous system (CNS). In opposition to primary CNS vasculitis, extraneurological involvement is common and is helpful in the diagnosis approach. AAV-related CNS involvement is rare, but serious, and is associated with a poor prognosis. The final diagnosis is often clinically based and relies on recognition of extraneurological symptoms and serologies consistent with a diagnosis of AAV [1]. However, CNS involvement can be a diagnosis challenge when neurological manifestations are inaugural or isolated. A large workup is thus required. Occurrence of CNS manifestations in a patient followed for a AAV questions whether the process is linked to a specific vasculitis-related involvement or to another process, such as infection, drug toxicity, or malignancy. Many features are common to the three AAV-related CNS involvement, but some specific characteristics have to be highlighted.

13.2 General Characteristics of AAV Affecting the Central Nervous System

In granulomatosis with polyangiitis (GPA), CNS is involved in 7–11% of patients and probably less frequently in other AAV [2, 3]. In the study from Pinching et al., a rate of 44% was observed but peripheral nervous system was included in neurological involvement [4].

H. de Boysson (✉)
Department of Internal Medicine, Caen University Hospital, Caen, France

University of Caen Basse Normandie, Caen, France
e-mail: deboysson-h@chu-caen.fr

R. A. Sinico, L. Guillevin (eds.), *Anti-Neutrophil Cytoplasmic Antibody (ANCA) Associated Vasculitis*, Rare Diseases of the Immune System,
https://doi.org/10.1007/978-3-030-02239-6_13

Different mechanisms have been described to explain GPA-related CNS involvement. Local extension from ophthalmological or sinus granulomatous lesions to the meninges, pituitary gland, or brain parenchyma is frequently reported. Otherwise, CNS vessels can be independently affected and/or isolated granulomatous lesions can develop within the brain or the spinal cord [1]. Isolated medullar involvement is exceptional [5]. Diagnosis of GPA-related CNS involvement is made in half of the patients at GPA onset and after diagnosis in other patients. In the study by de Luna et al., the median age at GPA diagnosis and onset of CNS involvement was 48 (range 2 78) and 51 (range 2 79) years, respectively, and 26 (74%) patients were male [6].

CNS involvement in eosinophilic granulomatosis with polyangiitis (EGPA) is rarer than in GPA, and may affect 4.6% of patients [7]. More than 85% of patients with EGPA-related CNS involvement showed neurological symptoms at diagnosis. Most cases regard patients in the fourth and fifth decade, and the sex ratio is 1 [7]. CNS involvement in EGPA is particularly associated with an increased mortality [7, 8]. In most patients, a vasculitic process affecting CNS vessels is responsible for neurological symptoms. CNS involvement could also be the consequence of eosinophil-mediated injury [7]. More rarely, myocardial fibrosis can lead to brain embolism, explaining the involvement of small perforant and subcortical arteries [9].

While peripheral neuropathy is common in microscopic polyangiitis (MPA), CNS involvement is rarely reported and no specific case series has been published. Affection of perforant arteries or intracranial hemorrhage has been described separately. Only few observations reported a biopsy-proven diagnosis, often in the setting of an important intracranial hemorrhage requiring a surgical treatment [10, 11].

13.3 Neurological Manifestations

Neurological symptoms in patients with AAV-related CNS involvement are widely polymorph and depend on the affected territory. Neurological onset can be acute in case of stroke or seizures. It can also be more chronic and insidious in patients with headaches, cognitive or vigilance disorders, or psychiatric manifestations.

Headaches are common and may affect 20–60% of the patients [6, 7]. Motor deficits are common (30–45% of patients) and are often explained by small to large brain infarction(s). Other neurological deficits can be observed, such as speech disorders (9% of patients), sensory deficits (16–43% of patients), or cerebellar ataxia (6% of patients) [6, 7]. Cranial nerve involvement may affect 20% of patients [7]. Encephalopathic presentations include confusion (11% of patients), psychiatric manifestations (mainly depression in 9–27% of patients), and vigilance troubles (rising from psychomotor slowdown to coma) [6, 7]. Seizures occur in 2% of patients with EGPA [7]. In the study by de Luna et al., two subgroups of GPA patients have been distinguished with different clinical presentations. Patients with granulomatous disease more likely suffered from headaches linked to pachymeningitis. Conversely, patients with predominant vascular pattern more likely developed neurovascular events with focal deficits linked to stroke on imaging [6]. Medullar involvement has been rarely described and affect less than 10% of patients with CNS involvement [12]. In patients with GPA, involvement of the pituitary gland can compress the optic chiasm, resulting in partial visual loss. In GPA and EGPA, visual loss can also be the consequence of an optic neuritis [6, 7].

Besides neurological examination, other extraneurological involvements frequently associated with neurological symptoms should be searched. In GPA, ENT involvement was present in 80% of patients, pulmonary disease in 57%, and peripheral nervous system involvement in 49% [6]. At the time of EGPA-related CNS involvement, asthma, peripheral neuropathy, and cardiac involvement were also observed in 98%, 55%, and 41% of patients, respectively [7].

13.4 Imaging

CT scan is often the first imaging performed, but has a poor sensitivity and specificity. Magnetic resonance imaging (MRI) is required in all patients, even in patients with abnormal CT scan. When available, vascular sequences should also be performed.

MRI analysis should include the following sequences: T1, T2, T2*, fluid-attenuated inversion recovery (FLAIR), diffusion-weighted imaging (DWI)/apparent diffusion coefficient mapping, and gadolinium-enhanced T1. Acute and subacute ischemic lesions appeared as hyperintense signal on DWI-weighted sequences, with corresponding restricted diffusion on apparent diffusion coefficient maps [13].

Different patterns of lesions can be observed. Ischemic lesions are common and observed in the three AAV. A vasculitic process should be searched in this setting. Leptomeningeal involvement is also described in the three AAV, but pachymeningitis is more likely secondary to GPA. In GPA, besides ischemic lesions and pachymeningitis, granulomatous or tumor-like lesions can be observed within brain or medullar parenchyma or in the pituitary gland. MRI sequences can also demonstrate orbital or sinus involvement, frequent in GPA.

13.4.1 MRI Findings Suggestive of CNS Vasculitis

Ischemic lesions can be isolated or disseminated. Subacute and chronic ischemic lesions are also observed, often associated with acute lesions. The presence of multiple ischemic lesions of different ages is suggestive of a vasculitic process but can be seen in atherosclerosis, infections, or other vasculopathies. Multiple patterns of acute ischemic lesions are observed, affecting grey and white matter (subcortical, peripheral, superficial, or deep lesions). In GPA and EGPA, unilateral or bilateral cerebral infarcts were observed in 60% and 52% of patients, respectively [6, 7].

Subcortical and white matter FLAIR hyperintense lesions are frequent and affect >90% of patients, but are nonspecific and are seen in other inflammatory and noninflammatory conditions. FLAIR lesions on the cortex or posterior areas are rare and more suspect. Gadolinium injection is required in the diagnosis workup of a CNS vasculitis and can demonstrate gadolinium-enhanced lesions, suggestive of inflammatory process. However, small infarctions can also be enhanced due to the rupture of the hematoencephalic barrier. Besides parenchyma, meningeal tissues can also be gadoliniium-enhanced [13].

Gradient echo sequences give information of hemosiderin deposits that can be linked to the rupture of small vessels (i.e., microbleeds). Microbleeds are small, round foci of hypointense signals in T2$*$ gradient-recalled echo-weighted images, $\leq$10 mm in brain parenchyma, and allocated to either deep or lobar locations. Hemorrhagic lesions can be within acute ischemic lesions indicating hemorrhagic transformation. However, spontaneous parenchymal or subarachnoid hemorrhages can be observed [13]. In GPA and EGPA, cerebral hemorrhagic lesions were observed in 6% and 24% of patients, respectively [6, 7].

The combination of different abnormalities on MRI is frequent and suggestive of vasculitis when showing multiple ischemic lesions along with small hemorrhages, FLAIR lesions, and gadolinium enhancements. Conversely, CNS vasculitis is not probable in a patient with normal MRI.

13.4.2 Other MRI Findings

Especially in GPA, MRI can demonstrate granulomatous lesions within the CNS, whose aspect can be tumor like. A gadolinium-enhanced ring around the lesions is often observed on T1 sequences with contrast [14]. Tumor-like lesions are more frequently described within the pituitary gland [15]. Spinal cord pachymeningitis is observed in 11% of GPA patients with CNS involvement [6].

13.4.3 Cerebral Angiography

In patients with demonstration of ischemic lesions on CNS imaging or with suspected AAV-related CNS vasculitis, angiography is required. Magnetic resonance angiography (MRA), brain CT angiography (CTA), and digital subtraction angiography (DSA) are the three main procedures used. DSA is the technique with the best spatial resolution, allowing to analyze vessels $\geq$500 μm. However, it remains an invasive procedure. MRA is limited to explore vessels <700 μm, but the development of 3Tesla units has increased the spatial resolution of the procedure.

Intracranial vessels can be classified into large-, medium-, and small-sized vessels [16]. Intracranial internal carotid artery and proximal anterior, middle, and posterior cerebral arteries are considered as large-sized vessels; second divisions and downstream vessels are considered as medium- and small-sized vessels, respectively. Small-sized vessels are beyond the detection capacity of DSA but can be demonstrated on biopsy. Large- and medium-sized vessels are seen on angiograms. In AAV-related CNS involvement, small-sized vessels are more likely affected resulting in frequent normal angiography (involvement of branches after A2, M2, and P2 divisions) in half of the patients [1]. However, in some patients, angiography can be pathologic and suggestive of CNS vasculitis. In GPA patients, more than half of the patients who underwent an angiography had negative results [6]. Typical vasculitis findings include multiple arterial segmental and focal stenoses (>80% of lumen narrowing), occlusions, or fusiform dilations [17, 18].

It is important to note that multiple arterial segmental and focal stenoses can be observed in other conditions such as atherosclerosis or reversible cerebral vasoconstriction syndrome. However, in the two latter conditions, lesions often diffuse and affect more vessels than vasculitis.

13.5 Distinctive Presentations of AAV-Related CNS Involvement

13.5.1 Meningeal Involvement

Among the three AAV, GPA is mainly associated with meningeal involvement. Pachymeningeal involvement is more frequent than the leptomininingeal involvement. In GPA and EGPA, pachymeningitis was observed in 46% and 2% of patients, respectively [6, 7]. Pachymeningitis has been associated with the granulomatous form of GPA, but rarely observed in the vasculitic form [6], and more frequently occurs at the onset than during follow-up [19]. Thickening of the dura is linked to the granulomatous inflammation and can cause headaches, seizures, cranial neuropathies, myelopathy, or neuro-ophthalmologic complications [1, 19].

No difference regarding clinical and radiological presentations was observed according to the ANCA anti-MPO or anti-PR3 specificity. Although treatments reported in anti-MPO or anti-PR3 pachymeningitis did not differ, patients with anti-PR3 disease relapsed more frequently [1, 19].

13.5.2 Pituitary Involvement

Pituitary involvement is rare and observed only in GPA. According to different series, it affects 1.1–1.3% of all GPA patients [20, 21]. Three mechanisms are described to explain pituitary involvement, similar to what is observed in other GPA-related CNS involvement. Development of a granulomatous inflammation within the gland and vasculitis of the gland's vessels are two rare mechanisms, whereas the invasion of granulomatous inflammation from neighboring sinus cavities remains the most frequent mechanism. Pituitary involvement can lead to partial or global pituitary dysfunction. Posterior involvement is responsible for diabetes insipidus, whereas anterior involvement leads more likely to secondary hypogonadism. Other hormonal dysfunctions have also been reported [1]. Visual loss can be observed in cases where pituitary enlargement compresses the optic chiasm [22].

MRI is mandated and abnormal in more than 90% of patients, showing an enlargement of the pituitary gland or a stellar mass with peripheral enhancement.

Other differential diagnoses should be evoked, especially when pituitary involvement is inaugural, such as tuberculosis, sarcoidosis, or histiocytosis [23–25].

Biopsy is rarely required in patients with other clinical manifestations of GPA. However, when isolated, biopsy should be discussed.

Treatment is common and relies on classical induction regimen for systemic vasculitis. Cyclophosphamide is probably preferred to rituximab [20]. Pituitary dysfunction often persists after treatment.

13.6 Cerebrospinal Fluid Analysis

Cerebrospinal fluid (CSF) analysis is rarely described in case reports or case series on AAV-related CNS involvement. In primary CNS vasculitis, more than half of the patients show abnormal CSF analysis [26]. In a cohort of GPA patients with CNS involvement, CSF analysis showed a protein level >0.40 g/l in 9/19 (47%) patients and a white blood cells count >10/mm^3 in 7/19 (37%) [6]. In a cohort of EGPA patients with CNS involvement, CSF analysis was abnormal in 44% of patients [7].

Normal CSF analysis does not exclude diagnosis. Pleocytosis is the most common finding, mainly lymphocytic. Increased protein level can be observed and can be >1 g/l. CSF analysis allows ruling out differential diagnoses such as infections (HSV, VZV, tuberculosis), malignancies (histological analysis, research of onconeuronal antibodies), or other inflammatory conditions (angiotensin-converting enzyme).

In the absence of signs of intracranial hypertension, CSF analysis should be performed.

13.7 Biopsy

The biopsy of meningeal and parenchymal tissue remains the gold standard to demonstrate vasculitis. However, given the invasive nature of this procedure, biopsy is rarely performed. Moreover, CNS involvement of AAV is mostly suspected when other extraneurologic symptoms specific of AAV exist. Biopsy is more frequently discussed in patients with isolated or inaugural involvement of CNS and when other diagnosis should be evoked besides AAV (e.g., tumor-like lesions). Image-guided biopsy increases the yield of the procedure. However, biopsy of the frontal lobe of the minor hemisphere can be done in the absence of easily accessible lesions. Biopsy can be stereotactic or open wedged [27].

Three different histological patterns are described [28] and can overlap: granulomatous lesions are more likely observed in GPA [3, 29]; otherwise lymphocytic or necrotizing lesions can be observed.

Histological samples allow ruling out other differential diagnoses such as infections or malignancies, especially lymphoma. Complementary analyses can be carried out such as culture or clonality testing.

13.8 Biological Analyses

In opposition to the systemic manifestations of AAV, inflammatory parameters (C-reactive protein level) are moderately increased in isolated CNS vasculitis.

Some studies suggested that CNS involvement more frequently occurred in patients with negative or atypical ANCA [30]. However, in a large cohort of GPA patients with CNS involvement, ANCA were positive in 90% of patients [6]. In EGPA patients, ANCA are positive in half of the patients [7].

Dosage of ANCA in CSF has been reported in a patient with pachymeningitis, but is still not validated in clinical practice [31].

Laboratory tests are also required to search other conditions that can affect CNS vessels, especially in patients with isolated or inaugural CNS involvement. A complete immunological screening is required (ANCA, antinuclear antibodies, complement dosage, research of cryoglobulin, antiphospholipid antibodies, angiotensin-converting enzyme). Exhaustive infective serologies have to be searched for HCV, HBV, HIV, CMV, EBV, syphilis, borrelia, tuberculosis (interferon-gamma release assays). Other laboratory tests can be carried out according to the context, such as toxicological screening.

13.9 Diagnosis Approach

In a patient with uncontrolled AAV, occurrence of a neurological event can indicate a specific CNS involvement. However, other frequent neurovascular diseases (atherosclerosis, infection, malignancy) should be eliminated before retaining the AAV as responsible.

In a patient with controlled disease, occurrence of CNS involvement may indicate a treatment-related complication or a relapse of the disease.

Isolated or inaugural CNS involvement in the absence of systemic AAV remains the most challenging presentation and many conditions have to be researched.

Whatever the situation, a complete workup is required, including a dosage of ANCA. MRI is helpful and should be completed by angiography.

Although required, angiography is often negative and biopsy is in practice rarely performed [32]. AAV-related specific CNS involvement is thus often retained on the systemic context, the ANCA positivity, and the exclusion of other differential diagnosis [1].

13.10 Differential Diagnosis

Many conditions, some of them more frequent than AAV, should be searched in the setting of a CNS involvement.

We described in Table 13.1, not exhaustively, some conditions mimicking CNS vasculitis, pachymeningitis, and CNS granulomatous lesions.

Table 13.1 Differential Diagnoses of AAV-Related CNS Involvement (Not Exhaustive)

Differential diagnoses of CNS vasculitis		
Vasculopathies	*Thrombotic conditions*	*Embolic conditions*
Reversible vasoconstriction syndrome	Antiphospholipid syndrome	Aortic arch atherosclerosis
Intracranial atherosclerosis	Disseminated intravascular coagulation	Intracardiac shunt
Intracranial arterial dissection	Thrombotic microangiopathy	Intracardiac myxoma
Fibromuscular dysplasia	Sneddon syndrome	Endocarditis
Moyamoya		
Other conditions		
Endovascular lymphoma	Fabry disease	Homocystinuria
CADASIL (cerebral autosomal dominant arteriopathy with subcortical infarcts and leukoencephalopathy)	MELAS (mitochondrial encephalomyopathy, lactic acidosis, and stroke-like episodes)	ADEM (acute disseminated encephalomyelitis)
Paraneoplastic syndrome		
Differential diagnoses of pachymeningitis		
Idiopathic pachymeningitis	Acute infective meningitis	Tuberculosis
Syphilis	Sarcoidosis	Intracranial hypotension
Primary diffuse leptomeningeal gliomatosis	Meningeal amylosis	Thrombophlebitis
Post neurosurgery	Other systemic vasculitis	Sjogren syndrome
Differential diagnoses of CNS granulomatous-like lesions		
Infections	*Tumoral lesions*	*Other*
Tuberculosis	Primitive tumor	Sarcoidosis
Intracranial abscesses	Secondary tumor	Behcet disease
Endocarditis	Lymphoma	Crohn disease
Mycosis (aspergillosis)	Lymphomatoid granulomatosis	
Parasites (toxoplasmosis)		

CNS central nervous system

13.11 Therapeutic Strategy (See Specific Chapter in This Book)

According to the new five-factor score, CNS involvement is no longer included in the five items given the rarity of this involvement [8]. However, CNS involvement is serious and is considered as an affection requiring an aggressive treatment.

Once the other differential diagnoses affecting CNS have been ruled out, treatment does not differ from an AAV with a FFS ≥ 1. Treatment relies on the combination of glucocorticoids (GC) and an immunosuppressant.

GC is the first step of the treatment and can rapidly improve clinical condition. In patients with severe neurological deterioration, intravenous pulses of methylprednisolone can be used (15 mg/kg for 1–5 days). Oral prednisone should be started at 1 mg/kg for at least 2–4 weeks and then progressively tapered.

Cyclophosphamide (CYC) remains the most used agent allowing to achieve remission in 80% of cases [33]. It can be administered by intravenous pulses or orally. In France and in most European countries, intravenous pulses are preferred. Both administration ways showed comparable remission rates, but higher cumulative doses were reached in patients with oral administration, increasing then the risk of toxicity.

Rituximab (RTX) is another option to achieve remission in combination with GC. RTX is approved in severe GPA. In AAV patients with CNS involvement, little information exists on the efficiency of RTX in this setting. In primary CNS vasculitis, RTX showed to be effective only in few case reports [34, 35]. Consequently, in CNS involvement of AAV, RTX should probably be used in patients with a contraindication for CYC or in relapsing patients who already received important cumulative doses of CYC (>20 g). Except CYC and RTX, other immunosuppressive agents, such as TNFα blockers, anti-IL1, or anti-IL6 biotherapy, should probably not be used as first intention for induction or should be discussed individually according to the situation.

Once remission has been achieved, a maintenance treatment is required, as in other form of AAV with a FFS ≥1. Experiences in primary CNS vasculitis showed better outcomes (better relapse-free survival with low damages) in patients who received maintenance therapy [26]. Azathioprine (AZA, 2–3 mg/kg/day) was the most used agent in the French PCNSV cohort, but other publications indicated good outcomes with mycophenolate mofetil (MMF, 2 g/day), especially in children [26]. In AAV, MMF showed poorer outcomes when compared to AZA [36]. Methotrexate is another option and can be used at 0.3 mg/kg/week [26, 37]. Few information exists on maintenance therapy with RTX in CNS involvement. The best duration of maintenance is not known, but probably should reach at least 2 years.

Finally, treatment relies in most patients with CNS involvement on a combination of GC and an immunosuppressant (mainly CYC) followed by a maintenance therapy.

13.12 Outcomes

In the study by de Luna et al., 30/35 patients with GPA-related CNS involvement achieved a response to treatment combining GC and immunosuppressant, mainly CYC in 34 patients. Among responders, 8/30 (27%) patients relapsed after a median time of 14 months (range 9–96). Thirteen relapsing patients required another induction regimen, RTX in 8 and CYC in 5 others. CYC showed improvement of neurological symptoms in 80% and stabilization in 20%, whereas RTX showed improvement in 50% and stabilization in 50%. Neurological sequelae assessed with the modified Rankin Scale indicated a score ≥2, in 18/35 (51%) patients. In this study, only one patient died from another cause than AAV [6].

In the study by André et al., all patients (n = 84) received GC combined with CYC in 63% of them. Follow-up information was available in 81 patients, and a complete response was observed in 43%, partial response in 43%, and no response in 14%. Relapse occurred in 14% (11/81) of patients, including CNS relapse in six cases. In this study, 11 (13%) patients died, mainly from cerebral hemorrhage. Of patients, 57% had persistence of neurological sequelae, including persistent visual impairment in 18/27 (67%) patients, motor and/or sensory deficiency in 21/45 (47%) patients with ischemic lesions and 8/16 (50%) patients with intracerebral hemorrhages, and persistent cranial nerve palsy in 4/16 (25%) patients [7].

References

1. Graf J. Central nervous system disease in antineutrophil cytoplasmic antibodies-associated vasculitis. Rheum Dis Clin N Am. 2017;43:573–8.
2. de Groot K, Schmidt DK, Arlt AC, Gross WL, Reinhold-Keller E. Standardized neurologic evaluations of 128 patients with Wegener granulomatosis. Arch Neurol. 2001;58:1215–21.
3. Seror R, Mahr A, Ramanoelina J, Pagnoux C, Cohen P, Guillevin L. Central nervous system involvement in Wegener granulomatosis. Medicine (Baltimore). 2006;85:54–65.
4. Pinching AJ, Lockwood CM, Pussell BA, et al. Wegener's granulomatosis: observations on 18 patients with severe renal disease. Q J Med. 1983;52:435–60.
5. Nishino H, Rubino FA, Parisi JE. The spectrum of neurologic involvement in Wegener's granulomatosis. Neurology. 1993;43:1334–7.
6. De Luna G, Terrier B, Kaminsky P, et al. Central nervous system involvement of granulomatosis with polyangiitis: clinical-radiological presentation distinguishes different outcomes. Rheumatology (Oxford). 2015;54:424–32.
7. Andre R, Cottin V, Saraux JL, et al. Central nervous system involvement in eosinophilic granulomatosis with polyangiitis (Churg-Strauss): Report of 26 patients and review of the literature. Autoimmun Rev. 2017;16:963–9.
8. Guillevin L, Pagnoux C, Seror R, et al. The Five-Factor Score revisited: assessment of prognoses of systemic necrotizing vasculitides based on the French Vasculitis Study Group (FVSG) cohort. Medicine (Baltimore). 2011;90:19–27.
9. Sairanen T, Kanerva M, Valanne L, Lyytinen J, Pekkonen E. Churg-Strauss syndrome as an unusual aetiology of stroke with haemorrhagic transformation in a patient with no cardiovascular risk factors. Case Rep Neurol. 2011;3:32–8.
10. Han S, Rehman HU, Jayaratne PS, Carty JE. Microscopic polyangiitis complicated by cerebral haemorrhage. Rheumatol Int. 2006;26:1057–60.
11. Sassi SB, Ghorbel IB, Mizouni H, Houman MH, Hentati F. Microscopic polyangiitis presenting with peripheral and central neurological manifestations. Neurol Sci. 2011;32:727–9.
12. Decker ML, Emery DJ, Smyth PS, Lu JQ, Lacson A, Yacyshyn E. Microscopic polyangiitis with spinal cord involvement: a case report and review of the literature. J Stroke Cerebrovasc Dis. 2016;25:1696–704.
13. Boulouis G, de Boysson H, Zuber M, et al. Primary angiitis of the central nervous system: magnetic resonance imaging spectrum of parenchymal, meningeal, and vascular lesions at baseline. Stroke. 2017;48:1248–55.
14. Murphy JM, Gomez-Anson B, Gillard JH, et al. Wegener granulomatosis: MR imaging findings in brain and meninges. Radiology. 1999;213:794–9.
15. Carpinteri R, Patelli I, Casanueva FF, Giustina A. Pituitary tumours: inflammatory and granulomatous expansive lesions of the pituitary. Best Pract Res Clin Endocrinol Metab. 2009;23:639–50.
16. MacLaren K, Gillespie J, Shrestha S, Neary D, Ballardie FW. Primary angiitis of the central nervous system: emerging variants. QJM. 2005;98:643–54.
17. Alhalabi M, Moore PM. Serial angiography in isolated angiitis of the central nervous system. Neurology. 1994;44:1221–6.

18. Kadkhodayan Y, Alreshaid A, Moran CJ, Cross DT 3rd, Powers WJ, Derdeyn CP. Primary angiitis of the central nervous system at conventional angiography. Radiology. 2004;233:878–82.
19. Shimojima Y, Kishida D, Hineno A, Yazaki M, Sekijima Y, Ikeda SI. Hypertrophic pachymeningitis is a characteristic manifestation of granulomatosis with polyangiitis: A retrospective study of anti-neutrophil cytoplasmic antibody-associated vasculitis. Int J Rheum Dis. 2017;20:489–96.
20. De Parisot A, Puechal X, Langrand C, et al. Pituitary involvement in granulomatosis with polyangiitis: report of 9 patients and review of the literature. Medicine (Baltimore). 2015;94:e748.
21. Kapoor E, Cartin-Ceba R, Specks U, Leavitt J, Erickson B, Erickson D. Pituitary dysfunction in granulomatosis with polyangiitis: the Mayo Clinic experience. J Clin Endocrinol Metab. 2014;99:3988–94.
22. Goyal M, Kucharczyk W, Keystone E. Granulomatous hypophysitis due to Wegener's granulomatosis. AJNR Am J Neuroradiol. 2000;21:1466–9.
23. Ates I, Katipoglu B, Copur B, Yilmaz N. A rare cause of hypophysitis: tuberculosis. Endocr Regul. 2017;51:213–5.
24. Huo Z, Lu T, Liang Z, et al. Clinicopathological features and BRAF(V600E) mutations in patients with isolated hypothalamic-pituitary Langerhans cell histiocytosis. Diagn Pathol. 2016;11:100.
25. Marques C, Roriz M, Chabriat H, Buffon-Porcher F, Cognat E. Differential diagnosis between sarcoidosis and granulomatosis with polyangiitis in a patient with leptomeningeal, cavernous sinus and pituitary lesions. QJM. 2017;110:691–2.
26. de Boysson H, Parienti JJ, Arquizan C, et al. Maintenance therapy is associated with better long-term outcomes in adult patients with primary angiitis of the central nervous system. Rheumatology (Oxford). 2017;56:1684–93.
27. de Boysson H, Pagnoux C. Letter by de Boysson and Pagnoux Regarding Article, "Diagnostic Yield and Safety of Brain Biopsy for Suspected Primary Central Nervous System Angiitis". Stroke. 2016;47:e256.
28. Miller DV, Salvarani C, Hunder GG, et al. Biopsy findings in primary angiitis of the central nervous system. Am J Surg Pathol. 2009;33:35–43.
29. Yajima R, Toyoshima Y, Wada Y, et al. A fulminant case of granulomatosis with polyangiitis with meningeal and parenchymal involvement. Case Rep Neurol. 2015;7:101–4.
30. Reinhold-Keller E, de Groot K, Holl-Ulrich K, et al. Severe CNS manifestations as the clinical hallmark in generalized Wegener's granulomatosis consistently negative for antineutrophil cytoplasmic antibodies (ANCA). A report of 3 cases and a review of the literature. Clin Exp Rheumatol. 2001;19:541–9.
31. Spranger M, Schwab S, Meinck HM, et al. Meningeal involvement in Wegener's granulomatosis confirmed and monitored by positive circulating antineutrophil cytoplasm in cerebrospinal fluid. Neurology. 1997;48:263–5.
32. Drachman DA, Winter TS 3rd, Karon M. Medulloblastoma with extracranial metastases. Arch Neurol. 1963;9:518–30.
33. Haubitz M, Busch T, Gerlach M, et al. Exhaled nitric oxide in patients with Wegener's granulomatosis. Eur Respir J. 1999;14:113–7.
34. De Boysson H, Arquizan C, Guillevin L, Pagnoux C. Rituximab for primary angiitis of the central nervous system: report of 2 patients from the French COVAC cohort and review of the literature. J Rheumatol. 2013;40:2102–3.
35. Salvarani C, Brown RD Jr, Huston J 3rd, Morris JM, Hunder GG. Treatment of primary CNS vasculitis with rituximab: case report. Neurology. 2014;82:1287–8.
36. Kallenberg CG. Treatment of ANCA-associated vasculitis, where to go? Clin Rev Allergy Immunol. 2012;43:242–8.
37. Pagnoux C, Mahr A, Hamidou MA, et al. Azathioprine or methotrexate maintenance for ANCA-associated vasculitis. N Engl J Med. 2008;359:2790–803.

Skin Involvement 14

Angelo Valerio Marzano, Simona Tavecchio,
and Emilio Berti

14.1 Introduction

Antineutrophil cytoplasmic antibodies (ANCA)-associated vasculitis (AAVs) encompass a spectrum of clinically distinct forms of vasculitis that share the predominant involvement of small-sized vessels and the serological profile consisting of ANCA positivity [1]. From a clinicopathological point of view, AAVs are classified in microscopic polyangiitis (MPA), granulomatosis with polyangiitis (GPA), and eosinophilic granulomatosis with polyangiitis (EGPA) on the basis of the distribution of vascular inflammation and the presence or absence of granulomatosis and asthma [2]. Concerning the serological profile, three main patterns of ANCAs are recognized by using indirect immunofluorescence [3]: the first, cytoplasmic (c)-ANCAs, are characterized by a diffuse cytoplasmic granular fluorescence most prominent centrally between the nuclear lobes; the antigen of this pattern is usually the leukocyte proteinase 3 (PR3) and this type of ANCAs is present in the majority of patients with GPA during the active phases of the disease [4]. The second type of ANCAs, perinuclear (p)-ANCAs, shows a perinuclear neutrophil staining pattern often with nuclear extension and its major target antigen is myeloperoxidase (MPO): p-ANCAs are typically detected in patients with MPA and EGPA [4]. The third type of ANCAs, atypical (a)-ANCAs, is rare and combines both cytoplasmic and perinuclear/nuclear staining, targeting different autoantigens [4]. Patients with c-ANCA and p-ANCA have different organ involvement, different response to treatment, and different risk of relapse [5]. The AAVs are rare diseases, with worldwide incidence

A. V. Marzano (✉) · S. Tavecchio · E. Berti
Dermatology Unit, Fondazione IRCCS Ca' Granda Ospedale Maggiore Policlinico, Milan, Italy

Department of Pathophysiology and Transplantation, Università degli Studi di Milano, Milan, Italy
e-mail: angelo.marzano@unimi.it

R. A. Sinico, L. Guillevin (eds.), *Anti-Neutrophil Cytoplasmic Antibody (ANCA) Associated Vasculitis*, Rare Diseases of the Immune System,
https://doi.org/10.1007/978-3-030-02239-6_14

ranging from 13 to 20 cases per million individuals per year and a prevalence of 46–184 cases per million individuals [6]. The incidence and prevalence of AAVs is increased over time probably due to the improvement in disease diagnosis. At disease onset, AAV can be limited to a single organ or involve multiple organs. Skin manifestations can occur frequently due to the vasculitic involvement of skin vessels. In a recently published multicenter, restrospective study on 1553 AAV patients, cutaneous manifestations were present in 45% of cases [7]. This prevalence is consistence with previous reports from Carlson et al. [8] and Guillevin et al. [9], which found skin manifestations in 50% and 44% of AAV patients, respectively. In the study of Frumholtz et al. [7], the prevalence of cutaneous involvement was higher in EGPA and MPA than in GPA, with different pattern of lesions among the three AAV entities, as discussed in more detail later in this chapter. Among the cutaneous manifestations, palpable purpura represents the most common vasculitis-related lesion, but the cutaneous picture of AAVs is typically polymorphic including also papules, nodules, urticarial lesions, livedo, pustules, blisters, and necrotic ulcers. Histologically, postcapillary venules are more often involved than arteries and capillaries in the skin lesions of the whole AAV group. This chapter is focused on the cutaneous manifestations of AAVs and their histopathological/immunofluorescence features. The differential diagnosis of these entities is discussed with an emphasis on the skin aspects and the main therapeutic approaches are briefly addressed.

14.2 Granulomatosis with Polyangiitis (Wegener's Granulomatosis)

According to the 2012 revised Chapel Hill criteria, GPA, previously known as Wegener's granulomatosis, is defined as a necrotizing granulomatous inflammation of the upper and lower respiratory tracts with necrotizing vasculitis of small and medium-sized vessels [2]. GPA has been associated with the presence of ANCA, which mainly have a cytoplasmic staining pattern in immunofluorescence, and with antibodies directed against PR3 in ELISA test [2]. GPA is a rare disease with an incidence evaluated between 7 and 12 new cases per million inhabitants per year [10]. The age at diagnosis is between 45 and 60 years, although pediatric cases have been described as well [11, 12]; in fact, GPA is the most frequent AAV form in the pediatric population, with incidence rates ranging from 0.03 and 3.2 per 100,000 children per year [13]. There are no differences in frequency between male and female and two different phenotypes of the disease have been described: localized and systemic GPA [14]. However, no general consensus was reached on this matter. GPA is a disease with specific multi-organ involvement and nonspecific constitutional symptoms that are present in around half of the cases. Ear, nose, and throat (ENT) manifestations are common and reported in about 70–100% of cases at the time of diagnosis [15]. Nasal-sinus involvement is the most common manifestation of GPA and may be the only sign observed in the localized form of the disease [15]. GPA can affect the lungs in about 50–90% of patients, causing alveolar hemorrhage and/or parenchymatous nodules [11, 14]. The kidney is often involved (40–100% of cases) generally with a segmental necrotizing glomerulonephritis, which may cause a wide range of clinical features, from isolated urinary abnormalities to rapidly progressive, potentially life-threatening kidney failure [16]. GPA may also affect the gastrointestinal system leading to ulcerative lesions with possible intestinal perforation, the urogenital tract with prostatitis, orchitis, epididymitis with possible ureteral stenosis, and the peripheral nervous system manifesting as mononeuritis multiplex or sensorimotor neuropathy. The eye involvement is rare but extremely characteristic of the disease presenting with the so-called eye socket (episcleritis, scleritis, corneal ulcerates, retinal vasculitis, granulomatous retro-orbital pseudotumor or dacryoadenitis) [11]. Skin involvement can be very frequent and various, as described in detail in this chapter. Data on disease course suggest that patients with GPA frequently experience relapse during treatment maintenance: one-quarter of patients within 2 years and about half of patients within 5 years from the diagnosis [17]. Some evidence reported that patients with ENT presentation and granulomatous manifestations, such as orbital pseudotumor or pulmonary nodules, go through relapse more frequently than patients with systemic form and kidney involvement [18]. Conversely, severity of renal involvement remains the major prognostic factor for both renal function and life-threatening potential of the disease [17]. Persistent ANCA positivity seems to be predictive of relapse, whereas variations in ANCA titres do not appear to be associated with new flares [11]. The main causes of mortality in patients with GPA are infections and kidney failure, especially in the first year following diagnosis. However, prognosis of untreated patients with AAV is poor with a mortality rate of about 90% after 1 year [19].

14.2.1 Cutaneous Features

Skin involvement is seen in around 50% of the patients with GPA (Table 14.1) [20, 21]. However, in a recent multicenter retrospective study of the French Vasculitis Group [7] on a large AAV cohort, the cutaneous manifestations were present only in 36.7% of patients with GPA. Interestingly, in GPA cutaneous involvement was associated with poorer prognosis, with poorer overall survival and relapse-free survival [7]. As confirmed by the aforementioned study, the most common lesion in GPA as well as in the whole group of AAVs is palpable purpura, but the cutaneous picture may be polymorphic, consisting of papules, nodules, vesicles, and blisters as well as necrotic-ulcerative lesions on a background of livedo reticularis. Livedo reticularis is an ischemic dermopathy characterized by a symmetric, violaceous reticular, or net-like mottling of the skin surrounding a pallorous conical core. All these cutaneous manifestations are similar to that of the cutaneous small vessel vasculitis, also known with the histological term of leukocytoclastic vasculitis, which is the most frequent form of vasculitis with predominant skin involvement. The skin lesions of GPA most commonly occur on the lower extremities, but may also appear on the face and scalp [20, 21]. The cutaneous features of GPA typically present with crops of lesions following a chronic-relapsing course; they manifest as recurrent episodes generally lasting from weeks to months and usually resolve with the treatment for

Table 14.1 Cutaneous and mucosal manifestations as well as histopathological features and direct immunofluorescence findings in GPA, EGPA, and MPA

	Skin	Oral mucosa	Upper respiratory airway mucosa	Histopathological aspects	Direct immunofluorescence findings
GPA	(10–50%) Palpable purpura, nodules, papules, vesiculobullous lesions, ulcers with possible necrosis, livedo reticularis, digital or penile ulceration/gangrene, PG-like ulcers	(10–50%) Erosive/ulcerative oral lesions, strawberry gingivitis	(70–100%) Sinusitis with purulent or hematic discharge; ulceration of the nasal mucosa and palate; nasal deformity with a saddle nose appearance, perforation of the septum	Leukocytoclastic vasculitis with fibrinoid necrosis and neutrophilic infiltration of the dermal small vessels; granulomatous inflammation around vessels; nonspecific perivascular lymphocytic infiltration	IgM and/or C3 deposits around dermal small vessels
EGPA	(40–52%) Palpable purpura, nodules, urticarial lesions, livedo reticularis, vesicles, aseptic pustules, ulcers with possible necrosis, EM-like lesions	(2.5%) Erosive/ulcerative oral lesions	Nasal polyposis, allergic rhinosinusitis, epistaxis	Leukocytoclastic vasculitis with fibrinoid necrosis and granulomatous inflammation involving venules; neutrophil-rich inflammatory infiltrate	IgM and/or C3 deposits around dermal small vessels
MPA	(30–60%) Palpable purpura, livedo reticularis, segmentary edema, nodules, urticarial lesions, ulcers with possible necrosis, bullae, EED-like nodules/plaques	(0.3%) Erosive/ulcerative oral lesions	–	Leukocytoclastic vasculitis with fibrinoid necrosis and neutrophilic infiltration of the dermal small vessels; nonspecific perivascular lymphocytic infiltration	Generally negative; sometimes IgM and/or C3 deposits around dermal small vessels

GPA granulomatosis with polyangiitis, *EGPA* eosinophilic granulomatosis with polyangiitis, *MPA* microscopic polyangiitis, *PG* pyoderma gangrenosum, *EM* erythema multiforme, *EED* erythema elevatum diutinum, *Ig* immunoglobulin, *C* complement
Reproduced with permission from [72]

the internal organ involvement. Ulceration and gangrene of the digits (Fig. 14.1a) or penis can rarely develop [11, 20]. Few cases of GPA manifesting as ulcerative lesions recalling pyoderma gangrenosum have also been reported (Fig. 14.1b) [11, 20, 22, 23]. In the study of the French Vasculitis group, pyoderma gangrenosum-like lesions, albeit rare, were specific of GPA since they were not found in the other AAVs [7]. A rare distinctive subset of GPA limited to the face and upper airway mucosa that shows a locally aggressive behavior with cartilage and bony disruption has recently been described [24, 25]; these cases represent a setting of localized GPA without systemic involvement after a prolonged follow-up. Oral lesions have been reported in 10–60% of patients and may be the presenting sign of GPA in around 5% of cases [26, 27]. Oral involvement usually presents with nonspecific

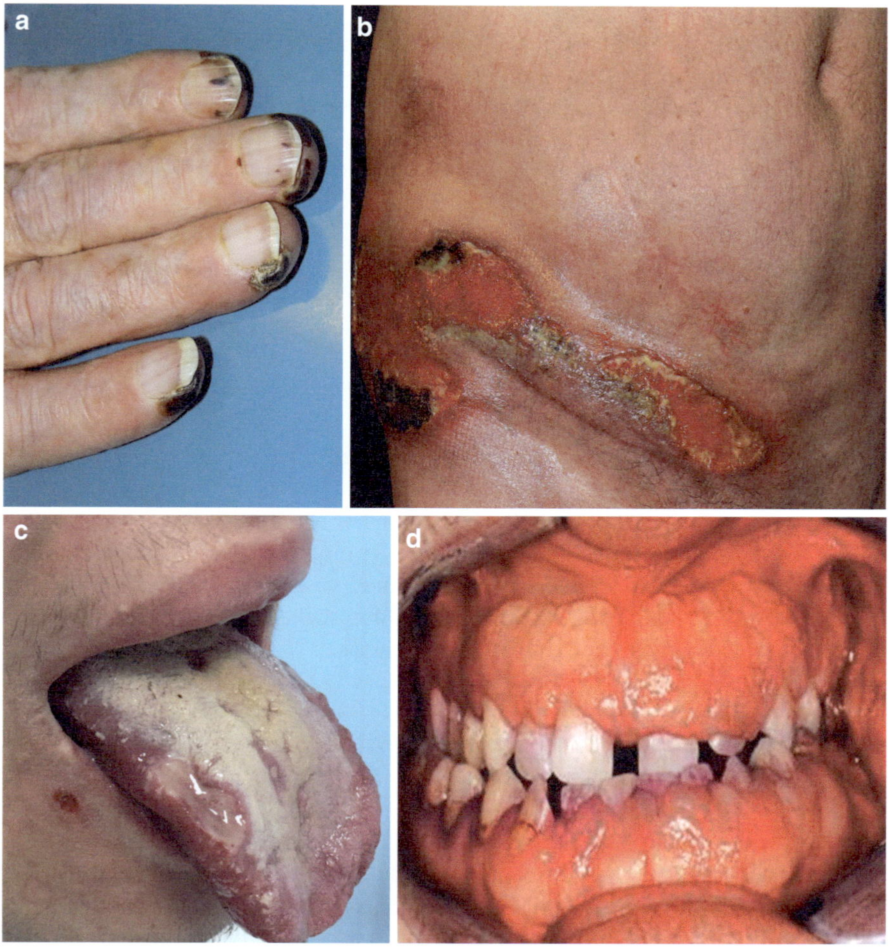

Fig. 14.1 Granulomatosis with polyangiitis. Gangrene of the digits (panel **a**); in (panel **b**), large pyoderma gangrenosum-like skin ulcer on the trunk. Oral ulcers on the tongue (panel **c**) and gingival hyperplasia (panel **d**)

erosive/ulcerative lesions (Fig. 14.1c), but can also manifest as strawberry gingivitis, which is a rare form of hyperplastic gingivitis nearly pathognomonic for GPA (Fig. 14.1d) [26, 27]. Indeed, in the recent multicenter study mentioned above oral ulcers were significantly more frequent in GPA than in the other AAVs and gingival hyperplasia proved to be specific for GPA, the latter being lacking in the other AAVs [7]. Nasal deformity with saddle nose features may rarely be seen in GPA, while frank perforation of the septum is less common [28]. No differences between adults and children have been reported concerning the morphology of skin lesions as well as their distribution [29, 30].

14.2.2 Histopathological Aspects

The histopathological pattern of GPA in skin lesions is represented by leukocytoclastic vasculitis in up to 50% of biopsies (Fig. 14.2a, b) [20]. The hallmark of leukocytoclastic vasculitis is the fibrinoid necrosis of the dermal small vessel wall; granulomatous features may be associated in a lesser percentage of GPA patients. Perivascular inflammatory infiltrates mainly consisting of neutrophils with lymphocytes and eosinophils as well as endothelial cell swelling, neutrophil fragmentation, nuclear dust, and red blood cell extravasation are also seen. Granulomatous inflammation surrounding vessels or palisading necrotizing granulomas, as observed in biopsy specimens taken from the internal organ infiltrates, are uncommonly demonstrated in skin lesions of GPA. Histology may also show only nonspecific perivascular lymphocytic infiltrates [20, 25].

14.2.3 Direct Immunofluorescence Studies

Direct immunofluorescence on GPA skin lesions of recent appearance (within few hours) usually demonstrates immunoglobulin (Ig), particularly IgM, and complement (C) three deposits around the wall of small vessels in the dermis in nearly 70% of cases [20, 31]. Thus, direct immunofluorescence represents an important adjuvant tool in diagnosis and differential diagnosis.

14.3 Eosinophilic Granulomatosis with Polyangiitis (Churg–Strauss Syndrome)

EGPA, previously called with the eponym Churg–Strauss syndrome, is a systemic disorder belonging to the AAV. According to the 2012 revised classification criteria, EGPA is defined as an eosinophil-rich and granulomatous inflammation involving the respiratory tract and necrotizing vasculitis predominantly affecting small- and medium-sized vessels, associated with asthma and eosinophilia [2]. The incidence of the disease is about 0.5–6.8 new cases per million inhabitants per year, with a presenting age between 40 and 60 years. ANCA positivity is present in about

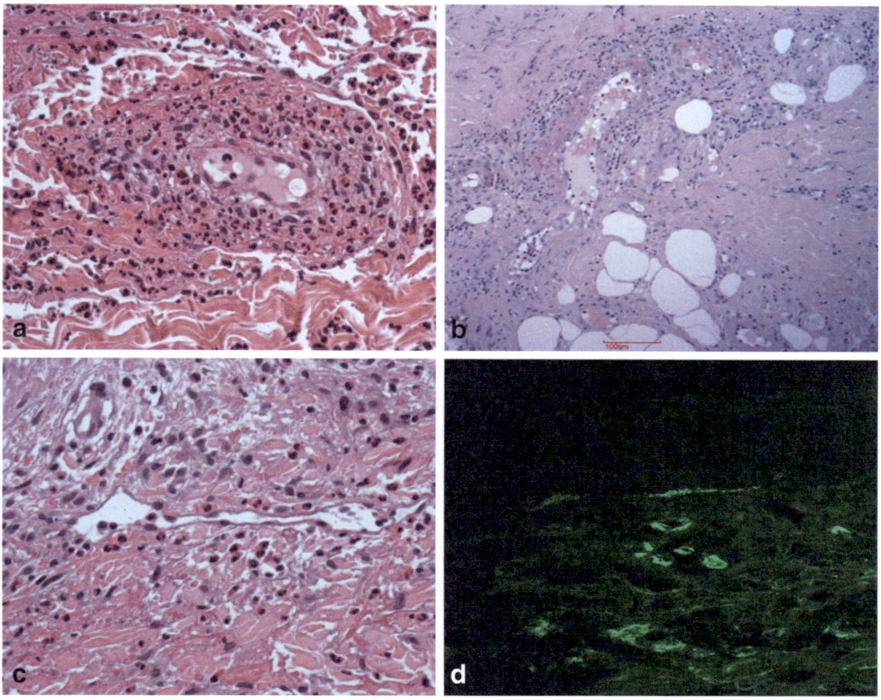

Fig. 14.2 (Panel **a**) Typical histological features of leukocytoclastic vasculitis with a sparse infiltrate of neutrophils and nuclear debris localized around dermal venules in skin specimens taken from palpable purpura in granulomatosis with polyangiitis (GPA). (Panel **b**) Histology of a pyoderma gangrenosum-like skin lesion of GPA showing necrotizing vasculitis with partial thrombosis, fibrinoid degeneration and infiltration of neutrophils with leukocytoclasia of a medium-sized vessel at the dermal-hypodermal junction (Courtesy of Prof. F. Rongioletti). (Panel **c**) Leukocytoclastic vasculitis with a sparse infiltrate of neutrophils and eosinophils in the dermis and around the venules associated with upper dermal edema in an urticarial lesion of a patient with eosinophilic granulomatosis with polyangiitis (EGPA). (Panel **d**) Direct immunofluorescence in EGPA revealing immunoglobulin M deposits around dermal small vessels

40–60% of patients, showing a perinuclear staining at the immunofluorescence analysis and a specificity for anti-MPO antibodies in solid phase immunoassays [32]. The clinical manifestations of EGPA may develop following three sequential phases. The prodromic or allergic phase is characterized by the occurrence of asthma (in about 95% of cases), allergic rhinitis, sinusitis, and nasal polyposis. The eosinophilic phase is characterized by a raise in the peripheral eosinophilic count (at least >1500 eosinophils/μL or >10% of the total white blood cells) and by possible eosinophilic multi-organ infiltrations. The third phase is characterized by a necrotizing vasculitis, usually associated with vascular or extravascular granulomatosis and constitutional symptoms [33]. Lung is the most frequently involved organ (more than 90% of patients with EGPA) followed by nervous system (about 70% of EGPA patients), principally manifesting as peripheral neuropathy [7]. Eosinophilic gastroenteritis as well as cardiac and renal involvement can also be present [33, 34]. A broad variety of skin lesions have been described, as reported below in this chapter. As for the other AAVs, patients with EGPA have an improved outcome when adequately treated. Indeed, a retrospective study of 383 EGPA patients enrolled in the French Vasculitis Study Group cohort showed 5- and 10-year survival rates of 88.9% and 78.6%, respectively, whereas vasculitis relapse-free survival rates were 64.8% and 54.4%, respectively [35].

14.3.1 Cutaneous Features

Skin involvement occurs in approximately 40–50% of patients with EGPA [7, 35, 36]. Palpable purpuric lesions (Fig. 14.3a) and nodules (Fig. 14.3b) arising on a background of purpura are the most common skin manifestations and are typically located on the limbs and scalp. Urticarial lesions are also frequent in EGPA (Fig. 14.3c). The French Vasculitis Group identified a peculiar pattern of

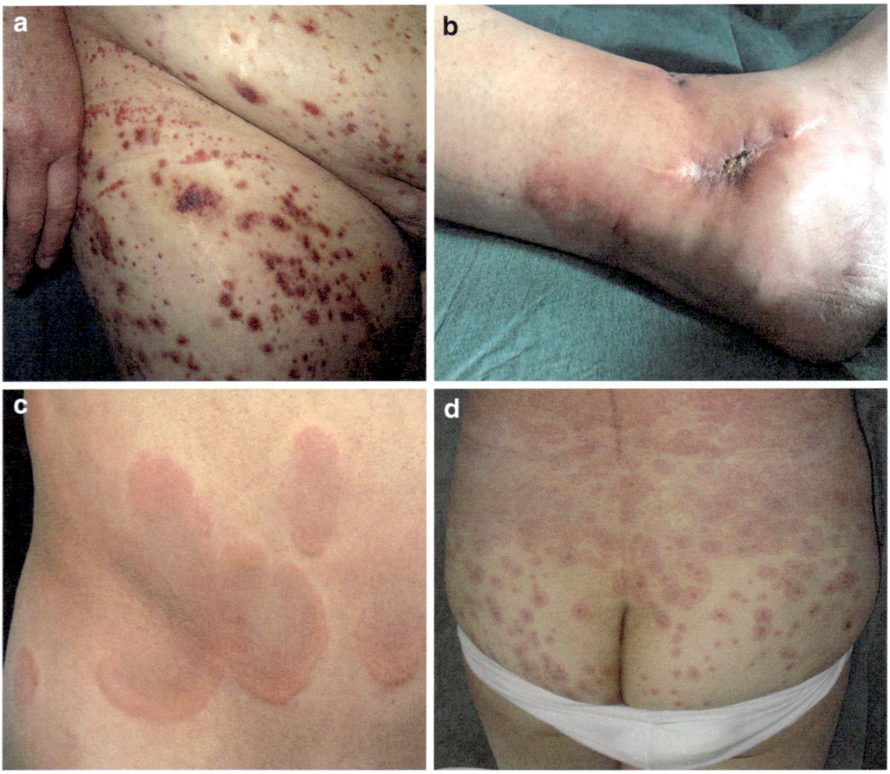

Fig. 14.3 Eosinophilic granulomatosis with polyangiitis. Palpable purpura (panel **a**) and erythematous nodules associated with necrotic-ulcerative lesions (panel **b**) on the lower extremities; urticarial lesions on the trunk (panel **c**); erythema multiforme-like lesions on the back (panel **d**)

EGPA cutaneous manifestations consisting of palpable purpura, nodules, and urticarial lesions, which were the most frequent skin features in the EGPA population of their AAV cohort [7]. Livedo reticularis, vesiculobullous lesions, and aseptic pustules can also develop at the same time or in different phases of the disease; papules and nodules may undergo a necrotic-ulcerative evolution [31]. A maculopapular erythematous eruption mimicking erythema multiforme (Fig. 14.3d) has also been described [20, 37]. Erythema multiforme is an immune-mediated skin disease presenting with targetoid lesions, symmetrically involving the extremities, particularly the palmar regions, and usually triggered by viral infections or, rarely, by drugs. Erosive/ulcerative oral lesions are present in 2.5% of patients with EGPA [7].

14.3.2 Histopathological Aspects

The skin biopsy shows a leukocytoclastic vasculitis mostly involving venules; in some cases, the fibrinoid necrosis of the vessel wall is associated with granulomatous changes. The diagnostic clue is the finding of numerous eosinophils in the inflammatory infiltrate, which consists also of neutrophils, lymphocytes and macrophages (Fig. 14.2c). A relevant number of eosinophils may also be present in the context of EGPA granulomas, where they are mixed with macrophages and multinucleated giant cells [20, 31].

14.3.3 Direct Immunofluorescence Studies

Direct immunofluorescence on recent onset skin lesions shows the presence of IgM and C3 deposits surrounding the wall of dermal small blood vessels in more than 50% of cases (Fig. 14.2d) [20, 31].

14.4 Microscopic Polyangiitis

MPA is a systemic vasculitis predominantly affecting small-sized blood vessels with absence of granuloma formation or hypereosinophilia [2]. In about 50–75% of cases, MPA is associated with ANCA positivity and generally with perinuclear staining at immunofluorescence evaluation due to antibodies directed against MPO [38]. MPA incidence is 2.7 to 94 new cases per million inhabitants per year [39]. The major organs involved in MPA are the lungs and the kidneys, although skin manifestations are also frequent, as reported below in this chapter. Renal involvement is present in almost 100% of patients and it is characterized by rapidly progressive glomerulonephritis [40]. Lung involvement can be seen in up to 90% of patients manifesting as a diffuse alveolar hemorrhage due to pulmonary capillaritis [38]. Neurological and gastrointestinal manifestations have also been reported with different frequency. The prognosis of MPA is poor if not promptly diagnosed and treated, especially due to alveolar hemorrhage and progressive glomerulonephritis that are life-threatening conditions [41].

14.4.1 Cutaneous Features

Skin lesions are found in 30–60% of patients [7, 8, 40, 42, 43] and are the initial presenting sign in 15–30% of patients [8]. Palpable purpura (Fig. 14.4a) is the most common manifestation and occurs in 30–40% of patients [8, 44]. Other manifestations include livedo reticularis (Fig. 14.4b), nodules, urticarial lesions, skin ulcers with necrosis, and segmentary edema [7, 8]. In the aforementioned multicenter study [7], livedo and segmentary edema were the most frequent cutaneous manifestations of MPA. Some patients present also bullae (Fig. 14.4c) or nodules and plaques recalling erythema elevatum diutinum (Fig. 14.4d) [45], a neutrophil-mediated skin disease presenting with erythematous-violaceous

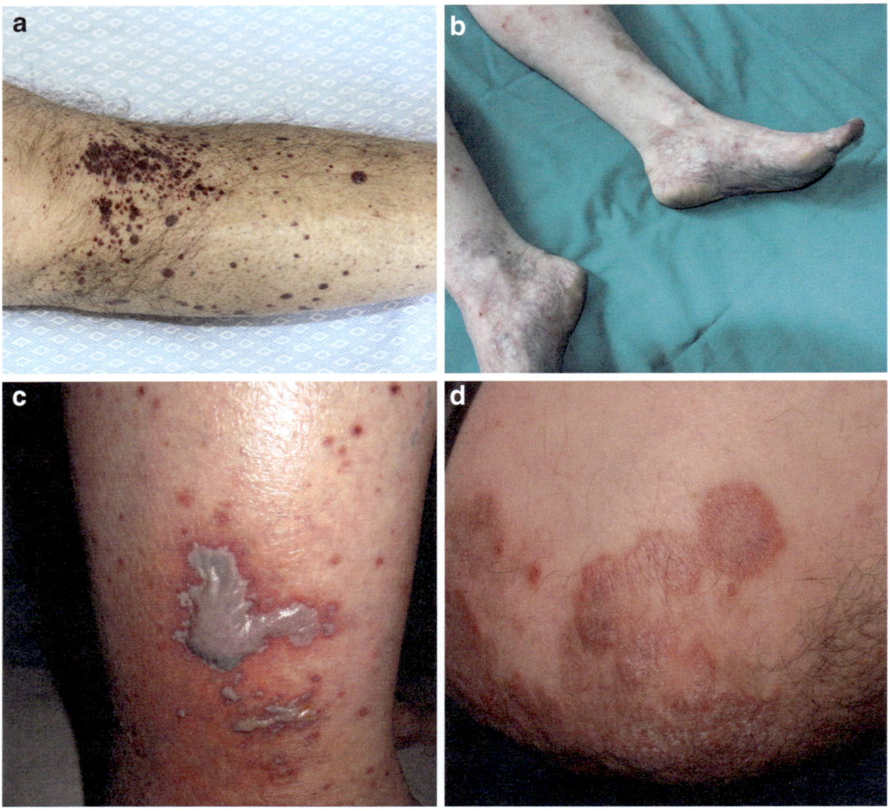

Fig. 14.4 Microscopic polyangiitis. Palpable purpura (panel **a**) and livedo reticularis (panel **b**) on the lower extremities. Bullous lesions on the legs (panel **c**); erythematous nodules and plaques resembling erythema elevatum diutinum on an elbow (panel **d**)

papules and nodules mainly located on the extensor aspects of the extremities, with a symmetrical distribution [46, 47]. The extremities are most commonly affected and the lesions usually appear at an early stage of microscopic polyangiitis [44]. Dermatologic manifestations are often associated with arthralgias [8]. No specific relationship between any skin eruption type and incidence of renal and/or pulmonary involvement has been shown [45]. Erosive/ulcerative oral lesions are rare, being present in only 0.3% of patients with MPA [7].

14.4.2 Histopathological Aspects

Biopsies of palpable purpura often show leukocytoclastic vasculitis, with fibrinoid necrosis, neutrophilic infiltration of the small vessels in the dermis and nuclear dust [44]. However, a nonspecific perivascular lymphocytic infiltration can also be seen [8, 48]. Biopsies of cutaneous nodules generally show vasculitis involving vessels of the deep dermis or subcutis [8].

14.4.3 Direct Immunofluorescence Studies

Immunofluorescence studies are generally negative or show few deposits of IgM and C3 [8, 48].

14.5 Diagnosis and Differential Diagnosis

Cutaneous manifestations commonly develop in patients with AAV with different frequency between EGPA, GPA, and MPA, as described in detail before [7, 28, 49, 50]. Different skin lesions may coexist in the same patient and occur in different occasions during the course of the vasculitis. Thus, the diagnosis of AAV is challenging and requires detailed medical history as well as accurate physical examination. This approach generally ends with the indication of a skin biopsy, whose histopathological analysis is essential for the diagnostic process. The ANCA serology does eventually support the diagnosis. As a first step for a correct differential diagnosis, drugs, infections, and other underlying systemic inflammatory diseases, such as systemic lupus erythematosus, must be excluded. This holds particularly true, if the first clinical presentation includes palpable purpura of the lower limbs, papules, nodules or plaques, ulcers and urticarial lesions, which together resemble the cutaneous small vessel vasculitis (CSVV) [51, 52]. In about 50% of CSVV cases, a triggering factor is recognized, being drugs or infections the main causes, whereas in the other half of patients, it is not possible to identify a specific etiology [20]. In AAV, CSVV can occur as component of the disease, thereby confusing the line between the two conditions. However, the characteristic internal organ involvement in AAV and the ANCA serology are crucial diagnostic clues to distinguish the two conditions. History of drug intake needs to be addressed, with specific attention to cocaine use. Indeed, midline destructive lesions induced by cocaine can mimic cases of limited GPA affecting ear, nose, and throat, potentially making the correct diagnosis difficult. However, inconsistent ANCA pattern and histological findings not suggestive for GPA can help in the diagnosis [53]. Indeed, the histology in cocaine-induced ulcerative lesions is characterized by a diffuse dermal infiltrate consisting mostly of neutrophils, without granulomas. Blastomycosis can cause skin lesions similar to those observed in AAV, and specifically in GPA [25]. Thus, microbiological analysis must be performed whenever an infection is suspected. Blastomycosis is a severe deep mycosis caused by *Blastomyces dermatitidis*, a dimorphic fungus endemic to the shore of lakes and rivers in Central and Southern North America. Infection usually occurs through inhalation and involves individuals coming from these areas with a history of recreational or occupational exposure to wooded areas or bodies of water. Another differential diagnosis for GPA is pyoderma gangrenosum (PG) involving the face, neck, and upper truncal region; these sites are atypical since this disease usually involves the lower extremities. PG is a neutrophil-mediated autoinflammatory disease presenting with single or multiple skin ulcers with undermined raised erythematous-violaceous borders often associated with pustules and possibly, albeit rarely, displaying internal organ involvement [54–56]. However, the typical histology of PG is characterized mainly by neutrophilic infiltrates, in the absence of frank vasculitis. On the other hand, it is important to highlight that some patients initially diagnosed as having PG were later reclassified as GPA, since they subsequently developed visceral involvement characteristic of GPA [22, 57]. Drug-induced PG, notably when it is triggered by propylthiouracil or by levamisole-adulterated cocaine [58, 59], should also be differentiated. However, clinical and histopathological findings recalling those of conventional PG, in combination with both disease resolution after trigger avoidance and the presence of atypical p-ANCA, help in differential diagnosis [43]. Extranodal natural killer/T-cell lymphoma should also be considered as a possible diagnosis alternative to GPA. However, the histopathological findings and the absence of clonality on molecular biology guaranty the exclusion of a neoplastic condition [28]. Livedo reticularis is a frequent expression of an underlying hypercoagulable or autoimmune disorder, including polyarteritis nodosa (PAN) and antiphospholipid syndrome. In analogy, urticarial lesions and targetoid lesions might lead to misdiagnosis of urticarial vasculitis and erythema multiforme, respectively. However, the presence of clinical manifestations suggesting a specific AAV, such as asthma, rhinitis, and sinusitis, as well as typical granuloma in different organs in association with the ANCA serology weigh the balance toward the diagnosis of a distinct form of AAV. Skin vasculitic lesions as well as kidney involvement are also typical manifestations of Henoch-Schönlein purpura, but a young presentation age and IgA deposition detectable by immunofluorescence help in the differential diagnosis [60]. Serology for hepatitis B and C should also be tested when cryoglobulinemia and PAN are suspected, especially if ulcerations or gangrene of digits or penis are present [31]. In conclusion, skin lesions might be observed in the course of several and different clinical conditions, not only including AAV. A global evaluation of the patient is mandatory for guiding the clinical judgment toward the correct diagnostic process. Medical and drug history and physical examination should be completed with blood tests and skin biopsy. Indeed, laboratory findings, including ANCA serology and peripheral blood eosinophilia, as well as histopathological aspects and direct immunofluorescence studies are pivotal for a correct diagnosis of AAV.

14.6 Treatment

The most recent published recommendations are multidisciplinary and based on an extensive literature search [61]. There is no specific therapeutic approach for cutaneous involvement, but the same patient-tailored algorithm used for systemic complications is suggested also for skin lesions. The updated recommendations provide a practical framework that may be applied to the majority of patients with AAV [61]. The first aim is the induction of remission of new-onset organ-threatening or life-threatening AAV. To this purpose, a combination of glucocorticoids (1 mg/kg/day with a maximum dose 80 mg daily with a target of 7.5–10 mg after 3–5 months of treatment) and either cyclophosphamide (2 mg/kg/day with a maximum 200 mg daily) or rituximab (375 mg/m^2 of body surface area, once a week for four infusions) is recommended. This approach is also suggested for major relapse of organ-threatening or life-threatening disease [61]. By contrast, for the induction of remission of non-organ-threatening disease, treatment with a combination of glucocorticoids and either methotrexate (20–25 mg/week, oral or parenteral) or mycophenolate mofetil is suggested [61]. It is known that complete remission may be achieved in nearly 70–90% of patients with AAV after induction therapy consisting of high-dose glucocorticoids combined with other immunosuppressive drugs [62–68]. Finally, for remission maintenance of AAV, a combination treatment of low-dose glucocorticoids and either azathioprine (starting at 2 mg/kg/day), rituximab, methotrexate, or mycophenolate mofetil (starting at 2000 mg/day) is possible [60]. In 2011, rituximab has been formally approved for the treatment of AAV [69]. The first randomized double-blind controlled trial (RAVE) showed that rituximab was not inferior to daily cyclophosphamide for induction of remission in severe AAV and it appeared to be superior in relapsing disease [70] and in maintenance of remissions in AAV [71].

14.7 Conclusions

In conclusion, AAVs are rare diseases but a high level of suspicion is necessary. Notably for skin manifestations, AAVs display many mimics that need to be excluded. Clinical features are frequently nonspecific thus requiring further laboratory tests such as the detection of ANCAs, as well as their antigen specificity. The categorization of patients by ANCA specificity seems to be an informative biomarker that is usually available at the time of AAV onset. Skin biopsy is always necessary to confirm the clinical diagnosis, particularly in the presence of skin manifestations that mimic other conditions such as pyoderma gangrenosum, erythema multiforme and erythema elevatum diutinum. Moreover, extravascular histopathological findings, such as an eosinophil-rich inflammatory infiltrate and/or granulomatous aspects, in addition to the presence of systemic symptoms and signs, may be important diagnostic clues to rule out a single-organ cutaneous vasculitis. Other important factors are the availability of recent data on safety profile, route of administration and cost of the new biologic treatments to be included in the physician's armamentarium.

References

1. Cornec D, Cornec-Le Gall E, Fervenza FC, Specks U. ANCA-associated vasculitis—clinical utility of using ANCA specificity to classify patients. Nat Rev Rheumatol. 2016;12(10):570–9.
2. Jennette JC, Falk RJ, Bacon PA, et al. 2012 revised International Chapel Hill Consensus Conference Nomenclature of vasculitides. Arthritis Rheum. 2013;65(1):1–11.
3. Csernok E, Moosig F. Current and emerging techniques for ANCA detection in vasculitis. Nat Rev Rheumatol. 2014;10(8):494–501.
4. Damoiseaux J, Csernok E, Rasmussen N, et al. Detection of antineutrophil cytoplasmic antibodies (ANCAs): a multicentre European Vasculitis Study Group (EUVAS) evaluation of the value of indirect immunofluorescence (IIF) versus antigen-specific immunoassays. Ann Rheum Dis. 2016;76(4):647–53.
5. Jennette JC, Falk RJ. Pathogenesis of antineutrophil cytoplasmic autoantibody-mediated disease. Nat Rev Rheumatol. 2014;10(8):463–73.
6. Watts RA, Mahr A, Mohammad AJ, Gatenby P, Basu N, Flores-Suarez LF. Classification, epidemiology and clinical subgrouping of antineutrophil cytoplasmic antibody (ANCA)-associated vasculitis. Nephrol Dial Transplant. 2015;30(Suppl 1):i14–22.
7. Frumholtz L, Laurent-Roussel S, Aumaître O, et al. Clinical and pathological significance of cutaneous manifestations in ANCA-associated vasculitides. Autoimmun Rev. 2017;16:1138–46.
8. Carlson JA, Chen KR. Cutaneous vasculitis update: small vessel neutrophilic vasculitis syndromes. Am J Dermatopathol. 2006;28(6):486–506.
9. Guillevin L, Pagnoux C, Seror R, et al. The five factor score revisited: assessment of prognoses of systemic necrotizing vasculitides based on the French Vasculitis Study Group (FVSG) cohort. Medicine (Baltimore). 2011;90:19–27.
10. Mohammad AJ, Jacobsson LT, Westman KW, Sturfelt G, Segelmark M. Incidence and survival rates in Wegener's granulomatosis, microscopic polyangiitis, Churg-Strauss syndrome and polyarteritis nodosa. Rheumatology (Oxford). 2009;48(12):1560–5.
11. Comarmond C, Cacoub P. Granulomatosis with polyangiitis (Wegener): clinical aspects and treatment. Autoimmun Rev. 2014;13(11):1121–5.
12. Calatroni M, Oliva E, Gianfreda D, et al. ANCA-associated vasculitis in childhood: recent advances. Ital J Pediatr. 2017;43(1):46.
13. Iudici M, Pagnoux C, Quartier P, et al. Childhood-versus adult-onset ANCA-associated vasculitides: a nested, matched case-control study from the French Vasculitis Study Group Registry. Autoimmun Rev. 2018;17(2):108–14.
14. Hoffman GS, Kerr GS, Leavitt RY, et al. Wegener granulomatosis: an analysis of 158 patients. Ann Intern Med. 1992;116(6):488–98.
15. Trimarchi M, Sinico RA, Teggi R, Bussi M, Specks U, Meroni PL. Otorhinolaryngological manifestations in granulomatosis with polyangiitis (Wegener's). Autoimmun Rev. 2013;12(4):501–5.
16. Chang DY, Wu LH, Liu G, Chen M, Kallenberg CG, Zhao MH. Re-evaluation of the histopathologic classification of ANCA-associated glomerulonephritis: a study of 121 patients in a single center. Nephrol Dial Transplant. 2012;27(6):2343–9.

17. Mukhtyar C, Flossmann O, Hellmich B, et al. Outcomes from studies of antineutrophil cytoplasm antibody associated vasculitis: a systematic review by the European league against rheumatism systemic vasculitis task force. Ann Rheum Dis. 2008;67(7):1004–10.
18. Stone JH. Wegener's Granulomatosis Etanercept Trial Research G. Limited versus severe Wegener's granulomatosis: baseline data on patients in the Wegener's granulomatosis etanercept trial. Arthritis Rheum. 2003;48(8):2299–309.
19. Luqmani R, Suppiah R, Edwards CJ, et al. Mortality in Wegener's granulomatosis: a bimodal pattern. Rheumatology (Oxford). 2011;50(4):697–702.
20. Marzano AV, Vezzoli P, Berti E. Skin involvement in cutaneous and systemic vasculitis. Autoimmun Rev. 2013;12(4):467–76.
21. Patten SF, Tomecki KJ. Wegener's granulomatosis: cutaneous and oral mucosal disease. J Am Acad Dermatol. 1993;28(5 Pt 1):710–8.
22. Tashtoush B, Memarpour R, Johnston Y, Ramirez J. Large pyoderma gangrenosum-like ulcers: a rare presentation of granulomatosis with polyangiitis. Case Rep Rheumatol. 2014;2014:850364.
23. Feighery C, Conlon N, Abuzakouk M. Skin ulcer presentation of Wegener's granulomatosis. BMJ Case Rep. 2010;2010:bcr0420102908.
24. Holle JU, Gross WL, Holl-Ulrich K, et al. Prospective long-term follow-up of patients with localised Wegener's granulomatosis: does it occur as persistent disease stage? Ann Rheum Dis. 2010;69(11):1934–9.
25. Marzano AV, Balice Y, Papini M, Testa R, Berti E, Crosti C. Localized Wegener's granulomatosis. J Eur Acad Dermatol Venereol. 2011;25(12):1466–70.
26. Ruokonen H, Helve T, Arola J, Hietanen J, Lindqvist C. Hagstrom. Strawberry-like gingivitis being the first sign of Wegener's granulomatosis. Eur J Intern Med. 2009;20(6):651–3.
27. Stewart C, Cohen D, Bhattacharyya I, et al. Oral manifestations of Wegener's granulomatosis: a report of three cases and a literature review. J Am Dent Assoc. 2007;138(3):338–48. quiz396,398
28. Marzano AV, Balice Y, Tavecchio S, Desimine C, Colombo A, Berti E. Granulomatous vasculitis. G Ital Dermatol Venereol. 2015;150(2):193–202.
29. Ozen S, Pistorio A, Iusan SM, et al. EULAR/PRINTO/PRES criteria for Henoch-Schönlein purpura, childhood polyarteritis nodosa, childhood Wegener granulomatosis and childhood Takayasu arteritis: Ankara 2008. Part II: final classification criteria. Ann Rheum Dis. 2010;69(5):798–806.
30. Gajic-Veljic M, Nikolic M, Peco-Antic A, Bogdanovic R, Andrejevic S, Bonaci-Nikolic B. Granulomatosis with polyangiitis (Wegener's granulomatosis) in children: report of three cases with cutaneous manifestations and literature review. Pediatr Dermatol. 2013;30(4):e37–42.
31. Decleva I, Marzano AV, Barbareschi M, Berti E. Cutaneous manifestations in systemic vasculitis. Clin Rev Allergy Immunol. 1997;15(1):5–20.
32. Mouthon L, Dunogue B, Guillevin L. Diagnosis and classification of eosinophilic granulomatosis with polyangiitis (formerly named Churg-Strauss syndrome). J Autoimmun. 2014;48–49:99–103.
33. Gioffredi A, Maritati F, Oliva E, Buzio C. Eosinophilic granulomatosis with polyangiitis: an overview. Front Immunol. 2014;5:549.
34. Sinico RA, Di Toma L, Maggiore U, et al. Renal involvement in Churg-Strauss syndrome. Am J Kidney Dis. 2006;47(5):770–9.
35. Comarmond C, Pagnoux C, Khellaf M, et al. Eosinophilic granulomatosis with polyangiitis (Churg-Strauss): clinical characteristics and long-term follow-up of the 383 patients enrolled in the French Vasculitis Study Group cohort. Arthritis Rheum. 2013;65(1):270–81.
36. Sable-Fourtassou R, Cohen P, Mahr A, et al. Antineutrophil cytoplasmic antibodies and the Churg-Strauss syndrome. Ann Intern Med. 2005;143(9):632–8.
37. Greco A, Rizzo MI, De Virgilio A, et al. Churg-Strauss syndrome. Autoimmun Rev. 2015;14(4):341–8.

38. Greco A, De Virgilio A, Rizzo MI, et al. Microscopic polyangiitis: advances in diagnostic and therapeutic approaches. Autoimmun Rev. 2015;14(9):837–44.
39. Mohammad AJ, Jacobsson LT, Mahr AD, Sturfelt G, Segelmark M. Prevalence of Wegener's granulomatosis, microscopic polyangiitis, polyarteritis nodosa and Churg-Strauss syndrome within a defined population in southern Sweden. Rheumatology (Oxford). 2007;46(8):1329–37.
40. Guillevin L, Durand-Gasselin B, Cevallos R, et al. Microscopic polyangiitis: clinical and laboratory findings in eighty-five patients. Arthritis Rheum. 1999;42(3):421–30.
41. Niles JL, Bottinger EP, Saurina GR, et al. The syndrome of lung hemorrhage and nephritis is usually an ANCA-associated condition. Arch Intern Med. 1996;156(4):440–5.
42. Savage CO, Winearls CG, Evans DJ, Rees AJ, Lockwood CM. Microscopic polyarteritis: presentation, pathology and prognosis. Q J Med. 1985;56(220):467–83.
43. Lhote F, Cohen P, Guillevin L. Polyarteritis nodosa, microscopi polyangiitis and Churg-Strauss syndrome. Lupus. 1998;7(4):238–58.
44. Kluger N, Pagnoux C, Guillevin L, Frances C. French Vasculitis Study G. Comparison of cutaneous manifestations in systemic polyarteritis nodosa and microscopic polyangiitis. Br J Dermatol. 2008;159(3):615–20.
45. Kawakami T, Soma Y, Saito C, et al. Cutaneous manifestations in patients with microscopic polyangiitis: two case reports and a minireview. Acta Derm Venereol. 2006;86(2):144–7.
46. Niiyama S, Amoh Y, Tomita M, Katsuoka K. Dermatological manifestations associated with microscopic polyangiitis. Rheumatol Int. 2008;28(6):593–5.
47. Wallach D, Vignon-Pennamen MD. From acute febrile neutrophilic dermatosis to neutrophilic disease: forty years of clinical research. J Am Acad Dermatol. 2006;55(6):1066–71.
48. Marzano AV, Menicanti C, Crosti C, Trevisan V. Neutrophilic dermatoses and inflammatory bowel diseases. G Ital Dermatol Venereol. 2013;148(2):185–96.
49. Seishima M, Oyama Z, Oda M. Skin eruptions associated with microscopic polyangiitis. Eur J Dermatol. 2004;14(4):255–8.
50. Chen KR. Skin involvement in ANCA-associated vasculitis. Clin Exp Nephrol. 2013;17(5):676–82.
51. Ishibashi M, Kawahara Y, Chen KR. Spectrum of cutaneous vasculitis in eosinophilic granulomatosis with polyangiitis (Churg- Strauss): a case series. Am J Dermatopathol. 2015;37(3):214–21.
52. Carlson JA. The histological assessment of cutaneous vasculitis. Histopathology. 2010;56(1):3–23.
53. Rachapalli SM, Kiely PD. Cocaine-induced midline destructive lesions mimicking ENT-limited Wegener's granulomatosis. Scand J Rheumatol. 2008;37(6):477–80.
54. Marzano AV, Ishak RS, Saibeni S, Crosti C, Meroni PL, Cugno M. Autoinflammatory skin disorders in inflammatory bowel diseases, pyoderma gangrenosum and Sweet's syndrome: a comprehensive review and disease classification criteria. Clin Rev Allergy Immunol. 2013;45(2):202–10.
55. Marzano AV, Cugno M, Trevisan V, et al. Role of inflammatory cells, cytokines and matrix metalloproteinases in neutrophil-mediated skin diseases. Clin Exp Immunol. 2010;162(1):100–7.
56. Marzano AV, Fanoni D, Antiga E, et al. Expression of cytokines, chemokines and other effector molecules in two prototypic autoinflammatory skin diseases, pyoderma gangrenosum and Sweet's syndrome. Clin Exp Immunol. 2014;178(1):48–56.
57. Gastman B, Hashem AM, Djohan R, et al. Malignant pyoderma associated with granulomatosis with polyangiitis (Wegener granulomatosis) as a unique indication for facial vascularized composite Allotransplantation: part I. Plast Reconstr Surg. 2016;137(6):1007e–15e.
58. Jeong HS, Layher H, Cao L, Vandergriff T, Dominguez AR. Pyoderma gangrenosum (PG) associated with levamisole adulterated cocaine: clinical, serologic, and histopathologic findings in a cohort of patients. J Am Acad Dermatol. 2016;74(5):892–8.
59. Jimenez-Gallo D, Albarran-Planelles C, Linares-Barrios M, et al. Pyoderma gangrenosum and Wegener granulomatosis-like syndrome induced by cocaine. Clin Exp Dermatol. 2013;38(8):878–82.

60. Saulsbury FT. Clinical update: Henoch-Schönlein purpura. Lancet. 2007;369(9566):976–8.
61. Yates M, Watts RA, Bajema IM, et al. EULAR/ERA-EDTA recommendations for the management of ANCA associated vasculitis. Ann Rheum Dis. 2016;75(9):1583–94.
62. Guillevin L, Cordier JF, Lhote F, et al. A prospective, multicenter, randomized trial comparing steroids and pulse cyclophosphamide versus steroids and oral cyclophosphamide in the treatment of generalized Wegener's granulomatosis. Arthritis Rheum. 1997;40(12):2187–98.
63. Jayne D, Rasmussen N, Andrassy K, et al. A randomized trial of maintenance therapy for vasculitis associated with antineutrophil cytoplasmic autoantibodies. N Engl J Med. 2003;349(1):36–44.
64. Hogan SL, Falk RJ, Chin H, et al. Predictors of relapse and treatment resistance in antineutrophil cytoplasmic antibody-associated small-vessel vasculitis. Ann Intern Med. 2005;143(9):621–31.
65. De Groot K, Rasmussen N, Bacon PA, et al. Randomized trial of cyclophosphamide versus methotrexate for induction of remission in early systemic antineutrophil cytoplasmic antibody associated vasculitis. Arthritis Rheum. 2005;52(8):2461–9.
66. Wegener's Granulomatosis Etanercept Trial Research G. Etanercept plus standard therapy for Wegener's granulomatosis. N Engl J Med. 2005;352(4):351–61.
67. Pagnoux C, Mahr A, Hamidou MA, et al. Azathioprine or methotrexate maintenance for ANCA-associated vasculitis. N Engl J Med. 2008;359(26):2790–803.
68. de Groot K, Harper L, Jayne DR, et al. Pulse versus daily oral cyclophosphamide for induction of remission in antineutrophil cytoplasmic antibody-associated vasculitis: a randomized trial. Ann Intern Med. 2009;150(10):670–80.
69. Food and Drug Administration. (2011). http://www.fda.gov/NewsEvents/Newsroom/PressAnnouncements/ucm251946.htm. Accessed October 10 2014.
70. Stone JH, Merkel PA, Spiera R, et al. Rituximab versus cyclophosphamide for ANCA-associated vasculitis. N Engl J Med. 2010;363(3):221–32.
71. Specks U, Merkel PA, Seo P, et al. Efficacy of remission induction regimens for ANCA-associated vasculitis. N Engl J Med. 2013;369(5):417–27.
72. Marzano AV, Raimondo MG, Berti E, Meroni PL, Ingegnoli F. Cutaneous Manifestations of ANCA-Associated Small Vessels Vasculitis. Clin Rev Allergy Immunol. 2017;53(3):428–38.

Miscellaneous Organ Involvement in ANCA-Associated Vasculitis

15

Giorgio Trivioli and Augusto Vaglio

Abbreviations

^{18}FDG	^{18}Fluorodeoxyglucose
AAV	ANCA-associated vasculitis
AKI	Acute kidney injury
ANA	Antinuclear antibody
ANCA	Antineutrophil cytoplasmic antibody
Anti-GBM	Anti-glomerular basal membrane
BD	Behcet's disease
CD	Crohn's disease
CK	Creatin kinase
CKD	Chronic kidney disease
CMR	Cardiac magnetic resonance
CT	Computed tomography
DVT	Deep venous thrombosis
ECG	Electrocardiography
EGPA	Eosinophilic granulomatosis with polyangiitis
EMB	Endomyocardial biopsy
EMG	Electromyography
ENT	Ear-nose-throat

G. Trivioli
Department of Biomedical Experimental and Clinical Sciences "Mario Serio", University of Florence, Florence, Italy
e-mail: giorgio.trivioli@unifi.it

A. Vaglio (✉)
Nephrology Unit, Meyer's Children Hospital, Florence, Italy

R. A. Sinico, L. Guillevin (eds.), *Anti-Neutrophil Cytoplasmic Antibody (ANCA) Associated Vasculitis*, Rare Diseases of the Immune System,
https://doi.org/10.1007/978-3-030-02239-6_15

EUVAS	European Vasculitis Study Group
FFS	Five-factor score
GI	Gastrointestinal
GPA	Granulomatosis with polyangiitis
HES	Hypereosinophilic syndrome
HLA	Human leukocyte antigen
IBD	Inflammatory bowel disease
IgAV	IgA vasculitis
IgG4-RD	IgG4-related disease
IHD	Ischemic heart disease
IMT	Intima-media thickening
LDH	Lactate dehydrogenase
LGE	Late gadolinium enhancement
MPA	Microscopic polyangiitis
MPO	Myeloperoxidase
MRI	Magnetic resonance imaging
NET	Neutrophil extracellular trap
PAN	Polyarteritis nodosa
PE	Pulmonary embolism
PET	Positron emission tomography
PNS	Peripheral nervous system
PR3	Proteinase 3
RA	Rheumatoid arthritis
RPF	Retroperitoneal fibrosis
RTX	Rituximab
SLE	Systemic lupus erythematosus
SOV	Single-organ vasculitis
SSc	Systemic sclerosis
STIR	Short-T1 inversion recovery
SVV	Small-vessel vasculitis
TF	Tissue factor
TNF	Tumor necrosis factor
UC	Ulcerative colitis
VTE	Venous thromboembolism

15.1 Introduction

ANCA-associated vasculitides (AAVs) are small-vessel vasculitides (SVV) that commonly affect the kidney, the lung, the ear-nose-throat (ENT) system, the skin, and peripheral nervous system (PNS) [1]. However, the spectrum of AAV manifestations is broader, since almost all organs and systems may be involved. The involvement of other organs, particularly gastrointestinal (GI), cardiovascular and urogenital systems, occurs only in a small proportion of patients, but its impact on morbidity and mortality may be profound. Moreover, the manifestations secondary to the involvement of such organ systems are often nonspecific, and may be attributed to more common diseases, with a significant delay in diagnosis and treatment. In exceptional cases, patients may even present with atypical single-organ involvement rather than with multisystemic disease, such as vasculitis limited to GI or urogenital tract. A deep knowledge of the possible manifestations is then of great value for proper recognition and management of patients with AAV.

In this chapter, we will present some of the various clinical manifestations that occur in patients with AAV, focusing on cardiac involvement and thrombotic events, GI involvement, musculoskeletal and urogenital disease. Finally, we will discuss unusual modalities of presentation of AAV, indeed, the possibility of overlap with other autoimmune or fibro-inflammatory diseases.

15.2 Cardiac Involvement

Cardiac abnormalities are common findings among AAV patients and may result from different mechanisms, mainly direct involvement of the heart by vasculitis and increased susceptibility to ischemic heart disease (IHD) [2]. Cardiac involvement may be a severe complication that usually occurs in a considerable proportion of patients with eosinophilic granulomatosis with polyangiitis (EGPA) whereas only in a small number of patients with granulomatosis with polyangiitis (GPA) and microscopic polyangiitis (MPA) [3–5]. The real prevalence has not yet been established, since results of clinical studies are highly varied, depending on diagnostic techniques and applied criteria [6–9]. In the last decades, cardiac magnetic resonance (CMR) has emerged as a gold-standard technique to evaluate heart anatomy and function and to characterize myocardial lesions [10]. The late gadolinium enhancement (LGE) technique allows the detection of fibrotic lesions or of active myocarditis, while STIR T2-weighted images and T1-mapping show respectively focal edema and diffuse fibrosis (Fig. 15.1). Recent studies have found that a considerable proportion of patients with normal clinical evaluation and absence of ECG and transthoracic echocardiographic abnormalities have subclinical lesions detected by CMR [11–13]. These observations have contributed to widen the concept of AAV-related cardiac involvement, from that of a serious but uncommon complication to that of a diffuse and insidious disease component.

Heart involvement has been identified as an independent predictor of overall and cardiovascular mortality in EGPA and GPA patients [3, 14, 15]. Moreover, the presence of cardiac symptoms at initial assessment further increases the risk of death. The pathologic process may affect all heart structures but the main form is endomyocarditis, resulting from white cell infiltration and possibly granulomatous inflammation. However, the clinical phenotype is highly variable, ranging from subclinical to life-threatening complications.

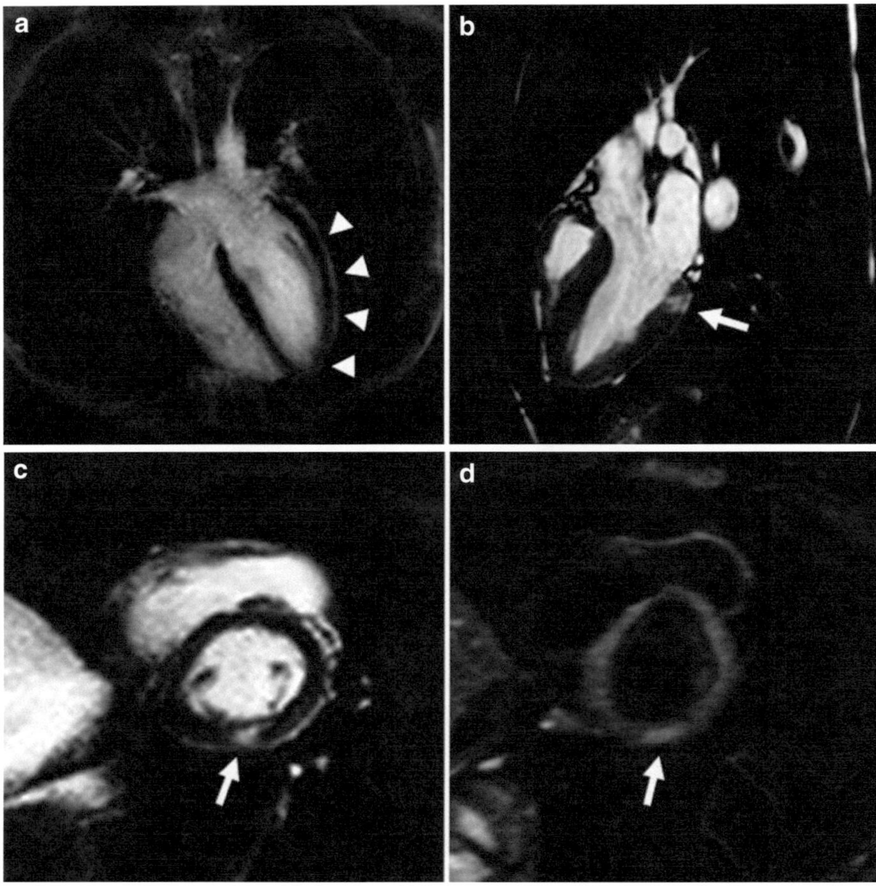

Fig. 15.1 Cardiac magnetic resonance (CMR) images of EGPA patients with cardiac involvement (courtesy of Dr. A. Palumbo). Images (**a**–**d**) refer to a 18-year-old female patient, with myo-pericarditis secondary to newly diagnosed EGPA. Laboratory tests showed hypereosinophilia, p-ANCA positivity, and elevated Troponin I, whereas echocardiography detected a minimal pericardial effusion and absence of wall motion abnormality. Four-chamber late gadolinium enhanced image (**a**) showing thickening of pericardium (*arrowheads*). Three-chamber contrast-based cine image (**b**) with focal enhancement in the basal wall of left ventricle (*arrow*), compatible with recent myocarditis. Short axis view (**c**) demonstrating late gadolinium enhancement in the postero-lateral wall of the left ventricle (*arrow*), corresponding to that seen in (**c**). Short axis T2-STIR-weighted image (**d**) showing epi-myocardial edema in the same area (*arrow*). Images (**e**) and (**f**) refer to a 41-year-old male patient admitted to hospital with acute pericarditis. Diagnosis of EGPA was made during hospitalization. CMR was performed because of elevation of cardiac markers (Troponin I and CK-MB) and ECG alterations (left bundle branch block). Four-chamber T2-weighted view (**e**) showing hypertrophy of the left ventricular wall and mild pericardial effusion (*arrows*). Short axis late gadolinium image (**f**) with mild enhancement of pericardium and epicardium (*arrows*)

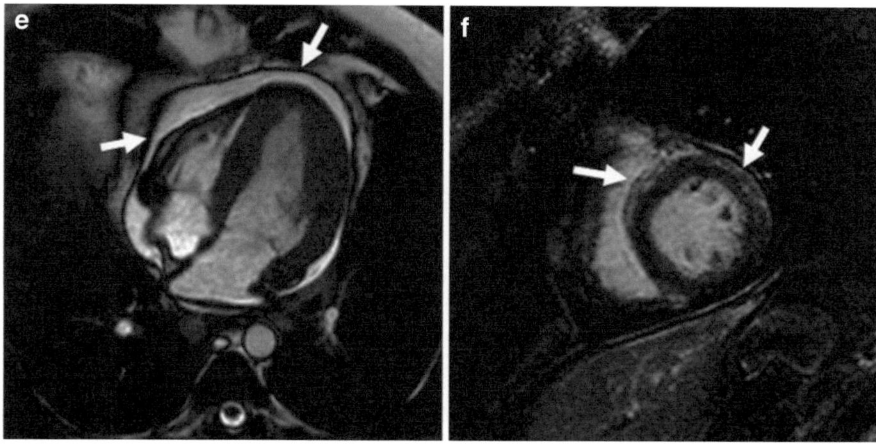

Fig. 15.1 (continued)

15.2.1 Cardiac Involvement in GPA and MPA

In GPA, clinically overt cardiac involvement has been reported to be rare. The frequency of cardiac symptoms was 3.3% in a cohort of 517 North American GPA patients followed up for more than 8 years [16]. The manifestations described were pericardial effusion, heart failure, conduction defects, and valvular involvement, with absence of a clearly dominant pattern. While symptomatic forms are less common, recent observations have suggested that subclinical forms could be more frequent and often overlooked. Hazebroek et al. have conducted a case–control study on a large cohort of GPA and EGPA patients in stable remission, carefully matched with the general population. ECG, transthoracic echocardiography, and CMR were performed in all patients, also in those without cardiac symptoms. Abnormalities, such as regional or global systolic dysfunction, valvular defects, pulmonary hypertension, pericardial effusion, or major rhythm alterations, were found in 64% of GPA patients and 71% of EGPA patients, but only in 20% of control subjects [14]. According to these results, cardiac involvement—mainly subclinical—may be quite frequent. To identify these forms, a multimodality screening should be encouraged, independently of the presence of related symptoms.

MPA-related cardiac involvement has been scarcely explored. However, large studies on Chinese and French cohorts reported high frequency of cardiac manifestations [4, 17]. The most common manifestations were pericardial effusion, chronic heart failure, and isolated cases of aortic incompetence and new-onset arrhythmia. Interestingly, a CMR study on a Dutch population detected a high prevalence of coronary ectasia and aneurysms among MPA but not among EGPA patients and rheumatois arthritis (RA) and systemic lupus erythematosus (SLE) controls [18]. These findings suggest that coronaritis with necrotizing changes and wall weakening may be an intrinsic component of MPA that contributes to increase the cardiovascular risk in these patients.

15.2.2 Cardiac Involvement in EGPA

Cardiac involvement in EGPA is by far more frequent than in other AAVs [3]. Since the original disease description in 1951 by Churg and Strauss, cardiac disease has been considered as a prominent disease manifestation, with a deep impact on morbidity and mortality [19]. The pathological process may affect all heart structures, resulting in a variable clinical phenotype. However, cardiomyopathy and pericardial effusion represent the main clinical patterns (Fig. 15.1), while valvular defects, conduction disturbances, and coronaritis occur less commonly.

In a study on 49 EGPA patients, 22 (45%) experienced acute or chronic heart failure and had clinical evidences of cardiac involvements, including conduction disturbances, elevated Troponin I, pericardial effusion, pulmonary hypertension and diastolic dysfunction, regional or global systolic dysfunction, and intraventricular thrombi [20]. Moreover, the majority of patients with available CMR had LGE in apical and mid-cavity left ventricular segments, particularly, in the subendocardial layer. This finding is suggestive of Loeffler endocarditis, a peculiar form of cardiomyopathy occurring in hypereosinophilic syndromes (HES), with a triphasic course [21]. The acute phase is the inflammatory stage, characterized by eosinophil infiltration of the myocardium and cellular necrosis due to eosinophil degranulation. Patients may often be clinically silent, although CMR and endomyocardial biopsy (EMB) can reveal corresponding abnormalities. The second phase is the so-called thrombotic stage, with the formation of intraventricular thrombi as consequence of endothelial disruption and hypercoagulability, which is a feature of EGPA [22]. The end-stage is the fibrotic phase, in which thrombus and necrosis are replaced by fibrosis. Subendocardial scarring leads to restrictive or dilated cardiomyopathy but also to progressive valvular incompetence. Neumann et al. found that most patients with subendocardial LGE had EMB findings compatible with Loeffler endocarditis. The majority of them had endomyocardial fibrosis, while only few patients had signs of acute eosinophilic myocarditis. These latter probably underwent early biopsy during the inflammatory stage, while most patients were diagnosed during the fibrotic stage. Moreover, patients with Loeffler endocarditis showed more severe heart failure, higher levels of Troponin I and a greater number of mural thrombi while little or no pericardial effusion.

The clinical phenotype of EGPA is highly variable, but can be broadly distinguished into two main disease subsets, differentiated on the basis of ANCA-positivity. ANCA-negative patients have predominance of eosinophilic manifestations, such as cardiac involvement, lung infiltrates, and GI disease, while ANCA-positive patients more commonly have vasculitic manifestations such as glomerulonephritis, peripheral neuropathy, and purpura [8, 23]. Thus, ANCA status can be regarded as a prognostic factor for the development of cardiac involvement and reduced survival [24]. The prognosis of EGPA has significantly improved over past decades, with 10-year survival rates of 81–92% [25, 26], but up to 50% of disease-specific mortality is related to cardiac involvement [3, 27]. Consistently, the Five-Factor Score (FFS), a tool designed to predict survival at diagnosis in patients with SVV, considers cardiac disease among the clinical parameters associated with negative outcome, such as age >65 years, renal insufficiency, and severe GI manifestations [28]. If one of them is present, the patient is generally treated with a combination of glucocorticoids and immunosuppressants. Immunosuppression can effectively prevent cardiac death and improve myocardial dysfunction in patients with cardiac involvement, as demonstrated by studies with CMR follow-up [29]. However, disease relapses at this level occur with high frequency.

Numerous studies have highlighted that clinical evaluation not including CMR may overlook subclinical abnormalities in a considerable proportion of EGPA but also MPA and GPA patients [12–14, 29, 30]. Since myocardial disease in Loeffler endocarditis progresses through clinically silent stages, early recognition and treatment initiation are central to improve prognosis. Hence, CMR evaluation of EGPA patients at initial assessment is strongly recommended and has become a standard examination in experienced centers. To date, most cases with cardiac involvement are recognized at a subclinical stage. On the contrary, routine assessment in GPA and MPA patients comprises only ECG and transthoracic echocardiography, whereas CMR is reserved to cases with suspected involvement. Further studies are warranted to determine whether subclinical forms may progress to clinically overt forms in these syndromes similarly to EGPA and require for this reason an early treatment.

15.2.3 Vascular Involvement

The immune and coagulation systems are closely related and a number of possible interactions may be implicated in the pathogenesis of thrombosis and hypercoagulability in AAV. Neutrophil activation triggered by ANCA is known to cause oxidative stress resulting in endothelial damage, that promotes platelet activation [31]. In addition, neutrophils may release prothrombotic factors such as tissue factor (TF) and platelet recruiting factors, facilitating thrombus formation. Neutrophil Extracellular Trap (NET) formation (NETosis) is a recently described further potential bridge between inflammatory response and coagulation, that has been implicated in thrombus formation [32, 33]. NETs are structures containing chromatin, TF, granule proteins, but also ANCA targets, such as MPO and PR3, in which microbes are trapped and killed. ANCA can induce NETosis, possibly creating a self-amplifying process, with increased ANCA production, more neutrophil activation and subsequent NET release that contribute to hypercoagulability. Moreover, antibodies directed against complementary PR3 (cPR3) can bind to plasminogen and delay the conversion from plasminogen to plasmin, impairing fibrinolysis and prolonging the dissolution time of fibrin clots [34]. In EGPA, an adjunctive thrombogenic effect may be related to eosinophil degranulation, with release of TF and other cationic proteins that initiate coagulation [35, 36]. These mechanisms could be responsible for the high rate of thrombotic events in AAV but their role as biomarker or therapeutic target is still unclear.

15.2.4 Arterial Involvement

With improvement of prognosis and prolongation of patient survival, several studies have investigated the burden of cardiovascular disease in AAV patients. Observations had shown an increased frequency of surrogate markers of atherosclerotic disease, such as impaired endothelium-dependent arterial vasodilatation [37], enhanced arterial stiffness [38], increased carotid artery intima-media thickening (IMT) [39, 40], high frequency of plaques [41] and altered ankle–brachial pressure indices [42]. Moreover, cardiovascular diseases account for the main cause of death in the period following the first year of AAV diagnosis [43]. AAV confers an increased risk of atherothrombotic events that is probably related to specific disease factors and not only due to impaired renal function. Morgan et al. showed that AAV patients have a twofold increase in the rate of cardiovascular events, as compared with a matched population of noninflammatory chronic kidney disease (CKD) patients [44]. Moreover, Faurschou et al. found that GPA patients are at higher risk of hospitalization for manifestations of IHD in the early period (5 years within diagnosis) but also in the late period since diagnosis (>10 years), as compared with a sex- and age-matched population [45]. Such bimodal pattern suggests that acute but also chronic inflammation contribute to increase cardiovascular risk. In addition, a subsequent study found that the cardiovascular manifestations are restricted to IHD events, since stroke frequency is not increased as compared to the general population [46].

Chronic inflammatory diseases such as RA and SLE are associated with high rates of atherosclerotic events. Increased cardiovascular risk seems to result from “accelerated atherosclerosis,” a condition of enhanced plaque formation promoted by chronic inflammation [47, 48]. Systemic inflammation may play a central role also in AAV, along with endothelial damage caused by ANCA-mediated neutrophil activation. Consistently, immunosuppression may reverse endothelial dysfunction [49]. However, the role of treatment, particularly of glucocorticoids, remains controversial. Although steroid therapy can effectively dampen systemic inflammation, it also increases the risk of arterial hypertension, atherogenic dyslipidemia, and diabetes mellitus, that are well-known cardiovascular risk factors [50, 51]. While in the short term the benefits resulting from anti-inflammatory effects prevail, glucocorticoid-related cardiovascular toxicity may emerge years after diagnosis. Accordingly, the atherothrombotic event excess reported in the first 5 years of diagnosis by Faurschou et al. may be caused by a sub-optimal suppression of systemic inflammation, whereas the high rates in the period following 10 years of disease may be related to high cumulative doses of glucocorticoids [45].

With improvement of patient prognosis, prevention of cardiovascular complications in AAV has become a major therapeutic challenge. The European Vasculitis Study Group (EUVAS) has recently performed a long-term follow-up study on 535 GPA and MPA patients with the aim of developing a statistical model to predict 5-year cardiovascular risk at first assessment. Diastolic dysfunction and advanced age were identified as adverse factors, while PR3-positive status has been considered a protective factor [52]. Strongly recommended is the careful assessment at presentation and during the whole follow-up, as well as the identification of potentially modifiable risk factors. Patients currently treated with glucocorticoids who have received a high cumulative dose represent the subset at highest risk and should be actively monitored [53]. They could also benefit of a treatment with simvastatin, since it has been observed to inhibit in vitro neutrophil degranulation induced by ANCA [54]. However, further studies are required to elucidate the optimal therapeutic strategy in AAV patients at high risk.

15.2.5 Venous Thromboembolism

Recent observations have shown that patients with AAV carry a high risk of venous thromboembolism (VTE). The WeCLOT study has reported an incidence rate of deep venous thrombosis (DVT) and/or pulmonary embolism (PE) of 7.0 per 100 person-years among GPA patients [55]. The frequency is significantly increased in comparison to the general population rate (0.31 per 100 person-years), SLE and RA patients (respectively 0.31 and 1 per 100 person-years), amounting to that of recurrent thrombosis among patients with recent VTE (7.20 per 100 person-years). Furthermore, most episodes occurred during periods of active disease or within few months of a documented disease flare, suggesting that VTE is due to disease-related factors. Subsequent studies have also found that MPA and EGPA share a similarly increased risk, while polyarteritis nodosa (PAN) has a lower VTE frequency [22, 35, 56]. These results suggest that VTE is a specific complication of AAV.

The high risk of VTE in AAV underscores the importance of a prolonged follow-up, with careful evaluation for thrombotic complications at occurrence of related symptoms. Moreover, some authors suggest a wide screening with ultrasound, since the rate of asymptomatic deep venous thrombosis (DVT) may be higher than the expected [57]. A further central question pertains to prophylaxis strategy. Results of the WeCLOT study may suggest preventive anticoagulation, similarly to patients with previous VTE, at least for subjects at high risk. Although criteria to define a patient at high risk are not fully understood, the analysis of a large dataset of GPA and MPA patients enrolled in EUVAS trials have found associations between VTE and high disease activity scores, cutaneous and GI involvement, impaired renal function and malignancy [58]. Thus, AAV patients with these features may represent a subset of patients at higher risk of VTE who need a more accurate follow-up and even prophylactic anticoagulation.

15.3 Gastrointestinal Involvement

As compared with other systemic vasculitides such as PAN, Behcet's Disease (BD) and IgA Vasculitis (IgAV), AAV have a lower rate of GI tract involvement [59]. However, the range of manifestations is extremely wide, since all organs can be affected, with mild to life-threatening complications. Severe GI manifestations, such as organ perforation, bleeding and pancreatitis, have been identified on the FFS as parameters suggestive of negative prognosis [15, 28]. Overall, GI involvement seems to be more frequent among EGPA patients, with reported rates of 20–50% versus 5–11% among GPA and MPA patients [60–62]. In EGPA, GI manifestations account for the fourth disease-related cause of death and usually predominate among ANCA-negative patients, as examples of eosinophilic manifestations.

Unlike cardiac involvement, research on GI disease in AAV has mainly focused on symptomatic forms and little is known about the prevalence of subclinical abnormalities [63]. In most reported cases, GI manifestations are already present at disease onset, rather than occurring subsequently as disease relapse. Moreover, a small proportion of AAV patients may have a single-organ vasculitis (SOV) limited to the GI tract [64, 65]. The diagnosis of GI-limited AAV is exceptional and must follow a careful differential diagnosis with other more common GI diseases, such as inflammatory bowel disease (IBD).

15.3.1 Clinical Manifestations and Treatment

GI manifestations are relatively nonspecific and highly variable. In a study on 62 patients affected by necrotizing vasculitis with GI involvement, almost all patients reported abdominal pain variably associated with nausea and vomiting, diarrhea and lower GI bleeding [63]. Endoscopic examination revealed gastroduodenal and colonic ulcers in most patients, while esophageal ulcers were detected only in GPA patients. Of note, although endoscopic appearance was suggestive, signs of vasculitis were found only in a minority of cases, perhaps, because of the superficial mucosal sampling. Symptomatic conditions not elucidated by endoscopy may be further investigated with capsule endoscopy or CT. This is often the case of EGPA with small bowel involvement. Possible capsule endoscopy findings are submucosal oedema with numerous lymphangiectasis, erythematous sites as well as large ulcers, whereas computed tomography (CT) can detect diffuse or multifocal bowel wall thickening, abnormal enhancement patterns of the bowel wall, dilatation of bowel segments and mesenteric vessel engorgement [63, 66] (Fig. 15.2).

A considerable proportion of patients (22–54%) may have severe manifestations potentially requiring surgery, such as bowel perforation or infarction, appendicitis, cholecystitis and acute pancreatitis [15, 67, 68]. The organ damage is probably due to ischemia caused by vasculitis. Patients with severe manifestations have a higher 5-year mortality rate in comparison to other patients with less severe GI lesions (44% vs. 18%), confirming that severe GI involvement is an adverse prognostic factor [63]. On the contrary, no significant difference in outcome has been observed between patients with less severe GI manifestations and those without GI involvement.

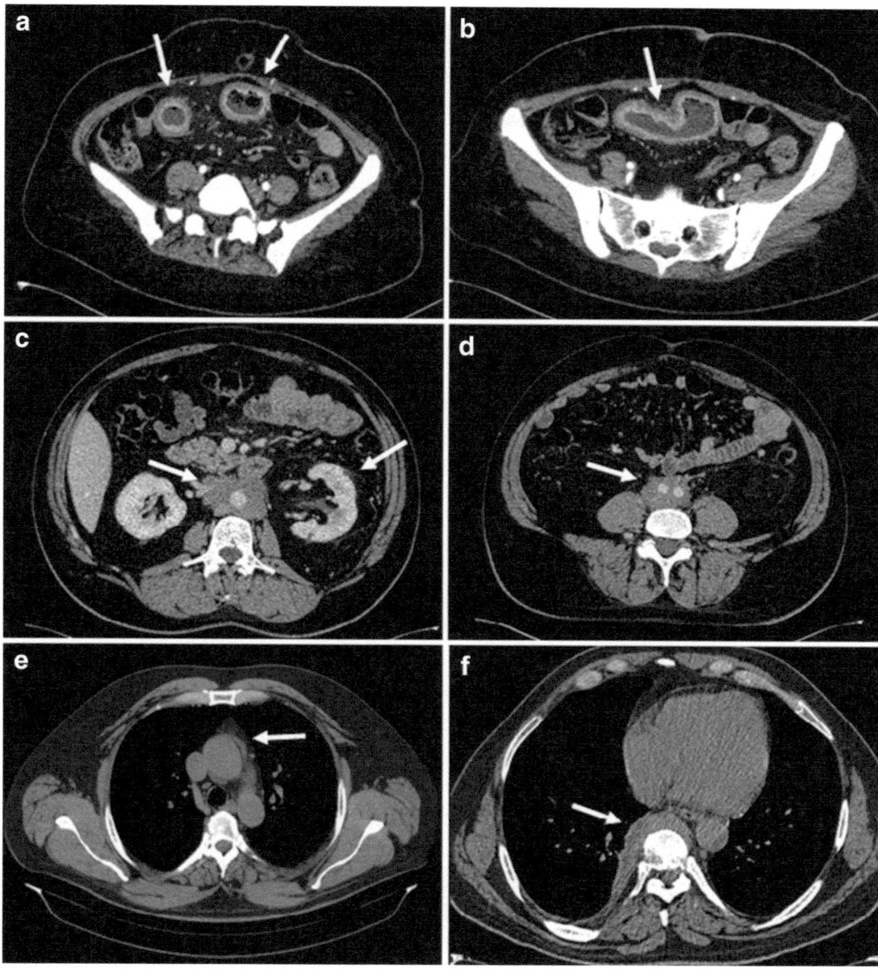

Fig. 15.2 Computed tomography (CT) findings of gastrointestinal involvement and fibro-inflammatory diseases in patients with AAV (courtesy of Dr. A. Palumbo). Contrast-enhanced abdominal CT (**a** and **b**) of a 43-year-old female patient with GPA, who experienced relevant weight loss and diarrhea. The scans show an ileal loop of augmented caliber (*arrows*), with thickened and enhanced bowel walls and stagnation of enteric material. The surrounding mesenteric tract is characterized by diffuse venous ectasia, inflammation of fat tissue, and enlarged lymph nodes, compatible with chronic mesenteritis. Images (**c** and **d**) refer to a 57-year-old male patient, who was admitted to a nephrology unit because of fever and marked worsening of renal function. Clinical and laboratory findings were suggestive of MPA. A contrast-enhanced abdominal CT (**c**) revealed a soft, homogeneous retroperitoneal tissue around the aorta (*arrow*) and left-sided hydronephrosis of moderate degree (*arrow*). The mass develops mainly around the anterior and lateral sides of the aorta and encircles also the iliac vessels (**d**). The findings were considered compatible with retroperitoneal fibrosis associated with AAV. Thoracic CT of a 51-year-old male patient with MPO-positive vasculitis involving the ENT tract. The images show the presence of hypodense tissue (*arrows*) surrounding the aortic arch (**e**) and the right-anterior side of the vertebral bodies (**f**). Histology examination of the prevertebral tissue revealed fibrosis with rare lymphocytes and IgG4-negative plasma cells. The lesions were considered manifestations of thoracic periaortitis (**e**) and fibrosing mediastinitis (**f**), respectively, in a patient with AAV

Similarly to other AAV manifestations, treatment of GI involvement is based on different combinations of glucocorticoids and immunosuppressants. Moreover, mild cases may benefit from mesalazine therapy. An effort should be made to limit glucocorticoid dose, since glucocorticoids could increase the risk of GI ulcers. Indeed, some authors have suggested that prolonged glucocorticoid treatment is a risk factor for the development of GI manifestations [69]. Severe AAV-related manifestations require a prompt initiation of potent immunosuppressant, mainly cyclophosphamide, and a careful investigation for surgical complications that should be immediately treated. In a previously mentioned study, four patients died before surgery could be performed, despite immunosuppressive treatment [63].

15.3.2 AAV and Associated Inflammatory Bowel Disease

A peculiar form of GI disease in course of AAV is related to the association between AAV and IBD, such as Crohn's Disease (CD) and Ulcerative Colitis (UC). This overlap is rare and few cases have been reported in the literature [70, 71]. In a retrospective study of the French Vasculitis Study Group, the association of IBD and AAV occurred in <1% of AAV patients [72]. The types of association seem to be limited to only two patterns: GPA with coexistent CD and EGPA with coexistent UC. No case of MPA with coexistent IBD was reported. According to these results, common pathogenic mechanisms may be shared by GPA and CD and by EGPA and UC. Cytokine patterns play a key role in the development of inflammatory diseases. Indeed, EGPA and UC are considered Th2-mediated diseases, with an increased production of IL-4, IL-5, and IL-10 that allows eosinophil recruitment [73–75]. Tissue eosinophilia is a key feature in EGPA, but increased levels of eosinophil in bowel mucosa have been also found in active UC[75]. On the contrary, GPA and CD have been described as Th1-mediated diseases, with increased amount of INFg- and of Th17-producing IL-17 that induce granulomas formation [76–78]. However, some studies have found forms of GPA with mixed polarization toward Th1/Th2 patterns, as well as patients with association between GPA and UC [79, 80]. In addition, 60–90% of the UC patients and 15–20% of CD patients have positive ANCA, mainly p-ANCA, with no specificity to common antigens such as MPO or PR3, but rather targeting other intracellular neutrophil enzymes [81].

Diagnosis of IBD preceded the onset of AAV in most reported cases, suggesting that IBD predisposes to AAV development. However, it seems likely that numerous cases with overlap are missed, since AAV-related GI manifestations often resemble those of IBD, for example, granulomatous colitis and ulcers. Moreover, one-third of IBD patients experience extra-intestinal manifestations that can mimic AAV manifestations, such as ocular complications, skin lesions, arthropathy, and nephrocalcinosis [82]. Hence, despite its rareness, the association between AAV and IBD should always be considered in AAV patients with GI symptoms and in IBD patients developing extra-intestinal manifestations.

15.4 Urogenital and Musculoskeletal Involvement

15.4.1 Urogenital Involvement

AAV may also be responsible for urogenital manifestations in a small proportion of patients (<1%) [7, 83–85]. In most cases, urogenital symptoms occur in GPA male patients at disease onset, as part of generalized systemic disease [86]. However, 12–18% in case series experienced isolated urogenital alterations preceding AAV diagnosis, when no other vasculitis manifestations were present [87]. These patients underwent biopsy of the lesions in the suspect of malignancy that revealed vasculitis or granulomatous inflammation and subsequently developed other vasculitic features.

GPA may affect all organs of the urogenital tract and prostatitis is the most common manifestation [86–88]. Related symptoms are nonspecific and comprise dysuria, urgency, purulent discharge, and acute urinary retention [89–91]. Physical examination may show a normal or enlarged gland, while imaging studies often reveal calcifications or abscess-like formations [92, 93]. Total prostate antigen may be slightly elevated, but the free fraction is usually within normal ranges [89, 94]. Histological findings are compatible with granulomatous prostatitis [86]. Thus, GPA-related involvement has to be distinguished from other granulomatous forms, such as sarcoidosis or infection caused by *Mycobacterium tuberculosis*. Immunosuppressive treatment is effective to control symptoms, but recurrences are frequent and intriguingly half of these episodes manifest as isolated prostate disease [87, 89]. Although it is the most common type of urogenital involvement, GPA-related prostatitis is rare among AAV patients and in general prostatitis series. However, postmortem studies on patients with severe GPA have revealed that 7% patients have findings of granulomatous prostatitis, indicating that the real prevalence of subclinical involvement may be considerable [95].

The ureters are most often involved in the distal tract, with the development of segmental thickening and subsequent obstruction and hydronephrosis [96–98]. Testicles and epididymis can be affected with a range of manifestations that comprise asymptomatic masses, pain, and infarction [99–101]. In addition, cases of destructive urethritis presenting with dysuria, urinary urgency, and other urinary symptoms have been reported [88, 102]. Some patients also have painless penis ulceration, possibly accompanied by regional lymphoadenopathy [103, 104]. A common urogenital finding during the course of AAV is micro-or macroscopic hematuria. Hematuria may be related to renal or bladder involvement by AAV, more rarely to ureter or prostate disease. Moreover, it is frequently consequence of cyclophosphamide toxicity, mediated by a metabolite called acrolein [105]. High cumulative dose and prolonged exposure to cyclophosphamide are associated with development of hemorrhagic cystitis and bladder carcinoma, whose modality of presentation is often asymptomatic hematuria [106–108]. Acrolein toxicity can be reduced by abundant fluid intake, in order to force diuresis, and concurrent administration of mesna (sodium 2-mercaptoethane sulfate) that inactivates acrolein in urine [109, 110]. Of note, these complications may also occur after cyclophosphamide discontinuation, requiring a prolonged follow-up, with urinalysis and urine cytology every 3–6 months.

15.4.2 Musculoskeletal Disease

Myalgia and joint pain or swelling are common symptoms in patients with AAV. More often, they occur at disease onset as prodromal manifestations, associated with fever, anorexia, and weight loss [1]. This group of symptoms is related to systemic inflammation and usually shows prompt regression after steroid therapy initiation. On the contrary, muscle weakness and atrophy, mostly regarding lower limbs, are much rarer and can be due to severe peripheral neuropathy, with axon damage caused by arteritis of vasa nervorum and subsequent muscle impairment [111, 112]. However, a small proportion of patients have myalgia and weakness as consequence of muscle ischemia and fiber degeneration caused by muscle vessel vasculitis. Some reports have described cases of EGPA presenting with myalgia, mild leg weakness, and CK elevation [113, 114]. Magnetic resonance imaging (MRI) showed mild muscle atrophy with diffuse hyperintense signal in STIR sequence, revealing the presence of muscle inflammation, while electromyography demonstrated myopathic recruitment pattern and fibrillations, with possible reduced nerve conduction amplitude. Muscle biopsy findings were perimyseal artery vasculitis with eosinophil infiltration and angulated atrophic fibers as a sign of denervation in cases with concomitant PNS involvement. Of note, this pattern differed from that of myositis for the absence of typical features, such as phagocytosis of non-necrotic fibers, dense endomysial infiltrates, and sarcolemmal overexpression of MHC-1. However, a first case of EGPA with typical myositic findings has been recently reported, indicating that AAV may associate with idiopathic inflammatory myopathies [115]. Precise medical history and neurological examination are necessary to distinguish AAV-related muscle involvement or idiopathic inflammatory myopathies from other more common causes, such as glucocorticoid- or statin-related myopathy. Laboratory findings usually reveal elevated levels of CK, LDH, and inflammatory markers; CK or LDH increase is usually absent in glucocorticoid-related myopathy. Moreover, myositis-related autoantibodies can be tested to accurately investigate the nature of muscle involvement. Electromyography (EMG) can differ between neuropathic or myopathic involvement and MRI can detect with high sensitivity muscle edema and atrophy, as consequence of muscle inflammation. However, definitive diagnosis is only achieved by muscle biopsy, which may distinguish between vasculitic and myositic patterns. Interestingly, all cases with muscle manifestations showed a prompt response to immunosuppressive therapy [113–115].

Other possible musculoskeletal manifestations during the course of AAV are paravertebral masses, detectable in a small number of GPA patients [116, 117].

Such lesions are often occasional findings on chest CT evaluation, although some patients may report back pain as a possible consequence. In one case, painful paravertebral mass was the initial presentation of GPA, subsequently followed by other manifestations [118]. The lesions are found on the right-anterior side of thoracic vertebrae and do not infiltrate surrounding tissues (Fig. 15.2). In addition, the [18]FDG uptake at PET is increased, indicating an active metabolism. For their rareness and unclear significance, paravertebral masses may be attributed to malignant or infectious conditions, especially tuberculosis, or to other inflammatory diseases, such as sarcoidosis, rather than to AAV. However, absence of invasiveness at radiological examination and stability or regression after immunosuppressive treatment are suggestive of a benign nature. The definitive diagnosis requires histologic examination of surgical or CT-guided biopsy, but the procedure should be carefully weighted for risk of complications and should be reserved for the most challenging cases. Where available, biopsy revealed fibrotic scars, calcification, and previously active inflammatory sites, with granuloma formation [117]. Paravertebral lesions in patients with back pain showed a prompt regression to immunosuppressive treatment initiation, while most asymptomatic lesions remained stable over whole follow-up. Consistently, histology of these latter was more characterized by fibrotic scars [117]. Some of these paravertebral lesions may also be part of fibro-inflammatory disorders such as IgG4-related disease (see paragraph below).

15.5 AAV in Overlap Syndromes

15.5.1 Association with Autoimmune Disorders

AAV are multisystemic diseases that may virtually cause all types of organ involvement. However, it must be kept in mind that some manifestations, particularly if less typical, may be due to coexistent diseases. Although co-occurrence is uncommon, AAV can be associated with a relevant number of immune-mediated diseases. In previous paragraphs, we mentioned the possibility of overlap with IBD and idiopathic inflammatory myopathies [72, 119]. Moreover, it has been reported that some female patients have a mixed pattern fulfilling both AAV (mainly MPA) and SLE classification criteria [120, 121], while a small number of RA patients may develop AAV features years after diagnosis [122, 123]. In addition, cases of association between AAV and systemic sclerosis (SSc) have been described and their genetic variants analyzed in details, revealing shared HLA haplotypes [124]. Finally, a subset of patients presenting with rapidly progressive renal failure and pulmonary hemorrhage have findings suggestive of overlap between AAV and Goodpasture syndrome (or anti-GBM disease) [125]. Reasons for co-occurrence of AAV with autoimmune syndromes are not fully understood, but probably pertain genetic predisposition to poly-autoimmunity involving HLA region. Studies on SLE have shown a shift and diversification of autoantibody targets occurring during disease course, a phenomenon defined as epitope spreading [126]. In such patients, a pathogenic ANCA response could emerge in the context of a progressive autoimmune dysfunction [120]. A further hypothesis is drug exposure inducing secondary vasculitis. An increasing number of patients developed MPA after TNF-targeted therapy for RA or CD [127]. To facilitate a quicker recognition of coexistent diseases and a prompt treatment initiation, AAV patients should receive an autoantibody screening at diagnosis and at occurrence of new manifestations, including Rheumatoid Factor, ANA, SSc-specific antibodies, and anti-GBM autoantibodies.

15.5.2 Association with Fibro-Inflammatory Disorders

In recent years, some authors have described cases of AAV with manifestations of associated fibro-inflammatory diseases, the most common being retroperitoneal fibrosis (RPF) [128–130]. RPF is a rare condition characterized by fibrosis and chronic inflammation in the retroperitoneum, spreading from the adventitia of aorta and iliac arteries, often encasing the ureters [131] (Fig. 15.2). Patients usually present with constitutional symptoms, abdominal or low back pain, and obstructive uropathy due to encased ureters that may progress to acute kidney injury (AKI). RPF is idiopathic in most cases (>75%), but some forms are secondary to infections, malignancy or drugs [132]. The differential diagnosis is usually made based on clinical data and radiologic aspects of the lesions, whereas unclear cases can be elucidated by tissue biopsy. The pathogenesis of idiopathic RPF is probably multifactorial, but immune-mediated mechanisms are likely to play a role [133, 134]. Treatment is immunosuppressive, with glucocorticoids as first-line agents, and has the primary goal of urinary obstruction and symptom relief. In a considerable proportion of patients, conservative urological procedures, such as ureteral stenting or nephrostomy, are often necessary, at least in the initial phase [135]. RPF mortality is low, but the disease is chronic-relapsing, with relapses occurring in up to 72% patients [136]. For refractory and relapsing forms, a number of conventional or biological immunosuppressant have been successfully used [137, 138]. Some forms of idiopathic RPF have been recently included in the spectrum of IgG4-related disease (IgG_4-RD) [139]. IgG4-RD is a newly recognized fibro-inflammatory disease that encompasses a number of fibrosing manifestations, previously considered as separate entities, such as salivary gland enlargement (Mikulicz's disease), tubulointerstitial nephritis, chronic sclerosing pancreatitis, Riedel's thyroiditis, orbital mass, pachymeningitis and RPF [140]. These conditions can occur isolated or in association and are characterized by distinctive histological features, namely dense lymphoplasmocytic infiltrates rich in IgG4-positive plasma cells, storiform fibrosis, and obliterative phlebitis. Serum IgG4 levels can also be high. Treatment is based on glucocorticoids too, usually with good response.

A recent European observational study has described 18 patients with evidence of both AAV and IgG4-RD [141]. In the majority of patients (72%), AAV and IgG4-RD were diagnosed simultaneously, but cases of metachronous development were also reported. Most patients (78%) were classified as GPA with severe systemic disease. Main IgG4-RD manifestations were chronic periaortitis (50%), comprising RPF, inflammatory aorta aneurysm and perianeurysmal fibrosis, tubulointerstitial nephritis (22%), and orbital masses (22%), although all types of organ involvement were observed. Most patients of the study were treated with a combination of glucocorticoids and rituximab (RTX) that proved effective for both vasculitic and IgG4-RD manifestations and may represent a preferential therapeutic option in cases of overlap syndrome.

Association between AAV and IgG4-RD is rare and difficult to diagnose, since both conditions have a variable spectrum of manifestations. However, overlap syndrome should be considered especially in GPA patients with RPF, orbital and sinonasal masses or pachymeningitis, although such manifestations could also be refractory granulomatous lesions related to GPA itself. Measuring serum IgG4 and IgG4/IgG ratio can be a useful test for screening, but sensitivity and specificity are insufficient. A subset of patients with biopsy-proven IgG4-RD have normal serum IgG4 titres, whereas elevated levels occur also in a number of malignant, infectious, and inflammatory diseases, among which are even vasculitides [142, 143]. Of note, high IgG4 are found in some GPA patients and to a greater extent in EGPA patients with active disease, but usually do not denote the coexistence of IgG4-related lesions [144]. Definitive diagnosis of pseudotumors requires histologic examination for recognition of distinctive microscopic features.

15.6 Conclusions

The clinical phenotype of patients with AAV is highly variable and relies on the combination of many possible manifestations. Miscellaneous organ involvement may represent a clinical dilemma, since manifestations are often nonspecific, and definitive diagnosis is not always available. On one side, AAV may be responsible of all kinds of organ involvement and manifestations. On the other side, concomitant diseases may be present, as indicated by cases of overlap with immune-mediated and fibro-inflammatory diseases. AAV patients should be carefully evaluated for all possible manifestations and should receive a serological screening to search for possible coexistent diseases. Furthermore, it should be kept in mind that uncommon manifestations may deeply affect morbidity and mortality. Overt cardiac and GI involvement are associated with poor prognosis, while urogenital and musculoskeletal disease may significantly decrease the quality of life. Recently, subclinical forms have raised much interest, since they may be diffuse in a considerable proportion of patients and possibly progress to overt forms. Thus, clinically silent lesions should be recognized and periodically evaluated to prevent severe organ damage.

References

1. Pagnoux C. Updates in ANCA-associated vasculitis. Eur J Rheumatol. 2016;3:122–33.
2. Knockaert DC. Cardiac involvement in systemic inflammatory diseases. Eur Heart J. 2007;28:1797–804.
3. Guillevin L, Cohen P, Gayraud M, Lhote F, Jarrousse B, Casassus P. Churg-Strauss syndrome. Clinical study and long-term follow-up of 96 patients. Medicine. 1999;78:26–37.

4. Guillevin L, Durand-Gasselin B, Cevallos R, et al. Microscopic polyangiitis: clinical and laboratory findings in eighty-five patients. Arthritis Rheum. 1999;42:421–30.
5. Reinhold-Keller E, Beuge N, Latza U, et al. An interdisciplinary approach to the care of patients with Wegener's granulomatosis: long-term outcome in 155 patients. Arthritis Rheum. 2000;43:1021–32.
6. Morelli S, Gurgo Di Castelmenardo AM, Conti F, et al. Cardiac involvement in patients with Wegener's granulomatosis. Rheumatol Int. 2000;19:209–12.
7. Holle JU, Gross WL, Latza U, et al. Improved outcome in 445 patients with Wegener's granulomatosis in a German vasculitis center over four decades. Arthritis Rheum. 2011;63: 257–66.
8. Sable-Fourtassou R, Cohen P, Mahr A, et al. Antineutrophil cytoplasmic antibodies and the Churg-Strauss syndrome. Ann Intern Med. 2005;143:632–8.
9. Comarmond C, Pagnoux C, Khellaf M, et al. Eosinophilic granulomatosis with polyangiitis (Churg-Strauss): clinical characteristics and long-term follow up of the 383 patients enrolled in the French Vasculitis Study Group cohort. Arthritis Rheum. 2013;65:270–81.
10. Cereda AF, Pedrotti P, De Capitani L, Giannattasio C, Roghi A. Comprehensive evaluation of cardiac involvement in eosinophilic granulomatosis with polyangiitis (EGPA) with cardiac magnetic resonance. Eur J Intern Med. 2017;39:51–6.
11. Marmursztejn J, Guillevin L, Trebossen R, et al. Churg-Strauss syndrome cardiac involvement evaluated by cardiac magnetic resonance imaging and positron-emission tomography: a prospective study on 20 patients. Rheumatology. 2013;52:642–50.
12. Miszalski-Jamka T, Szczeklik W, Sokolowska B, et al. Standard and feature tracking magnetic resonance evidence of myocardial involvement in Churg-Strauss syndrome and granulomatosis with polyangiitis (Wegener's) in patients with normal electrocardiograms and transthoracic echocardiography. Int J Cardiovasc Imaging. 2013;29:843–53.
13. Miszalski-Jamka T, Szczeklik W, Sokolowska B, et al. Cardiac involvement in Wegener's granulomatosis resistant to induction therapy. Eur Radiol. 2011;21:2297–304.
14. Hazebroek MR, Kemna MJ, Schalla S, et al. Prevalence and prognostic relevance of cardiac involvement in ANCA-associated vasculitis: eosinophilic granulomatosis with polyangiitis and granulomatosis with polyangiitis. Int J Cardiol. 2015;199:170–9.
15. Guillevin L, Lhote F, Gayraud M, et al. Prognostic factors in polyarteritis nodosa and Churg-Strauss syndrome. A prospective study in 342 patients. Medicine. 1996;75:17–28.
16. McGeoch L, Carette S, Cuthbertson D, et al. Cardiac involvement in granulomatosis with polyangiitis. J Rheumatol. 2015;42:1209–12.
17. Shuai ZW, Lv YF, Zhang MM, Hu ZY. Clinical analysis of patients with myeloperoxidase antineutrophil cytoplasmic antibody-associated vasculitis. Genet Mol Res. 2015;14:5296–303.
18. Mavrogeni S, Manoussakis MN, Karagiorga TC, et al. Detection of coronary artery lesions and myocardial necrosis by magnetic resonance in systemic necrotizing vasculitides. Arthritis Rheum. 2009;61:1121–9.
19. Churg J, Strauss L. Allergic granulomatosis, allergic angiitis, and periarteritis nodosa. Am J Pathol. 1951;27:277–301.
20. Neumann T, Manger B, Schmid M, et al. Cardiac involvement in Churg-Strauss syndrome: impact of endomyocarditis. Medicine. 2009;88:236–43.
21. Curtis C, Ogbogu P. Hypereosinophilic syndrome. Clin Rev Allergy Immunol. 2016;50:240–51.
22. Allenbach Y, Seror R, Pagnoux C, et al. High frequency of venous thromboembolic events in Churg-Strauss syndrome, Wegener's granulomatosis and microscopic polyangiitis but not polyarteritis nodosa: a systematic retrospective study on 1130 patients. Ann Rheum Dis. 2009;68:564–7.
23. Sinico RA, Di Toma L, Maggiore U, et al. Prevalence and clinical significance of antineutrophil cytoplasmic antibodies in Churg-Strauss syndrome. Arthritis Rheum. 2005;52:2926–35.
24. Mavrogeni S, Karabela G, Gialafos E, et al. Cardiac involvement in ANCA (+) and ANCA (−) Churg-Strauss syndrome evaluated by cardiovascular magnetic resonance. Inflamm Allergy Drug Targets. 2013;12:322–7.

25. Cohen P, Pagnoux C, Mahr A, et al. Churg-Strauss syndrome with poor-prognosis factors: a prospective multicenter trial comparing glucocorticoids and six or twelve cyclophosphamide pulses in forty-eight patients. Arthritis Rheum. 2007;57:686–93.
26. Ribi C, Cohen P, Pagnoux C, et al. Treatment of Churg-Strauss syndrome without poor-prognosis factors: a multicenter, prospective, randomized, open-label study of seventy-two patients. Arthritis Rheum. 2008;58:586–94.
27. Bourgarit A, Le Toumelin P, Pagnoux C, et al. Deaths occurring during the first year after treatment onset for polyarteritis nodosa, microscopic polyangiitis, and Churg-Strauss syndrome: a retrospective analysis of causes and factors predictive of mortality based on 595 patients. Medicine. 2005;84:323–30.
28. Guillevin L, Pagnoux C, Seror R, et al. The Five-Factor Score revisited: assessment of prognoses of systemic necrotizing vasculitides based on the French Vasculitis Study Group (FVSG) cohort. Medicine. 2011;90:19–27.
29. Szczeklik W, Miszalski-Jamka T, Mastalerz L, et al. Multimodality assessment of cardiac involvement in Churg-Strauss syndrome patients in clinical remission. Circ J. 2011;75: 649–55.
30. Dennert RM, van Paassen P, Schalla S, et al. Cardiac involvement in Churg-Strauss syndrome. Arthritis Rheum. 2010;62:627–34.
31. Halbwachs L, Lesavre P. Endothelium-neutrophil interactions in ANCA-associated diseases. J Am Soc Nephrol. 2012;23:1449–61.
32. Kambas K, Chrysanthopoulou A, Vassilopoulos D, et al. Tissue factor expression in neutrophil extracellular traps and neutrophil derived microparticles in antineutrophil cytoplasmic antibody associated vasculitis may promote thromboinflammation and the thrombophilic state associated with the disease. Ann Rheum Dis. 2014;73:1854–63.
33. Engelmann B, Massberg S. Thrombosis as an intravascular effector of innate immunity. Nat Rev Immunol. 2013;13:34–45.
34. Bautz DJ, Preston GA, Lionaki S, et al. Antibodies with dual reactivity to plasminogen and complementary PR3 in PR3-ANCA vasculitis. J Am Soc Nephrol. 2008;19:2421–9.
35. Ames PR, Margaglione M, Mackie S, Alves JD. Eosinophilia and thrombophilia in churg strauss syndrome: a clinical and pathogenetic overview. Clin Appl Thromb Hemost. 2010;16: 628–36.
36. Maino A, Rossio R, Cugno M, Marzano AV, Tedeschi A. Hypereosinophilic syndrome, Churg-Strauss syndrome and parasitic diseases: possible links between eosinophilia and thrombosis. Curr Vasc Pharmacol. 2012;10:670–5.
37. Filer AD, Gardner-Medwin JM, Thambyrajah J, et al. Diffuse endothelial dysfunction is common to ANCA associated systemic vasculitis and polyarteritis nodosa. Ann Rheum Dis. 2003;62:162–7.
38. Booth AD, Wallace S, McEniery CM, et al. Inflammation and arterial stiffness in systemic vasculitis: a model of vascular inflammation. Arthritis Rheum. 2004;50:581–8.
39. de Leeuw K, Kallenberg C, Bijl M. Accelerated atherosclerosis in patients with systemic autoimmune diseases. Ann N Y Acad Sci. 2005;1051:362–71.
40. de Leeuw K, Sanders JS, Stegeman C, Smit A, Kallenberg CG, Bijl M. Accelerated atherosclerosis in patients with Wegener's granulomatosis. Ann Rheum Dis. 2005;64:753–9.
41. Chironi G, Pagnoux C, Simon A, et al. Increased prevalence of subclinical atherosclerosis in patients with small-vessel vasculitis. Heart. 2007;93:96–9.
42. Sangle SR, Davies RJ, Mora M, Baron MA, Hughes GR, D'Cruz DP. Ankle-brachial pressure index: a simple tool for assessing cardiovascular risk in patients with systemic vasculitis. Rheumatology. 2008;47:1058–60.
43. Flossmann O, Berden A, de Groot K, et al. Long-term patient survival in ANCA-associated vasculitis. Ann Rheum Dis. 2011;70:488–94.
44. Morgan MD, Turnbull J, Selamet U, et al. Increased incidence of cardiovascular events in patients with antineutrophil cytoplasmic antibody-associated vasculitides: a matched-pair cohort study. Arthritis Rheum. 2009;60:3493–500.

45. Faurschou M, Mellemkjaer L, Sorensen IJ, Svalgaard Thomsen B, Dreyer L, Baslund B. Increased morbidity from ischemic heart disease in patients with Wegener's granulomatosis. Arthritis Rheum. 2009;60:1187–92.
46. Faurschou M, Obel N, Baslund B. High risk of pulmonary embolism and deep venous thrombosis but not of stroke in granulomatosis with polyangiitis (Wegener's). Arthritis Care Res. 2014;66:1910–4.
47. Bacon PA, Stevens RJ, Carruthers DM, Young SP, Kitas GD. Accelerated atherogenesis in autoimmune rheumatic diseases. Autoimmun Rev. 2002;1:338–47.
48. Gasparyan AY, Stavropoulos-Kalinoglou A, Mikhailidis DP, Toms TE, Douglas KM, Kitas GD. The rationale for comparative studies of accelerated atherosclerosis in rheumatic diseases. Curr Vasc Pharmacol. 2010;8:437–49.
49. Raza K, Thambyrajah J, Townend JN, et al. Suppression of inflammation in primary systemic vasculitis restores vascular endothelial function: lessons for atherosclerotic disease? Circulation. 2000;102:1470–2.
50. Hafstrom I, Rohani M, Deneberg S, Wornert M, Jogestrand T, Frostegard J. Effects of low-dose prednisolone on endothelial function, atherosclerosis, and traditional risk factors for atherosclerosis in patients with rheumatoid arthritis—a randomized study. J Rheumatol. 2007;34:1810–6.
51. Wei L, MacDonald TM, Walker BR. Taking glucocorticoids by prescription is associated with subsequent cardiovascular disease. Ann Intern Med. 2004;141:764–70.
52. Suppiah R, Judge A, Batra R, et al. A model to predict cardiovascular events in patients with newly diagnosed Wegener's granulomatosis and microscopic polyangiitis. Arthritis Care Res. 2011;63:588–96.
53. Souverein PC, Berard A, Van Staa TP, et al. Use of oral glucocorticoids and risk of cardiovascular and cerebrovascular disease in a population based case-control study. Heart. 2004;90:859–65.
54. Al-Ani B. Simvastatin inhibits neutrophil degranulation induced by anti-neutrophil cytoplasm auto-antibodies and N-formyl-methionine-leucine-phenylalanine (fMLP) peptide. Saudi Med J. 2013;34:477–83.
55. Merkel PA, Lo GH, Holbrook JT, et al. Brief communication: high incidence of venous thrombotic events among patients with Wegener granulomatosis: the Wegener's Clinical Occurrence of Thrombosis (WeCLOT) Study. Ann Intern Med. 2005;142:620–6.
56. Weidner S, Hafezi-Rachti S, Rupprecht HD. Thromboembolic events as a complication of antineutrophil cytoplasmic antibody-associated vasculitis. Arthritis Rheum. 2006;55:146–9.
57. Novikov P, Makarov E, Moiseev S, Meshkov A, Strizhakov L. Venous thromboembolic events in systemic vasculitis. Ann Rheum Dis. 2015;74:e27.
58. Kronbichler A, Leierer J, Leierer G, et al. Clinical associations with venous thromboembolism in anti-neutrophil cytoplasm antibody-associated vasculitides. Rheumatology. 2017;56:704–8.
59. Bailey M, Chapin W, Licht H, Reynolds JC. The effects of vasculitis on the gastrointestinal tract and liver. Gastroenterol Clin N Am. 1998;27:747–82, v-vi
60. Fraioli P, Barberis M, Rizzato G. Gastrointestinal presentation of Churg Strauss syndrome. Sarcoidosis. 1994;11:42–5.
61. Pinkney JH, Clarke G, Fairclough PD. Gastrointestinal involvement in Wegener's granulomatosis. Gastrointest Endosc. 1991;37:411–2.
62. Gayraud M, Guillevin L, le Toumelin P, et al. Long-term followup of polyarteritis nodosa, microscopic polyangiitis, and Churg-Strauss syndrome: analysis of four prospective trials including 278 patients. Arthritis Rheum. 2001;44:666–75.
63. Pagnoux C, Mahr A, Cohen P, Guillevin L. Presentation and outcome of gastrointestinal involvement in systemic necrotizing vasculitides: analysis of 62 patients with polyarteritis nodosa, microscopic polyangiitis, Wegener granulomatosis, Churg-Strauss syndrome, or rheumatoid arthritis-associated vasculitis. Medicine. 2005;84:115–28.
64. Le Thi Huong D, Wechsler B, Grand d'Esnon A, et al. Severe digestive vasculitis: value of bolus of cyclophosphamide. Gastroenterol Clin Biol. 1988;12:402–4.

65. Vaglio A, Corradi D, Ronda N, Garini G, Buzio C. Large bowel obstruction heralding Churg-Strauss syndrome. Am J Gastroenterol. 2004;99:562–3.
66. Beye B, Lesur G, Claude P, Martzolf L, Kieffer P, Sondag D. Small bowel involvement documented by capsule endoscopy in Churg-Strauss syndrome. Pan Afr Med J. 2015;22:41.
67. Camilleri M, Pusey CD, Chadwick VS, Rees AJ. Gastrointestinal manifestations of systemic vasculitis. Q J Med. 1983;52:141–9.
68. Desbazeille F, Soule JC. Digestive manifestations of vasculitis. Gastroenterol Clin Biol. 1986;10:405–14.
69. Matolo NM, Garfinkle SE, Wolfman EF Jr. Intestinal necrosis and perforation in patients receiving immunosuppressive drugs. Am J Surg. 1976;132:753–4.
70. Vaszar LT, Orzechowski NM, Specks U, et al. Coexistent pulmonary granulomatosis with polyangiitis (Wegener granulomatosis) and Crohn disease. Am J Surg Pathol. 2014;38:354–9.
71. Jozwiak L, Lawnicka I, Ksiazek A. Coexistence of granulomatosis with polyangiitis (GPA) and Crohn's disease or multiorgan manifestation of the same disease? Reumatologia. 2016;54:86–90.
72. Humbert S, Guilpain P, Puechal X, et al. Inflammatory bowel diseases in anti-neutrophil cytoplasmic antibody-associated vasculitides: 11 retrospective cases from the French Vasculitis Study Group. Rheumatology. 2015;54:1970–5.
73. Kiene M, Csernok E, Muller A, Metzler C, Trabandt A, Gross WL. Elevated interleukin-4 and interleukin-13 production by T cell lines from patients with Churg-Strauss syndrome. Arthritis Rheum. 2001;44:469–73.
74. Jakiela B, Szczeklik W, Plutecka H, et al. Increased production of IL-5 and dominant Th2-type response in airways of Churg-Strauss syndrome patients. Rheumatology. 2012;51:1887–93.
75. Fuss IJ, Neurath M, Boirivant M, et al. Disparate CD4+ lamina propria (LP) lymphokine secretion profiles in inflammatory bowel disease. Crohn's disease LP cells manifest increased secretion of IFN-gamma, whereas ulcerative colitis LP cells manifest increased secretion of IL-5. J Immunol. 1996;157:1261–70.
76. Sanders JS, Stegeman CA, Kallenberg CG. The Th1 and Th2 paradigm in ANCA-associated vasculitis. Kidney Blood Press Res. 2003;26:215–20.
77. Csernok E, Trabandt A, Muller A, et al. Cytokine profiles in Wegener's granulomatosis: predominance of type 1 (Th1) in the granulomatous inflammation. Arthritis Rheum. 1999;42:742–50.
78. Fuss IJ, Becker C, Yang Z, et al. Both IL-12p70 and IL-23 are synthesized during active Crohn's disease and are down-regulated by treatment with anti-IL-12 p40 monoclonal antibody. Inflamm Bowel Dis. 2006;12:9–15.
79. Fagin U, Csernok E, Muller A, et al. Distinct proteinase 3-induced cytokine patterns in Wegener s granulomatosis, Churg-Strauss syndrome, and healthy controls. Clin Exp Rheumatol. 2011;29:S57–62.
80. Balding CE, Howie AJ, Drake-Lee AB, Savage CO. Th2 dominance in nasal mucosa in patients with Wegener's granulomatosis. Clin Exp Immunol. 2001;125:332–9.
81. Nakamura RM, Matsutani M, Barry M. Advances in clinical laboratory tests for inflammatory bowel disease. Clin Chim Acta. 2003;335:9–20.
82. Ardizzone S, Puttini PS, Cassinotti A, Porro GB. Extraintestinal manifestations of inflammatory bowel disease. Dig Liver Dis. 2008;40(Suppl 2):S253–9.
83. Anderson G, Coles ET, Crane M, et al. Wegener's granuloma. A series of 265 British cases seen between 1975 and 1985. A report by a sub-committee of the British Thoracic Society Research Committee. Q J Med. 1992;83:427–38.
84. Fauci AS, Haynes BF, Katz P, Wolff SM. Wegener's granulomatosis: prospective clinical and therapeutic experience with 85 patients for 21 years. Ann Intern Med. 1983;98:76–85.
85. Hoffman GS, Kerr GS, Leavitt RY, et al. Wegener granulomatosis: an analysis of 158 patients. Ann Intern Med. 1992;116:488–98.
86. Dufour JF, Le Gallou T, Cordier JF, et al. Urogenital manifestations in Wegener granulomatosis: a study of 11 cases and review of the literature. Medicine. 2012;91:67–74.

87. Huong DL, Papo T, Piette JC, et al. Urogenital manifestations of Wegener granulomatosis. Medicine. 1995;74:152–61.
88. Davenport A, Downey SE, Goel S, Maciver AG. Wegener's granulomatosis involving the urogenital tract. Br J Urol. 1996;78:354–7.
89. Gunnarsson R, Omdal R, Kjellevold KH, Ellingsen CL. Wegener's granulomatosis of the prostate gland. Rheumatol Int. 2004;24:120–2.
90. Yalowitz PA, Greene LF, Sheps SG, Carlin MR. Wegener's granulomatosis involving the prostate gland: report of a case. J Urol. 1966;96:801–4.
91. Murty GE, Powell PH. Wegener's granulomatosis presenting as prostatitis. Br J Urol. 1991;67:107–8.
92. Stillwell TJ, DeRemee RA, McDonald TJ, Weiland LH, Engen DE. Prostatic involvement in Wegener's granulomatosis. J Urol. 1987;138:1251–3.
93. Vaught WW, Wilson TM, Raife MJ, Horne DW. Wegener granulomatosis: prostatic involvement and bladder outlet obstruction. Urology. 1989;34:43–5.
94. Middleton G, Karp D, Lee E, Cush J. Wegener's granulomatosis presenting as lower back pain with prostatitis and ureteral obstruction. J Rheumatol. 1994;21:566–9.
95. Walton EW. Giant-cell granuloma of the respiratory tract (Wegener's granulomatosis). Br Med J. 1958;2:265–70.
96. Lillaz J, Bernardini S, Algros MP, Bittard H, Kleinclauss F. Wegener's granulomatosis: a rare cause of hydronephrosis. Case Rep Med. 2011;2011:814794.
97. Le Thi Huong D, De Gennes C, Wechsler B, Etienne SD, Godeau P. Anuria caused by bilateral ureteral stenosis in Wegener's granulomatosis. Presse Med. 1988;17:870.
98. Plaisier EM, Mougenot B, Khayat R, Gattegno B, Mignon F, Ronco PM. Ureteral stenosis in Wegener's granulomatosis. Nephrol Dial Transplant. 1997;12:1759–61.
99. Agraharkar M, Gokhale S, Gupta R. Wegener's granulomatosis diagnosed by testicular biopsy. Int Urol Nephrol. 2002;34:559–64.
100. Lee SS, Tang SH, Sun GH, Yu CP, Jin JS, Chang SY. Limited Wegener's granulomatosis of the epididymis and testis. Asian J Androl. 2006;8:737–9.
101. Barber TD, Al-Omar O, Poulik J, McLorie GA. Testicular infarction in a 12-year-old boy with Wegener's granulomatosis. Urology. 2006;67:846 e9–10.
102. Dore B, Duriez P, Grange P, Aubert J. Wegener's granulomatosis with urethral-penile location. Apropos of a case. Ann Urol. 1990;24:256–8.
103. Bories N, Becuwe C, Marcilly MC, Wolf F, Balme B, Thomas L. Glans penis ulceration revealing Wegener's granulomatosis. Dermatology. 2007;214:187–9.
104. Al Rajabi W, Venturini M, Sala R, Calzavara-Pinton P. Wegener's granulomatosis of the penis: genital presentation of systemic disease. Dermatology. 2006;212:370–2.
105. Cox PJ. Cyclophosphamide cystitis—identification of acrolein as the causative agent. Biochem Pharmacol. 1979;28:2045–9.
106. Stillwell TJ, Benson RC Jr. Cyclophosphamide-induced hemorrhagic cystitis. A review of 100 patients. Cancer. 1988;61:451–7.
107. Knight A, Askling J, Granath F, Sparen P, Ekbom A. Urinary bladder cancer in Wegener's granulomatosis: risks and relation to cyclophosphamide. Ann Rheum Dis. 2004;63:1307–11.
108. Talar-Williams C, Hijazi YM, Walther MM, et al. Cyclophosphamide-induced cystitis and bladder cancer in patients with Wegener granulomatosis. Ann Intern Med. 1996;124:477–84.
109. Hows JM, Mehta A, Ward L, et al. Comparison of mesna with forced diuresis to prevent cyclophosphamide induced haemorrhagic cystitis in marrow transplantation: a prospective randomised study. Br J Cancer. 1984;50:753–6.
110. Lapraik C, Watts R, Bacon P, et al. BSR and BHPR guidelines for the management of adults with ANCA associated vasculitis. Rheumatology. 2007;46:1615–6.
111. Hattori N, Ichimura M, Nagamatsu M, et al. Clinicopathological features of Churg-Strauss syndrome-associated neuropathy. Brain. 1999;122(Pt 3):427–39.
112. Hattori N, Mori K, Misu K, Koike H, Ichimura M, Sobue G. Mortality and morbidity in peripheral neuropathy associated Churg-Strauss syndrome and microscopic polyangiitis. J Rheumatol. 2002;29:1408–14.

113. Uehara M, Hashimoto T, Sasahara E, Higuchi K, Matsubara K, Ikeda S. Churg-Strauss syndrome presenting as myositis following unaccustomed exercise. J Clin Neurosci. 2009;16:1232–3.
114. Della Rossa A, Baldini C, Tavoni A, et al. Churg-Strauss syndrome: clinical and serological features of 19 patients from a single Italian centre. Rheumatology. 2002;41:1286–94.
115. Parent ME, Larue S, Ellezam B. Eosinophilic granulomatosis with polyangiitis (Churg-Strauss syndrome) presenting as diffuse myositis. BMC Musculoskelet Disord. 2014;15:388.
116. Barreto P, Pagnoux C, Luca L, et al. Dorsal prevertebral lesions in Wegener granulomatosis: report on four cases. Joint Bone Spine. 2011;78:88–91.
117. Ramirez GA, Della-Torre E, Campochiaro C, et al. Juxta-vertebral lesions in granulomatosis with polyangiitis. Semin Arthritis Rheum. 2016;46:356–60.
118. Cardenal-Urdampilleta J, Gorospe L, Marquez C, Segur V, Romera B. Wegener's granulomatosis mimicking a thoracic spondylodiscitis. J Rheumatol. 2007;34:1779–81.
119. Lazzarin P, Presotto F, Polo A. Churg-Strauss syndrome presenting as polymyositis: report of a case. Reumatismo. 2009;61:140–4.
120. Jarrot PA, Chiche L, Hervier B, et al. Systemic lupus erythematosus and antineutrophil cytoplasmic antibody-associated vasculitis overlap syndrome in patients with biopsy-proven glomerulonephritis. Medicine. 2016;95:e3748.
121. Nasr SH, D'Agati VD, Park HR, et al. Necrotizing and crescentic lupus nephritis with antineutrophil cytoplasmic antibody seropositivity. Clin J Am Soc Nephrol. 2008;3:682–90.
122. Draibe J, Salama AD. Association of ANCA associated vasculitis and rheumatoid arthritis: a lesser recognized overlap syndrome. Springerplus. 2015;4:50.
123. Gaber LW, Wall BM, Cooke CR. Coexistence of anti-neutrophil cytoplasmic antibody-associated glomerulonephritis and membranous glomerulopathy. Am J Clin Pathol. 1993;99:211–5.
124. Derrett-Smith EC, Nihtyanova SI, Harvey J, Salama AD, Denton CP. Revisiting ANCA-associated vasculitis in systemic sclerosis: clinical, serological and immunogenetic factors. Rheumatology. 2013;52:1824–31.
125. Kalluri R, Meyers K, Mogyorosi A, Madaio MP, Neilson EG. Goodpasture syndrome involving overlap with Wegener's granulomatosis and anti-glomerular basement membrane disease. J Am Soc Nephrol. 1997;8:1795–800.
126. Vanderlugt CL, Miller SD. Epitope spreading in immune-mediated diseases: implications for immunotherapy. Nat Rev Immunol. 2002;2:85–95.
127. Ramos-Casals M, Brito-Zeron P, Soto MJ, Cuadrado MJ, Khamashta MA. Autoimmune diseases induced by TNF-targeted therapies. Best Pract Res Clin Rheumatol. 2008;22:847–61.
128. Vaglio A, Manenti L, Allegri L, Ferrozzi F, Corradi D, Buzio C. ANCA-positive periaortic vasculitis: does it fall within the spectrum of vasculitis? J Intern Med. 2002;251:268–71.
129. ter Maaten JC, Franssen CF, Daenekindt AA, Hoorntje SJ. Triple Wegener's granulomatosis in the urogenital tract. Nephron. 1993;63:358–9.
130. Blockmans D, Baeyens H, Van Loon R, Lauwers G, Bobbaers H. Periaortitis and aortic dissection due to Wegener's granulomatosis. Clin Rheumatol. 2000;19:161–4.
131. Vaglio A, Maritati F. Idiopathic Retroperitoneal Fibrosis. J Am Soc Nephrol. 2016;27:1880–9.
132. Urban ML, Palmisano A, Nicastro M, Corradi D, Buzio C, Vaglio A. Idiopathic and secondary forms of retroperitoneal fibrosis: a diagnostic approach. Rev Med Interne. 2015;36:15–21.
133. Ceresini G, Urban ML, Corradi D, et al. Association between idiopathic retroperitoneal fibrosis and autoimmune thyroiditis: a case-control study. Autoimmun Rev. 2015;14:16–22.
134. Vaglio A, Salvarani C, Buzio C. Retroperitoneal fibrosis. Lancet. 2006;367:241–51.
135. Mertens S, Zeegers AG, Wertheimer PA, Hendriksz TR, van Bommel EF. Efficacy and complications of urinary drainage procedures in idiopathic retroperitoneal fibrosis complicated by extrinsic ureteral obstruction. Int J Urol. 2014;21:283–8.
136. van Bommel EF, Siemes C, Hak LE, van der Veer SJ, Hendriksz TR. Long-term renal and patient outcome in idiopathic retroperitoneal fibrosis treated with prednisone. Am J Kidney Dis. 2007;49:615–25.

137. Jois RN, Kerrigan N, Scott DG. Mycophenolate mofetil for maintenance of remission in idiopathic retroperitoneal fibrosis. Rheumatology. 2007;46:717–8.
138. Alberici F, Palmisano A, Urban ML, et al. Methotrexate plus prednisone in patients with relapsing idiopathic retroperitoneal fibrosis. Ann Rheum Dis. 2013;72:1584–6.
139. Khosroshahi A, Carruthers MN, Stone JH, et al. Rethinking Ormond's disease: "idiopathic" retroperitoneal fibrosis in the era of IgG4-related disease. Medicine. 2013;92:82–91.
140. Stone JH, Zen Y, Deshpande V. IgG4-related disease. N Engl J Med. 2012;366:539–51.
141. Danlos FX, Rossi GM, Blockmans D, et al. Antineutrophil cytoplasmic antibody-associated vasculitides and IgG4-related disease: a new overlap syndrome. Autoimmun Rev. 2017;16:1036–43.
142. Carruthers MN, Khosroshahi A, Augustin T, Deshpande V, Stone JH. The diagnostic utility of serum IgG4 concentrations in IgG4-related disease. Ann Rheum Dis. 2015;74:14–8.
143. Perez Alamino R, Martinez C, Espinoza LR. IgG4-associated vasculitis. Curr Rheumatol Rep. 2013;15:348.
144. Vaglio A, Strehl JD, Manger B, et al. IgG4 immune response in Churg-Strauss syndrome. Ann Rheum Dis. 2012;71:390–3.

Prognosis and Outcomes of ANCA-Associated Vasculitis

16

David Jayne

16.1 Introduction

In the modern therapeutic era the outcome of systemic vasculitis has changed from a usually fatal course to a chronic relapsing disorder [1]. During this period, the ANCA vasculitides have been defined and have received the most research attention, especially concerning treatment regimens and the longer term consequences of disease. Achievement of initial disease control, and removal of a direct threat to life or further organ damage, is now considered routine and physicians are concerned with their patients' longer term health, prevention of further disease flares and comorbidities, minimizing the toxic consequences of treatment, and improving quality of life. From a research perspective, this has meant development of disease state definitions and objective quantification of disease activity and long-term outcome parameters, such as damage and glucocorticoid toxicity [2, 3]. The Birmingham Vasculitis Activity Score (BVAS) and its subsequent modifications are routinely used for activity assessment, while the vasculitis damage index (VDI) has been developed to assess all-cause damage after the vasculitis diagnosis. Disease-specific quality-of-life tools are in development and approaches to economic evaluation are at an early stage [4, 5].

Identification of comorbidity risks, including thromboembolic disease and cardiovascular risk, has posed new research questions of relevance to the pathogenicity of vasculitis itself that largely remain unanswered [6, 7]. Concern over cyclophosphamide-induced malignancy has dominated discussion over optimal treatments but is now a fading issue with lower dose regimens and the availability of rituximab as an alternative [8]. Similarly, newer therapeutic targets, such as the

D. Jayne (✉)
Department of Medicine, University of Cambridge, Cambridge, UK
e-mail: Dj106@cam.ac.uk

R. A. Sinico, L. Guillevin (eds.), *Anti-Neutrophil Cytoplasmic Antibody (ANCA) Associated Vasculitis*, Rare Diseases of the Immune System,
https://doi.org/10.1007/978-3-030-02239-6_16

alternative complement pathway, are providing opportunities for anti-inflammatory strategies that permit glucocorticoid sparing [9].

Data concerning prognosis and outcomes are derived from inclusive single-center and multicenter registries and from clinical trials. Prospective studies provide higher quality data but are often of limited duration and subject to bias inherent on the eligibility of patients for the studies [10]. Since the 1980s, collaborative research networks have supported the data acquisition, initially single country then international. However, these have focused on Western Europe, North America, and Japan, and with the exception of Japan, have necessarily focused on Caucasian patients [11]. They have also included patients cared for in expert centers rather than being population based, although this is changing as the networks enlarge [12]. This has the implication that the literature may reflect better practice, and better outcomes, than the routine patient might experience.

ANCA vasculitis is characterized by heterogeneity, age at presentation, organ distribution and severity, response to treatment, and susceptibility to morbidities. Certain subgroups, such as eosinophilic granulomatosis with polyangiitis (EGPA), have received less research effort, while others—for example, nephritis—are much better studied. This chapter will review the dimensions of prognosis and outcomes as the literature permits, will identify changes where these are occurring, and the gaps in our understanding (Fig. 16.1).

16.2 Disease Activity

Control of the presenting episode of ANCA vasculitis is achieved in 80–90% with current therapies, and those with refractory disease have poor long-term outcomes. A recent analysis of European Vasculitis Society (EUVAS) data has demonstrated that achieving a BVAS of zero in 3 months is associated with better survival, lower risk of end-stage renal disease, and less damage as assessed by VDI. Those achieving remission in 3 months and maintaining this to at least 6 months have the best outcome suggesting the use of this parameter as an end point for interventional studies. PR3-ANCA and higher baseline disease activity are associated with a failure to achieve remission [13]. Refractory disease confers a high mortality risk with 11/32 patients in one report dying within 3 months, alveolar hemorrhage and renal failure being key predictors [14]. Patients with severe disease requiring intensive care unit (ITU) admission due to alveolar hemorrhage or other severe organ failure have carried a mortality of 50%, but survival rates have been improving with contributions from advanced intensive therapy unit (ITU) care and ventilator support, extracorporeal membrane oxygenation (ECMO), and newer treatment regimens [15, 16].

While it has been assumed that return of disease activity, relapse, would be associated with mortality, this has not proved the case overall as the majority of relapses occur in GPA and involve the upper respiratory tract [17]. Although this drives increased local damage, reduced quality of life, and cumulative drug exposure, it does not increase mortality risk. In contrast, the less frequent renal relapses are more important with respect to survival and end-stage renal failure risk, especially

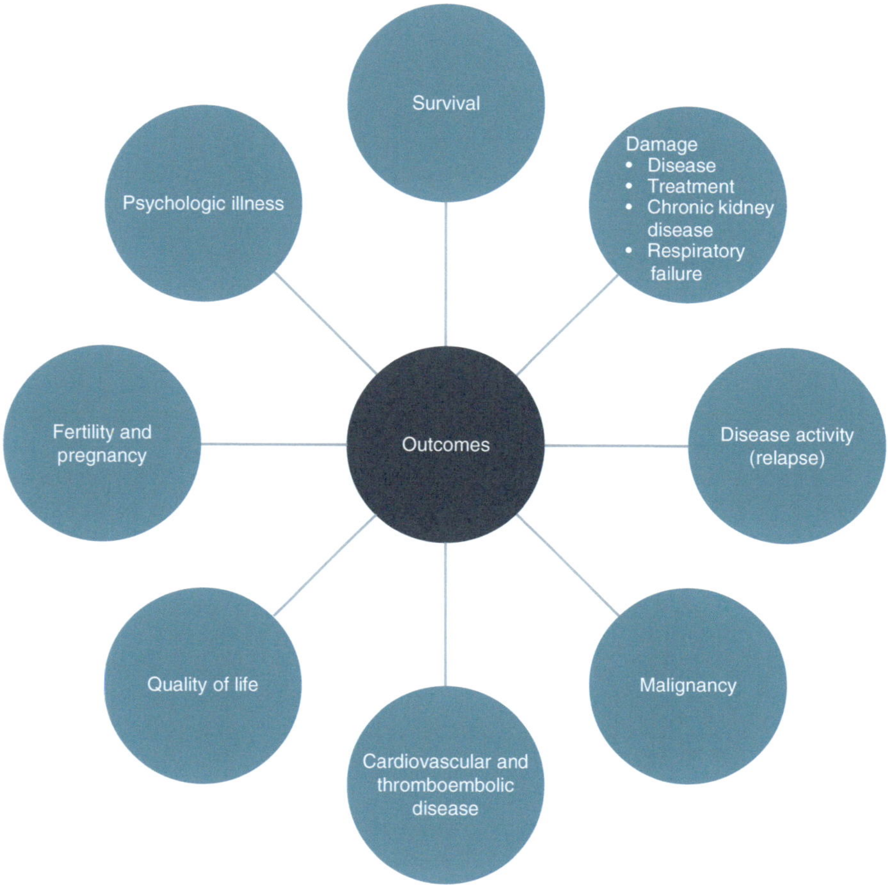

Fig. 16.1 The dimensions of outcome in AAV

as they are likely to occur in patients with previous episodes of nephritis and chronic kidney disease [18].

ANCA vasculitis is a relapsing disorder with around 50% relapsing by 5 years after diagnosis. Many factors have been associated with relapse (summarized in Table 16.1). The duration of immunosuppressive therapy and use of ANCA in relapse prediction have been the more controversial areas. Longer treatment with azathioprine and glucocorticoids, for 4 years from diagnosis, was associated with fewer relapses and a reduced rate of progression to end-stage renal disease than stopping maintenance therapy at 2 years [19]. However, opinion on when to withdraw glucocorticoids has been particularly variable, a systematic review of clinical trials where data on glucocorticoid dosing were available has demonstrated that glucocorticoid withdrawal is a strong predictor of relapse [20]. Comparative studies have found no difference in efficacy or safety between azathioprine and methotrexate when used to prevent relapse, and mycophenolate mofetil was not found to be

Table 16.1 Factors associated with relapse in ANCA-associated vasculitis

Factors increasing relapse risk		
Clinical presentation	Serology	Treatment related
Diagnosis of GPA	PR3-ANCA > MPO-ANCA	Glucocorticoid withdrawal
Ear, nose, and throat involvement	ANCA positive after induction	Immunosuppressive or rituximab withdrawal
Better renal function (creatinine < 200 μmol/l)	Rise in ANCA, in particular after treatment reduction	Lower cyclophosphamide exposure and noncyclophosphamide induction
Higher BVAS and failure to achieve BVAS zero		Rituximab induction

more effective than azathioprine [21, 22]. Repeat-dose rituximab was more effective than azathioprine in the one completed maintenance trial [23].

The availability of rituximab is changing the approach to relapse management. Given as an induction therapy, relapse is at least as frequent as with conventional cyclophosphamide/azathioprine therapy, and the risk of relapse following rituximab was specifically highlighted in the license for AAV [24]. Approaches to managing this relapse risk have varied from watchful waiting to use of an oral immunosuppressive, or repeat-dose rituximab either following a fixed interval or guided by ANCA and B-cell counts [25]. Even after a 2-year course of repeat-dose rituximab, a relapse risk persists, although it may be lower than after a single course [26].

Multiple studies have provided evidence for and against a role of ANCA in predicting relapse [27, 28]. Many are confounded by concurrent therapy, but the persistence of ANCA after induction therapy appears to predict a higher relapse risk and the return of ANCA after treatment withdrawal, especially after rituximab, also predicts relapse [29]. However, ANCA itself is not sufficiently sensitive to be a reliable biomarker in this setting with many relapses occurring without change in ANCA [26].

16.3 Survival

In a study from the 1950s, 80% of GPA patients had died without therapy, with renal failure being the main cause of death [1]. The introduction of cyclophosphamide and glucocorticoids has dramatically changed the high mortality [30]. In a survey of clinical trials recruited between 1995 and 2003, there was a threefold excess mortality, compared to a matched control population [31]. Older age, renal impairment, and MPO-ANCA positivity were negative predictors for survival. Although not observed in this study, others have reported a higher BVAS at diagnosis as being associated with worse survival probably related to cardiovascular comorbidity [32, 33]. Selection of higher risk patients in the original trials may have influenced these results and prevalent AAV cohorts have much better survival risk [10]. A recent population-based study from Southern Sweden has confirmed the high overall

Table 16.2 Predictive factors for end - stage renal disease

Baseline	After induction therapy
Low GFR	Low GFR
MPO-ANCA or ANCA negative	Persisting proteinuria
"Mixed" or "sclerotic" histological classification	Persisting or return of hematuria
Tubulointerstitial inflammation and fibrosis	Nephritis relapse
Extraglomerular arteritis	Failure to achieve BVAS zero after induction

mortality risk for AAV, but this was driven by the presence of renal, cardiovascular, or gastrointestinal involvement, and those without these complications had similar survival to the background population [12, 34, 35] (Table 16.2). These results reflect previous work by the French Vasculitis Study Group and their development of a five-factor score for survival prediction in AAV. They and others have shown that the presence of ear, nose, and throat involvement in GPA is associated with a lower risk of renal involvement; renal disease follows a milder course if it occurs and survival is better [36]. The Swedish study also confirmed a worse outcome with the MPO-ANCA subgroup. The elderly have a different pattern of organ involvement that confers a worse prognosis over and above their age, with more severe renal disease and less frequent ear, nose, and throat disease [37].

Early mortality is strongly influenced by the adverse effects of therapy. A "therapy burden" tool has been developed to quantify these effects and a high score strongly predicts early mortality risk [38]. Other factors early in the course of disease that predict death are low GFR, cumulative cyclophosphamide exposure, and infection.

16.4 Renal Outcomes

About 70% of AAV patients have renal involvement and the renal outcome is dependent largely on the speed with which the diagnosis is made and the serum creatinine at diagnosis. Those with GPA present earlier due to extrarenal disease, while those with renal-limited vasculitis present late, often with symptoms of renal failure. Furthermore, ear, nose, and throat involvement is associated with milder nephritis [36]. Reductions in diagnostic delay, facilitated by ANCA testing and greater awareness of vasculitis, are the most important factors in the improved renal outcomes that have been observed over the last 20 years [39]. EUVAS data from the 1990s suggested that 20% of survivors developed end-stage renal failure, but this figure may have been inflated by selection criteria for the EUVAS trials [31]. A glomerular filtration rate of 50 ml/min split the prognosis for patient and renal survival, being very good for those with a higher GFR, while 50% of those below 50 ml/min had either died or were on dialysis for 5 years [40].

The PR3-ANCA subgroup have a better prognosis, serum creatinine is lower at diagnosis, the renal histology contains more acute and reversible glomerular and tubular lesions, and less fibrosis [41]. In contrast, the MPO-ANCA and

ANCA-negative subgroups have a worse renal prognosis, the renal scarring suggesting chronicity to the disease prior to diagnosis. Using inception renal biopsies from the EUVAS trials, a histologic score, the "Berden" score, had categorized glomerular involvement into four groups that correlate with the risk of renal failure [42]. Multiple confirmatory studies have been performed and the predictive value of the Berden system enhanced by inclusion of tubulointerstitial fibrosis and ANCA subtype [43]. Most structures within the kidney can be affected in ANCA vasculitis and tubulointerstitial inflammation, T-cell tubulitis and extraglomerular vasculitis have all been associated with worse renal outcomes [44]. A predictive formula for GFR 12 months after diagnosis has been developed based on renal histology and baseline GFR [45]. About 5% of AAV patients with renal involvement have antiglomerular basement membrane (GBM) antibodies and histologic features of anti-GBM disease [46]. Their renal prognosis is worse than for patients without anti-GBM antibodies, and many progress to end-stage renal disease [47].

Hematuria with proteinuria is almost universal at diagnosis and persists in up to 50% after apparent disease control has been established. The level of proteinuria rises during the recovery phase in severe renal vasculitis and persistent proteinuria, especially as assessed by IgM excretion, associates with a lower long-term GFR, reflecting renal damage [48]. The significance of persistent hematuria is more controversial with an observational study pointing to an increased risk of renal relapse, while a EUVAS study found no predictive value of hematuria [49]. However, the return of or increase in hematuria may indicate renal relapse. Patients presenting with impaired renal function are at lower risk of relapse, but the consequences of renal relapses when they occur are severe, with many progressing to end-stage renal failure (Table 16.3). Other factors that have been associated with worse renal outcome include lower complement C3 levels at diagnosis and the presence of antiplasminogen antibodies [50, 51].

AAV patients on dialysis may continue to suffer relapses and are less tolerant to conventional therapies. Once transplanted, the relapse risk drops, vasculitis recurrence can occur in the renal allograft but is rare, less than 2% although usually

Table 16.3 Survival predictors in ANCA-associated vasculitis

Negative survival predictors	Positive survival predictors
Older age	Ear, nose, and throat involvement
Low GFR < 15 ml/min	Remission of disease activity, BVAS zero by 3 months
MPO-ANCA or ANCA negative	
Higher cyclophosphamide exposure	
Severe infection	
Higher BVAS at diagnosis	
Cardiovascular or gastrointestinal involvement	
Intensive care unit admission	
Lower hemoglobin and higher white blood cell count	

results in loss of the graft when it occurs. Transplant patients with a history of vasculitis carry a higher risk of opportunistic infection, but otherwise their transplant outcomes are similar to those of other nondiabetic causes of renal disease [52, 53]. ANCA positivity at the time of transplant does not appear to influence outcome but has been associated with vasculopathy in the graft of uncertain significance [54].

16.5 Damage

Vasculitic inflammation can result in irreversible tissue damage and this is more likely to occur with relapsing disease [55]. Damage is also caused by adverse effects of therapy and by the development of comorbidities. The accrual of damage not only is a stronger mortality predictor than disease activity but also directly impacts on a patient's function and quality of life. Most damage is acquired early, in the first 6 to 12 months, but there is then a continued slower addition of damage driven by relapsing disease and therapy. Long-term damage in the AAVs may be associated with the severity of initial disease, age, number of relapses, and duration of glucocorticoid use [55, 56]. Children tend to have more severe disease activity, a higher relapse rate, and acquire more damage than adults with AAV [57].

Respiratory insufficiency can result from differing pulmonary manifestations of vasculitis including pulmonary fibrosis, bronchial stenosis, and chronic infection [58, 59]. However, lung cavities, seen in GPA, resolve with treatment and do not influence pulmonary outcome or survival [60]. Rarely, they can be complicated by aspergilloma with serious consequences [61]. Alveolar hemorrhage is potentially life threatening when it occurs but does not cause long-term respiratory disease unless it occurs on a background of preexisting fibrotic lung disease [62]. Vasculitic neuropathy, occurring in 20%, causes chronic morbidity due to impaired function and neuropathic pain, but is not associated with an increased frequency of vital organ damage or reduced survival [63].

The overlap between interstitial lung disease (ILD) and ANCA-associated vasculitis is an active topic of investigation. At least 20% of AAV patients have ILD at diagnosis and many ILD patients have MPO-ANCA without vasculitis [64]. ILD can progress regardless of therapy in AAV patients and dominates prognosis. Whether its course is modified by vasculitis therapy is unclear. Silicosis is associated with MPO-ANCA vasculitis but is not the explanation for the majority of patients with ILD [65].

16.5.1 Treatment-Related Toxicity

In long-term follow-up, the frequency of damage items caused by treatment rivals that caused by the disease, with glucocorticoid-related toxicity predominating [56]. A glucocorticoid toxicity index has recently been developed to more accurately quantify these effects [3]. The impact of immunosuppression on malignancy risk is discussed below, but other chronic toxic effects which are uncommon include cyclophosphamide-induced cardiomyopathy, azathioprine-associated hepatic cirrhosis, and myelodysplasia. Oral cyclophosphamide delivers a higher cyclophosphamide exposure and has consistently been shown to be more toxic, with more frequent cytopenias and infection and higher mortality risk [66].

16.6 Comorbidities

Preexisting disease may predispose to ANCA vasculitis, and overlaps occur between ANCA vasculitis and other autoimmune diseases (Table 16.4); in these settings, prognosis and outcomes will be influenced by the prior or concomitant disease.

16.6.1 Malignancy

An increase in malignancy has been consistently reported with cyclophosphamide-based regimens. Urothelial malignancy is dose dependent with markedly increased frequency after a cumulative exposure of 25 g of cyclophosphamide and over 60-fold frequency with exposures over 100 g [67]. There are likely to be increased risks with lower doses, but the sample size of published studies have been too small

Table 16.4 Comorbidities associated with the diagnosis of ANCA vasculitis or developing during the course of ANCA vasculitis

Prior to, or at the time of, AAV onset	During AAV course
Malignancy	Malignancy • Urothelial carcinoma related to cyclophosphamide • Lymphoproliferative malignancy • Nonmelanoma skin cancer
Infection • Endocarditis • Tuberculosis • Chronic viral infection	Chronic or recurrent infection
Drugs • Penicillamine • Hydralazine	Immunodeficiency
Chronic lung disease (associated with MPO-ANCA) • Interstitial lung disease • Bronchiectasis • Silicosis	Cardiovascular disease • Thromboembolic disease • Myocardial infarction • Stroke
Other autoimmune disease • Rheumatoid arthritis • Anti-GBM disease • SLE	Psychological morbidity
	Other drug toxicities • Glucocorticoid damage • Cytopenias

to detect an increase at cyclophosphamide doses below 15 g [68]. The increased risk of these malignancies increases with the length of observation highlighting the need to minimize cyclophosphamide exposure in the young. Bladder malignancy is much more common in those who have had hemorrhagic cystitis, an adverse event almost never seen with current intravenous dosing and hydration. Whether or not bladder protection exerts a useful role with current regimens is unclear. Lymphoproliferative malignancy is also cyclophosphamide dose dependent but may also be influenced by other immunosuppressives and chronic inflammation. Nonmelanoma skin cancer rates are elevated, both caused by nonspecific immunosuppression and azathioprine. An increase in other solid organ cancers has been linked to cyclophosphamide, but is less notable than the other malignancies [68].

Rituximab was introduced as a treatment for B-cell lymphoma and has been predicted to reduce malignancy rates in AAV by minimizing cyclophosphamide and immunosuppressive exposure and improving control of disease activity. One, single-center study found no increased malignancy risk in a rituximab-exposed AAV population whether or not they had received cyclophosphamide, but found a standardized incidence ratio over 3 in the group that had not received rituximab consistent with previous literature [69].

16.6.2 Infection

An increased susceptibility to infection results from immunosuppression and glucocorticoid use, chronic damage, and microbial colonization of the respiratory tract [58, 70]. There is no specific pattern to the infections, with bacterial respiratory infections and herpes zoster being most frequent, but opportunistic infection including *Cytomegalovirus* and *Pneumocystis jirovecci* (PJP) seen [71]. A population-based study examining hospitalization reports found an increased rate of fourfold in admissions in the AAV group compared to the background population [59]. Sulfamethoxazole–trimethoprim used in a PJP prophylactic dose has reduced overall infection rates and is advised after either cyclophosphamide or rituximab, but the optimal duration is uncertain [72]. A randomized trial of high-dose sulfamthoxazole–trimethoprim in GPA reported lower respiratory tract relapse rates associated with better infection control [73].

Glucocorticoids may be the major contributor to early infective risk, there was no difference in infection rates between cyclophosphamide and rituximab treatment groups in the RAVE trial, all patients receiving glucocorticoids, and data from lupus nephritis demonstrate a dose-dependent severe infection risk with glucocorticoids [74, 75]. Age-adjusted dose reductions of cyclophosphamide and glucocorticoids have reduced serious infection rates without compromising efficacy [76, 77]. Cyclophosphamide-induced neutropenia confers a high risk of infection and infection-related death, but has become an uncommon occurrence with modern dosing regimens [78]. A rare complication of rituximab is progressive multifocal leukoencephalopathy caused by JC virus reactivation. It can be fatal or causes chronic disability in survivors [79].

Respiratory tract damage in GPA affects epithelial barrier function and normal host defense. Chronic infection of damaged upper respiratory tract tissues with *Staphylococcus aureus* progressively rises with disease duration and is hard to eradicate [80]. The normally sterile lower respiratory tract becomes colonized with bacteria, fungi, and viruses, with infection being more common when there is structural damage such as bronchiectasis or bronchial stenosis [81]. There is a complex interplay between infection, disease activity, and vasculitis therapy that can dominate the management of GPA patients late in their disease course and may require long-term antibiotics to control.

16.6.3 Immunodeficiency

Prior to rituximab, hypogammaglobulinemia and lymphopenia were occasionally noted with immunosuppressive drugs, but were not perceived as a major problem and were potentially reversible. For unknown reasons, AAV patients are susceptible to sustained hypogammaglobulinemia after rituximab with 5% requiring immunoglobulin replacement [82–85]. This does not appear to be a dose-dependent phenomenon or to be dependent on prior cyclophosphamide exposure. A low IgG level at the time of first rituximab has been identified as a predictor for the development of hypogammaglobulinemia [83]. Immunoglobulin replacement is effective at reducing infection rates in these patients and has been well tolerated. Although there can be considerable variability in IgG levels in a particular patient, it is unclear to what extent they can recover immunoglobulin production. Babies born to mothers who have received rituximab during pregnancy have low or no detectable B cells or IgM, but appear to recover by 6 months of age.

16.6.4 Cardiovascular Disease

A high rate of deep venous thrombosis and pulmonary embolism was noted in the WEGET study of etanercept in GPA and has been subsequently confirmed in the EUVAS and other datasets [6, 86]. Long-term EUVAS data reported an incidence of 10%, and although more common at times of disease activity, the risk of these events continued during the remission period. Thrombosis at a microvascular level is a component of vasculitis pathogenesis, but classical prothrombotic factors are normal apart from platelet counts, which can be elevated especially in GPA. Antiplasminogen antibodies have been associated with thrombosis in AAV, but this remains to be confirmed [51, 87]. The interplay between alternative complement pathway activation and platelet aggregation and thrombosis is an emerging field [88].

Myocardial infarction and stroke are also more common in AAV patients than the background population with an increase of 65% similar to that seen in other chronic inflammatory diseases [89]. Higher disease activity and not being PR3-ANCA positive confers an increased risk [7]. Again, the mechanism for this risk is not clear and is probably not explained by transient changes in classical risk factors, such as hypertension, hyperlipidemia, and hyperglycemia, that occur early in the course of the disease. Carotid intima-media thickness is increased in AAV patients compared to matched controls reflecting an acceleration of atheromatous disease [7, 90]. No interventional studies have yet reported for cardiovascular complications of vasculitis, but there is preliminary evidence that rituximab may be beneficial [91]. Both thromboprophylaxis and statin use have scientific rationale that await further investigation.

16.7 Quality of Life

Sequential studies of quality of life using the short form 36 (SF-36) have been performed in parallel with interventional drug trials [92]. They have consistently demonstrated depressed mental and physical functioning when the disease is active with recovery of mental domains to control population levels, indicating a low level of long-term psychological morbidity in ANCA-associated vasculitis. In contrast, physical domains, especially pain and vitality, remain depressed during the remission phase and are reflected by reduced physical activity. The level of depressed physical function is equivalent to that seen in rheumatoid arthritis and chronic kidney disease and is not associated with baseline disease or demographic factors [93]. Depressed physical SF-36 domains at diagnosis were associated with older age and neurologic involvement with vasculitis, while mental domains were particularly influenced by pulmonary disease [94, 95].

Elevated frequency of depression and anxiety was demonstrated using the Hospital Anxiety and Depression Scale (HADS) in a single-center study, affecting 43% and 25%, respectively [96]. Chronic pain, fatigue, neuropathy, and high glucocorticoid dosing were associated with these psychological symptoms [96]. Furthermore, depression was associated with an increase in physical symptoms and was more common in those with ear, nose, and throat disease [97]. Cross-sectional studies of prevalent AAV clinic patient populations have replicated these findings and have associated low physical dimension scores with C-reactive protein and serum albumin levels [94]. Both are nonspecific inflammatory markers, but whether the inflammation reflects underlying vasculitis activity, infection, or another cause is unclear. Fatigue is a frequently reported symptom that has been associated with interrupted sleep patterns, but has otherwise not been systematically investigated [98]. A magnetic resonance imaging study using blood-oxygen-level- dependent (BOLD) signals revealed greater activation in the right thalamus, left paracentral lobule, left medial frontal gyrus, and right medial globus pallidus in GPA patients with fatigue compared to those without, suggesting a neurophysiologic basis to fatigue [99]. Potential contributions to fatigue include disease activity, irreversible tissue damage, fibromyalgia, vitamin deficiency, drug toxicity, and anemia. As some of these factors are modifiable, there is a direction for future research to address fatigue.

Over 25% of those employed prior to their diagnosis become long-term unemployed, with higher associated depression levels, fatigue, unexplained symptomatology, weight gain, and demand on healthcare services [100, 101]. The interaction between physical and mental symptoms, employment, and healthcare demand requires further investigation and the involvement of specialists beyond internal medicine. Physical rehabilitation programs copied from other rheumatic diseases are currently being explored.

Generic quality-of-life tools, such as SF-36, have been of little value in discriminating between treatment groups in randomized controlled trials, though have broadly correlated with measures of vasculitic disease activity and damage. There have been two exceptions: with rituximab proving superior to azathioprine in the MAINRITSAN trial and improvements in vitality and physical domains with avacopan when compared to glucocorticoids in a Phase II trial [9, 102]. A disease-specific patient-reported outcome, AAV-PRO, has been developed which may offer greater sensitivity [5]. The Health Assessment Questionnaire (HAQ) demonstrated greater improvement in the rituximab as compared to the azathioprine group in the MAINRITSAN trial of remission maintenance therapy, but this result conflicted with the SF-36 data, where greater improvement in the mental domains were seen in the azathioprine group [102].

16.8 Fertility and Pregnancy

Vasculitis activity and its therapy are potential threats to the fertility of patients with vasculitis. Loss of fertility is an important consequence of the disease, but the risks of this occurring can be considerably reduced with newer forms of treatment. As a chronic disease, vasculitis also causes psychosexual and relationship problems due to effects on self-esteem and mental well-being. Chronic kidney disease is a common consequence of renal vasculitis and the depressed kidney function itself affects fertility in both women and men. Primary ovarian failure is related to the total amount of cyclophosphamide administered and to the age of the patient. Data from lupus nephritis suggest that a total cyclophosphamide exposure of 14–20 g results in infertility in over 50% of women aged over 32 years [103]. These risks can also be reduced by using short-term regimens or by intravenous pulse as opposed to daily oral administration. Three months of oral cyclophosphamide leads to an exposure of 9–14 g, and an equivalent six-dose course of intravenous pulse cyclophosphamide, 5–7 g. Even if infertility is not induced, less severe ovarian damage leads to earlier menopause. Direct damage to the ovaries or female reproductive tract by vasculitis is rare but has occurred.

Cyclophosphamide directly affects sperm production in men, but there is more potential for recovery by the generation of new sperm forming cells when cyclophosphamide is withdrawn. An alternative immunosuppressive used in vasculitis, methotrexate, also reduces sperm formation, but has a lower risk of sustained effects after drug withdrawal [103]. Testosterone therapy has also been used to protect the testes from cyclophosphamide toxicity. The testicles can be directly attacked by vasculitis in polyarteritis nodosa causing pain and swelling and subsequent loss of function, and rarely in GPA, which can also affect the prostate gland, but the effects on fertility are not well understood.

Pregnancy success in AAV is influenced by the presence of organ damage, in particular, chronic kidney disease. Immunosuppressive drugs, including cyclophosphamide, mycophenolate mofetil, and methotrexate are teratogenic, especially in the first trimester, while rituximab in the second or third trimester depress B-cell and IgM levels in the newborn baby [104–106].

16.9 Health Economics

The introduction of higher cost drugs has inspired research into the health economic impact of AAV. A US study has revealed first year all-cause health costs in GPA (2013 costs) of $30,682 in those without relapse and $88,065 in those with relapse, which rose to $136,007 and $89,721 for the two subgroups in 24 months. Costs were higher for MPA patients at $56,642, reflecting worse renal disease. It was noted that a second hospitalization after diagnosis was a major driver of heath costs and occurred in 42% of patients in their first year after diagnosis and 22% of prevalent patients in a 12-month period. Serious adverse events were a more frequent cause of hospitalization than disease relapse. These data highlight the high cost of ANCA vasculitis and the need for safer, more effective treatments. No reliable studies have been performed of indirect health costs to the individual patient and society associated with their disease and employment.

16.10 Conclusions

The various aspects of outcome of vasculitis have been reviewed together with factors predictive of these outcomes. Knowledge of drug toxicities, such as cyclophosphamide-induced malignancy, has been a major incentive in the development of newer therapies and will become a minor issue with increasing use of rituximab. The frequency of adverse outcomes, including death and end-stage renal disease, is declining due to earlier diagnosis and advances in therapy [107]. Unfortunately, rituximab has introduced its own long-term problem of immunodeficiency. Glucocorticoids are now the major modifiable cause of drug-induced damage, and newer targeted therapeutics, such as complement factor 5 receptor blockade, are being evaluated as an alternative to glucocorticoids. Rituximab has also been shown to be steroid sparing and the combination of rituximab with cyclophosphamide may permit lower glucocorticoid dosing in severe disease [108, 109].

Demographic variables such as age and sex have been studied, but there are little data on different ethnicities or geographic regions. Chinese and Japanese patients are more likely to be MPO-ANCA positive and have interstitial lung disease, both adverse predictors of survival, and one study from North Carolina found worse outcomes in Black patients [110–112]. Genomic studies have identified associations with ANCA subtype, but have not otherwise explored prognosis [113]. A transcriptomic study has identified an expression signature indicative of T-cell senescence that associates with a reduced relapse risk. This requires confirmation and development as a clinical tool [114].

Delayed diagnosis and disease relapse are potentially avoidable contributors to vasculitis-associated damage and better strategies are needed for both components. The multiple dimensions of ANCA vasculitis demand an expert approach to management and access to a range of specialty advice to manage organ-specific manifestations. The development of longer term clinical trials and registries is providing better data on the long-term outcomes of vasculitis.

References

1. Walton EW. Giant-cell granuloma of the respiratory tract (Wegener's granulomatosis). Br Med J. 1958;2:265–70.
2. Bacon PA, Moots RJ, Exley A, Luqmani R, Rasmussen N. VITAL (Vasculitis Integrated Assessment Log) assessment of vasculitis. Clin Exp Rheumatol. 1995;13:275–8.
3. Miloslavsky EM, Naden RP, Bijlsma JW, et al. Development of a Glucocorticoid Toxicity Index (GTI) using multicriteria decision analysis. Ann Rheum Dis. 2017;76(3):543–6.
4. Robson JC, Tomasson G, Milman N, et al. OMERACT endorsement of patient-reported outcome instruments in antineutrophil cytoplasmic antibody-associated vasculitis. J Rheumatol. 2017;44:1529–35.
5. Robson JC, Dawson J, Cronholm PF, et al. Health-related quality of life in ANCA-associated vasculitis and item generation for a disease-specific patient-reported outcome measure. Patient Relat Outcome Meas. 2018;9:17–34.
6. Merkel PA, Lo GH, Holbrook JT, et al. Brief communication: high incidence of venous thrombotic events among patients with Wegener granulomatosis: the Wegener's Clinical Occurrence of Thrombosis (WeCLOT) Study. Ann Intern Med. 2005;142:620–6.
7. Suppiah R, Judge A, Batra R, et al. A model to predict cardiovascular events in patients with newly diagnosed Wegener's granulomatosis and microscopic polyangiitis. Arthritis Care Res (Hoboken). 2011;63:588–96.
8. Hoffman GS, Kerr GS, Leavitt RY, et al. Wegener granulomatosis: an analysis of 158 patients. Ann Intern Med. 1992;116:488–98.
9. Jayne DR, Bruchfeld AN, Harper L, et al. Randomized trial of C5a receptor inhibitor avacopan in ANCA-associated vasculitis. J Am Soc Nephrol. 2017;28(9):2756–67.
10. Pagnoux C, Carette S, Khalidi NA, et al. Comparability of patients with ANCA-associated vasculitis enrolled in clinical trials or in observational cohorts. Clin Exp Rheumatol. 2015;33:77–83.
11. Jayne D, Rasmussen N. Twenty-five years of European Union collaboration in ANCA-associated vasculitis research. Nephrol Dial Transplant. 2015;30:i1–7.
12. Heijl C, Mohammad AJ, Westman K, Höglund P. Long-term patient survival in a Swedish population-based cohort of patients with ANCA-associated vasculitis. RMD Open. 2017;3:e000435.
13. Miloslavsky E, Specks U, Merkel P, et al. Clinical outcomes of remission induction therapy for severe ANCA-Associated vasculitis. Arthritis Rheum. 2013;65(9):2441–9.
14. Seror R, Pagnoux C, Ruivard M, et al. Treatment strategies and outcome of induction-refractory Wegener's granulomatosis or microscopic polyangiitis: analysis of 32 patients with first-line induction-refractory disease in the WEGENT trial. Ann Rheum Dis. 2010;69:2125–30.
15. Gallagher H, Kwan JT, Jayne DR. Pulmonary renal syndrome: a 4-year, single-center experience. Am J Kidney Dis. 2002;39:42–7.
16. Pagnoux C, Hogan SL, Chin H, et al. Predictors of treatment resistance and relapse in antineutrophil cytoplasmic antibody-associated small-vessel vasculitis: comparison of two independent cohorts. Arthritis Rheum. 2008;58:2908–18.

17. Walsh M, Flossmann O, Berden A, et al. Risk factors for relapse of ANCA associated vasculitis. Arthritis Rheum. 2012;64(2):542–8.
18. Göçeroğlu A, Berden AE, Fiocco M, et al. ANCA-associated glomerulonephritis: risk factors for renal relapse. PLoS One. 2016;11:e0165402.
19. Karras A, Pagnoux C, Haubitz M, et al. European VS. Randomised controlled trial of prolonged treatment in the remission phase of ANCA-associated vasculitis. Ann Rheum Dis. 2017;76(10):1662–8.
20. Walsh M, Merkel PA, Mahr A, Jayne D. The effects of duration of glucocorticoid therapy on relapse rate in anti-neutrophil cytoplasm antibody associated vasculitis: a meta-analysis. Arthritis Care Res (Hoboken). 2010;62:1166–73.
21. Pagnoux C, Mahr A, Hamidou MA, et al. Azathioprine or methotrexate maintenance for ANCA-associated vasculitis. N Engl J Med. 2008;359:2790–803.
22. Hiemstra TF, Walsh M, Mahr A, et al. Mycophenolate mofetil vs azathioprine for remission maintenance in antineutrophil cytoplasmic antibody-associated vasculitis: a randomized controlled trial. JAMA. 2010;304(21):2381–8.
23. Guillevin L, Pagnoux C, Karras A, et al. Rituximab versus azathioprine for maintenance in ANCA-associated vasculitis. N Engl J Med. 2014;371:1771–80.
24. Specks U, Merkel PA, Seo P, et al. Efficacy of remission-induction regimens for ANCA-associated vasculitis. N Engl J Med. 2013;369:417–27.
25. Smith RM, Jones RB, Guerry MJ, et al. Rituximab for remission maintenance in relapsing ANCA-associated vasculitis. Arthritis Rheum. 2012;64(11):3760–9.
26. Alberici F, Smith RM, Jones RB, et al. Long-term follow-up of patients who received repeat-dose rituximab as maintenance therapy for ANCA-associated vasculitis. Rheumatology (Oxford). 2015;54(7):1153–60.
27. Rasmussen N, Wiik A, Jayne DR. A historical essay on detection of anti-neutrophil cytoplasmic antibodies. Nephrol Dial Transplant. 2015;30:i8–i13.
28. Morgan MD, Szeto M, Walsh M, et al. Negative anti-neutrophil cytoplasm antibody at switch to maintenance therapy is associated with a reduced risk of relapse. Arthritis Res Ther. 2017;19:129.
29. Sanders JS, Huitma MG, Kallenberg CG, Stegeman CA. Prediction of relapses in PR3-ANCA-associated vasculitis by assessing responses of ANCA titres to treatment. Rheumatology (Oxford). 2006;45:724–9.
30. Novack SN, Pearson CM. Cyclophosphamide therapy in Wegener's granulomatosis. N Engl J Med. 1971;284:938–42.
31. Flossmann O, Berden A, de Groot K, et al. Long-term patient survival in ANCA-associated vasculitis. Ann Rheum Dis. 2011;70:488–94.
32. Gayraud M, Guillevin L, le Toumelin P, et al. French VSG. Long-term followup of polyarteritis nodosa, microscopic polyangiitis, and Churg-Strauss syndrome: analysis of four prospective trials including 278 patients. Arthritis Rheum. 2001;44:666–75.
33. Bai YH, Li ZY, Chang DY, Chen M, Kallenberg CG, Zhao MH. The BVAS is an independent predictor of cardiovascular events and cardiovascular disease-related mortality in patients with ANCA-associated vasculitis: a study of 504 cases in a single Chinese center. Semin Arthritis Rheum. 2018;47:524–9.
34. Guillevin L, Pagnoux C, Seror R, Mahr A, Mouthon L, Le Toumelin P. The Five-Factor Score revisited: assessment of prognoses of systemic necrotizing vasculitides based on the French Vasculitis Study Group (FVSG) cohort. Medicine (Baltimore). 2011;90:19–27.
35. Mahr A, Katsahian S, Varet H, et al. Revisiting the classification of clinical phenotypes of anti-neutrophil cytoplasmic antibody-associated vasculitis: a cluster analysis. Ann Rheum Dis. 2012;72(6):1003–10.
36. Rahmattulla C, de Lind van Wijngaarden RA, Berden AE, et al. Renal function and ear, nose, throat involvement in anti-neutrophil cytoplasmic antibody-associated vasculitis: prospective data from the European Vasculitis Society clinical trials. Rheumatology (Oxford). 2015;54(5):899–907.
37. Krafcik SS, Covin RB, Lynch JP, Sitrin RG. Wegener's granulomatosis in the elderly. Chest. 1996;109:430–7.

38. Little MA, Nightingale P, Verburgh CA, et al. Early mortality in systemic vasculitis: relative contribution of adverse events and active vasculitis. Ann Rheum Dis. 2010;69(6):1036–43.
39. Houben E, Groenland SL, van der Heijden JW, Voskuyl AE, Doodeman HJ, Penne EL. Relation between duration of the prodromal phase and renal damage in ANCA-associated vasculitis. BMC Nephrol. 2017;18:378.
40. Walsh M, Merkel PA, Peh CA, et al. Plasma exchange and glucocorticoid dosing in the treatment of anti-neutrophil cytoplasm antibody associated vasculitis (PEXIVAS): protocol for a randomized controlled trial. Trials. 2013;14:73.
41. Hauer HA, Bajema IM, van Houwelingen HC, et al. Renal histology in ANCA-associated vasculitis: differences between diagnostic and serologic subgroups. Kidney Int. 2002;61:80–9.
42. Berden AE, Ferrario F, Hagen EC, et al. Histopathologic classification of ANCA-associated glomerulonephritis. J Am Soc Nephrol. 2010;21:1628–36.
43. Quintana LF, Perez NS, De Sousa E, et al. ANCA serotype and histopathological classification for the prediction of renal outcome in ANCA-associated glomerulonephritis. Nephrol Dial Transplant. 2014;29(9):1764–9.
44. Berden AE, Jones RB, Erasmus DD, et al. Tubular lesions predict renal outcome in antineutrophil cytoplasmic antibody-associated glomerulonephritis after rituximab therapy. J Am Soc Nephrol. 2012;23:313–21.
45. Vergunst CE, van Gurp E, Hagen EC, et al. An index for renal outcome in ANCA-associated glomerulonephritis. Am J Kidney Dis. 2003;41:532–8.
46. Jayne DR, Marshall PD, Jones SJ, Lockwood CM. Autoantibodies to GBM and neutrophil cytoplasm in rapidly progressive glomerulonephritis. Kidney Int. 1990;37:965–70.
47. Alchi B, Griffiths M, Sivalingam M, Jayne D, Farrington K. Predictors of renal and patient outcomes in anti-GBM disease: clinicopathologic analysis of a two-centre cohort. Nephrol Dial Transplant. 2015;30(5):814–21.
48. Bakoush O, Segelmark M, Torffvit O, Ohlsson S, Tencer J. Urine IgM excretion predicts outcome in ANCA-associated renal vasculitis. Nephrol Dial Transplant. 2006;21:1263–9.
49. Rhee RL, Davis JC, Ding L, et al. The utility of urinalysis in determining the risk of renal relapse in ANCA-associated vasculitis. Clin J Am Soc Nephrol. 2018;13:251–7.
50. Crnogorac M, Horvatic I, Kacinari P, Ljubanovic DG, Galesic K. Serum C3 complement levels in ANCA associated vasculitis at diagnosis is a predictor of patient and renal outcome. J Nephrol. 2018;31:257–62.
51. Berden AE, Nolan SL, Morris HL, et al. Anti-plasminogen antibodies compromise fibrinolysis and associate with renal histology in ANCA-associated vasculitis. J Am Soc Nephrol. 2010;21:2169–79.
52. Moiseev S, Novikov P, Jayne D, Mukhin N. End-stage renal disease in ANCA-associated vasculitis. Nephrol Dial Transplant. 2017;32(2):248–53.
53. Hruskova Z, Stel VS, Jayne D, et al. Characteristics and outcomes of granulomatosis with polyangiitis (Wegener) and microscopic polyangiitis requiring renal replacement therapy: results from the European Renal Association-European dialysis and transplant association registry. Am J Kidney Dis. 2015;66(4):613–20.
54. Little MA, Hassan B, Jacques S, et al. Renal transplantation in systemic vasculitis: when is it safe? Nephrol Dial Transplant. 2009;24:3219–25.
55. Robson J, Doll H, Suppiah R, et al. Damage in the ANCA-associated vasculitides: long-term data from the European Vasculitis Study group (EUVAS) therapeutic trials. Ann Rheum Dis. 2013;74(1):177–84.
56. Robson J, Doll H, Suppiah R, et al. Glucocorticoid treatment and damage in the anti-neutrophil cytoplasm antibody-associated vasculitides: long-term data from the European Vasculitis Study Group trials. Rheumatology (Oxford). 2015;74(1):177–84.
57. Iudici M, Pagnoux C, Quartier P, et al. Childhood- versus adult-onset ANCA-associated vasculitides: A nested, matched case-control study from the French Vasculitis Study Group Registry. Autoimmun Rev. 2018;17:108–14.

58. Mohammad AJ, Mortensen KH, Babar J, et al. Pulmonary Involvement in Antineutrophil Cytoplasmic Antibodies (ANCA)-associated vasculitis: the influence of ANCA subtype. J Rheumatol. 2017;44(10):1458–67.
59. Mohammad AJ, Segelmark M, Smith R, et al. Severe infection in antineutrophil cytoplasmic antibody-associated vasculitis. J Rheumatol. 2017;44(10):1468–75.
60. Russell BA, Mohan S, Chahal R, Carette S, Pagnoux C, Canadian VNC. Prognostic significance of cavitary lung nodules in granulomatosis with polyangiitis—a clinical and imaging study of 225 patients. Arthritis Care Res (Hoboken). 2017;70(7):1082–9.
61. Frankel SK, Jayne D. The pulmonary vasculitides. Clin Chest Med. 2010;31:519–36.
62. Hruskova Z, Casian A, Konopasek P, et al. Long-term outcome of severe alveolar haemorrhage in ANCA-associated vasculitis: a retrospective cohort study. Scand J Rheumatol. 2013;42(3):211–4.
63. Suppiah R, Hadden RD, Batra R, et al. Peripheral neuropathy in ANCA-associated vasculitis: outcomes from the European Vasculitis Study Group trials. Rheumatology (Oxford). 2011;50(12):2214–22.
64. Arulkumaran N, Periselneris N, Gaskin G, et al. Interstitial lung disease and ANCA-associated vasculitis: a retrospective observational cohort study. Rheumatology (Oxford). 2011;50:2035–43.
65. Bartunkova J, Pelclova D, Fenclova Z, et al. Exposure to silica and risk of ANCA-associated vasculitis. Am J Ind Med. 2006;49:569–76.
66. La-Crette J, Royle J, Lanyon PC, Ferraro A, Butler A, Pearce FA. Long-term outcomes of daily oral vs. pulsed intravenous cyclophosphamide in a non-trial setting in ANCA-associated vasculitis. Clin Rheumatol. 2018;37(4):1085–90.
67. Westman KW, Bygren PG, Olsson H, Ranstam J, Wieslander J. Relapse rate, renal survival, and cancer morbidity in patients with Wegener's granulomatosis or microscopic polyangiitis with renal involvement. J Am Soc Nephrol. 1998;9:842–52.
68. Heijl C, Harper L, Flossmann O, et al. Incidence of malignancy in patients treated for anti-neutrophil cytoplasm antibody-associated vasculitis: follow-up data from European Vasculitis Study Group clinical trials. Ann Rheum Dis. 2011;70:1415–21.
69. van Daalen EE, Rizzo R, Kronbichler A, et al. Effect of rituximab on malignancy risk in patients with ANCA-associated vasculitis. Ann Rheum Dis. 2017;76(6):1064–9.
70. Kronbichler A, Jayne DR, Specks U. Con: should all patients with anti-neutrophil cytoplasmic antibody-associated vasculitis be primarily treated with rituximab? Nephrol Dial Transplant. 2015;30(7):1075–81.
71. Ognibene FP, Shelhamer JH, Hoffman GS, et al. Pneumocystis carinii pneumonia: a major complication of immunosuppressive therapy in patients with Wegener's granulomatosis. Am J Respir Crit Care Med. 1995;151:795–9.
72. Kronbichler A, Jayne DR, Mayer G. Frequency, risk factors and prophylaxis of infection in ANCA-associated vasculitis. Eur J Clin Investig. 2015;45(3):346–68.
73. Stegeman CA, Tervaert JW, de Jong PE, Kallenberg CG. Trimethoprim-sulfamethoxazole (co-trimoxazole) for the prevention of relapses of Wegener's granulomatosis. Dutch Co-Trimoxazole Wegener Study Group. N Engl J Med. 1996;335:16–20.
74. Stone JH, Merkel PA, Spiera R, et al. Rituximab versus cyclophosphamide for ANCA-associated vasculitis. N Engl J Med. 2010;363:221–32.
75. Zeher M, Doria A, Lan J, et al. Efficacy and safety of enteric-coated mycophenolate sodium in combination with two glucocorticoid regimens for the treatment of active lupus nephritis. Lupus. 2011;20(14):1484–93.
76. de Groot K, Harper L, Jayne DR, et al. Pulse versus daily oral cyclophosphamide for induction of remission in antineutrophil cytoplasmic antibody-associated vasculitis: a randomized trial. Ann Intern Med. 2009;150:670–80.
77. Pagnoux C, Quéméneur T, Ninet J, et al. Treatment of systemic necrotizing vasculitides in patients aged sixty-five years or older: results of a multicenter, open-label, randomized controlled trial of corticosteroid and cyclophosphamide-based induction therapy. Arthritis Rheumatol. 2015;67:1117–27.

78. Booth AD, Almond MK, Burns A, et al. Outcome of ANCA-associated renal vasculitis: a 5-year retrospective study. Am J Kidney Dis. 2003;41:776–84.
79. Agarwal S, Patrick J, Jones J, Smith R, Coles A, Jayne D. Progressive multifocal leucoencephalopathy with Behçet's disease: an insight into pathophysiology. Rheumatology (Oxford). 2017;56(4):668–70.
80. Salmela A, Rasmussen N, Tervaert JW, Jayne DR, Ekstrand A, European VSG. Chronic nasal Staphylococcus aureus carriage identifies a subset of newly diagnosed granulomatosis with polyangiitis patients with high relapse rate. Rheumatology (Oxford). 2017;56(6):965–72.
81. Néel A, Espitia-Thibault A, Arrigoni PP, et al. Bronchiectasis is highly prevalent in anti-MPO ANCA-associated vasculitis and is associated with a distinct disease presentation. Semin Arthritis Rheum. 2018;48(1):70–6.
82. Marco H, Smith RM, Jones RB, et al. The effect of rituximab therapy on immunoglobulin levels in patients with multisystem autoimmune disease. BMC Musculoskelet Disord. 2014;15:178.
83. Roberts DM, Jones RB, Smith RM, et al. Rituximab-associated hypogammaglobulinemia: incidence, predictors and outcomes in patients with multi-system autoimmune disease. J Autoimmun. 2015;57:25–9.
84. Roberts DM, Jones RB, Smith RM, et al. Immunoglobulin G replacement for the treatment of infective complications of rituximab-associated hypogammaglobulinemia in autoimmune disease: a case series. J Autoimmun. 2016;57:75–9.
85. Cortazar FB, Pendergraft WF, Wenger J, Owens CT, Laliberte K, Niles JL. Effect of continuous B cell depletion with rituximab on pathogenic autoantibodies and total IgG levels in antineutrophil cytoplasmic antibody-associated vasculitis. Arthritis Rheumatol. 2017;69:1045–53.
86. Kronbichler A, Leierer J, Leierer G, European VS, et al. Clinical associations with venous thromboembolism in anti-neutrophil cytoplasm antibody-associated vasculitides. Rheumatology (Oxford). 2017;56(5):704–8.
87. Bautz DJ, Preston GA, Lionaki S, et al. Antibodies with dual reactivity to plasminogen and complementary PR3 in PR3-ANCA vasculitis. J Am Soc Nephrol. 2008;19:2421–9.
88. Chen M, Jayne DR, Zhao MH. Complement in ANCA-associated vasculitis: mechanisms and implications for management. Nat Rev Nephrol. 2017;13(6):359–67.
89. Houben E, Penne EL, Voskuyl AE, et al. Cardiovascular events in anti-neutrophil cytoplasmic antibody-associated vasculitis: a meta-analysis of observational studies. Rheumatology (Oxford). 2018;57:555–62.
90. Sherer Y, Pagnoux C, Chironi G, et al. Carotid artery intima-media thickness, heat shock proteins and oxidized LDL autoantibodies in systemic necrotizing vasculitis. Rheumatol Int. 2008;28:1099–103.
91. Kerekes G, Soltesz P, Der H, et al. Effects of rituximab treatment on endothelial dysfunction, carotid atherosclerosis, and lipid profile in rheumatoid arthritis. Clin Rheumatol. 2009;28:705–10.
92. Walsh M, Mukhtyar C, Mahr A, et al. Health related quality of life in patients with newly diagnosed anti-neutrophil cytoplasm antibody associated vasculitis. Arthritis Care Res (Hoboken). 2011;63(7):1055–61.
93. Basu N, Jones GT, Fluck N, et al. Fatigue: a principal contributor to impaired quality of life in ANCA-associated vasculitis. Rheumatology (Oxford). 2010;49:1383–90.
94. Basu N, McClean A, Harper L, et al. The characterisation and determinants of quality of life in ANCA associated vasculitis. Ann Rheum Dis. 2014;73(1):207–11.
95. Faurschou M, Sigaard L, Bjorner JB, Baslund B. Impaired health-related quality of life in patients treated for Wegener's granulomatosis. J Rheumatol. 2010;37:2081–5.
96. Koutantji M, Harrold E, Lane SE, Pearce S, Watts RA, Scott DG. Investigation of quality of life, mood, pain, disability, and disease status in primary systemic vasculitis. Arthritis Rheum. 2003;49:826–37.
97. Srouji I, Lund V, Andrews P, Edwards C. Rhinologic symptoms and quality-of-life in patients with Churg-Strauss syndrome vasculitis. Am J Rhinol. 2008;22:406–9.
98. Basu N, McClean A, Harper L, et al. Explaining fatigue in ANCA-associated vasculitis. Rheumatology (Oxford). 2013;52(9):1680–5.

99. Basu N, Murray AD, Jones GT, Reid DM, Macfarlane GJ, Waiter GD. Neural correlates of fatigue in granulomatosis with polyangiitis: a functional magnetic resonance imaging study. Rheumatology (Oxford). 2014;53:2080–7.
100. Basu N, McClean A, Harper L, et al. Markers for work disability in anti-neutrophil cytoplasmic antibody-associated vasculitis. Rheumatology (Oxford). 2014;53(5):953–6.
101. Barra L, Borchin RL, Burroughs C, Vasculitis clinical research consortium and the vasculitis patient-powered research network, et al. Impact of vasculitis on employment and income. Clin Exp Rheumatol. 2018;36(Suppl 111(2)):58–64.
102. Pugnet G, Pagnoux C, Terrier B, et al. Rituximab versus azathioprine for ANCA-associated vasculitis maintenance therapy: impact on global disability and health-related quality of life. Clin Exp Rheumatol. 2016;34:S54–9.
103. Hickman RA, Gordon C. Causes and management of infertility in systemic lupus erythematosus. Rheumatology (Oxford). 2011;50:1551–8.
104. Chakravarty EF, Murray ER, Kelman A, Farmer P. Pregnancy outcomes after maternal exposure to rituximab. Blood. 2011;117:1499–506.
105. Sangle SR, Lutalo PM, Davies RJ, Khamashta MA, D'Cruz DP. B-cell depletion therapy and pregnancy outcome in severe, refractory systemic autoimmune diseases. J Autoimmun. 2013;43:55–9.
106. Conduit C, Yew S, Jose M, Jayne D, Kirkland G. A case of de novo diagnosis anti-neutrophil cytoplasmic antibody-negative pauci-immune necrotising glomerulonephritis in pregnancy. [letter]. Intern Med J. 2017;47(5):600–1.
107. Hilhorst M, Wilde B, van Paassen P, et al. Improved outcome in anti-neutrophil cytoplasmic antibody (ANCA)-associated glomerulonephritis: a 30-year follow-up study. Nephrol Dial Transplant. 2013;28:373–9.
108. Miloslavsky EM, Niles JL, Wallace ZS, et al. Reducing glucocorticoid duration in ANCA-associated vasculitis: a pilot trial. Semin Arthritis Rheum. 2018;48(2):288–92.
109. McAdoo SP, Medjeral-Thomas N, Gopaluni S, et al. Long-term follow-up of a combined rituximab and cyclophosphamide regimen in renal anti-neutrophil cytoplasm antibody-associated vasculitis. Nephrol Dial Transplant. 2018;33(5):899.
110. Furuta S, Chaudhry AN, Hamano Y, et al. Comparison of phenotype and outcome in microscopic polyangiitis between Europe and Japan. J Rheumatol. 2014;41:325–33.
111. Fujimoto S, Watts RA, Kobayashi S, et al. Comparison of the epidemiology of anti-neutrophil cytoplasmic antibody-associated vasculitis between Japan and the UK. Rheumatology (Oxford). 2011;50(10):1916–20.
112. Hogan SL, Nachman PH, Wilkman AS, Jennette JC, Falk RJ. Prognostic markers in patients with antineutrophil cytoplasmic autoantibody-associated microscopic polyangiitis and glomerulonephritis. J Am Soc Nephrol. 1996;7:23–32.
113. Lyons PA, Rayner TF, Trivedi S, et al. Genetically distinct subsets within ANCA-Associated Vasculitis. N Engl J Med. 2012;367:214–23.
114. McKinney EF, Lee JC, Jayne DR, Lyons PA, Smith KG. T-cell exhaustion, co-stimulation and clinical outcome in autoimmunity and infection. Nature. 2015;523(7562):612–6.

Treatment of ANCA-Associated Vasculitides

17

Loïc Guillevin, Loïc Raffray, Yann Nguyen, Benjamin Chaigne, and Benjamin Terrier

17.1 Introduction

A subgroup of systemic necrotizing vasculitides, antineutrophil cytoplasm antibody (ANCA)-associated vasculitides (AAVs), are known to have circulating ANCA in >30–90% of the affected patients. Granulomatosis with polyangiitis (GPA, formerly Wegener's granulomatosis), eosinophilic granulomatosis with polyangiitis (EGPA, formerly Churg–Strauss syndrome), and microscopic polyangiitis (MPA) are AAVs [1]. Renal-limited vasculitis, another AAV, is a bit of a question mark, as it is a disease that initially affects the kidney but could then evolve to become MPA or GPA. All AAVs affect small-sized vessels, and ANCA are thought to play a role in their pathogeneses. Due to our improved understanding of AAV pathophysiological mechanisms and identification of their cellular and molecular targets, AAV treatments are now more specific than they had been in the past.

AAV treatments, too, are now changing, with the long-standing conventional treatments, based on the combination of corticosteroids (CS) and immunosuppressants, being challenged by biotherapies targeting cytokines or lymphocytes that are thought to be involved in the pathogeneses of these entities.

L. Guillevin (✉) · Y. Nguyen · B. Chaigne · B. Terrier
Department of Internal Medicine, Referral Center for Rare Systemic and Autoimmune Diseases, Hôpital Cochin, Université Paris Descartes, Paris, France
e-mail: loic.guillevin@aphp.fr; yann.nguyen@aphp.fr; benjamin.chaigne@aphp.fr; benjamin.terrier@aphp.fr

L. Raffray
Department of Internal Medicine, Félix-Guyon University Hospital of La Réunion, Saint Denis, Réunion Island, France

R. A. Sinico, L. Guillevin (eds.), *Anti-Neutrophil Cytoplasmic Antibody (ANCA) Associated Vasculitis*, Rare Diseases of the Immune System,
https://doi.org/10.1007/978-3-030-02239-6_17

17.2 General Principles

Although ANCA can be detected in GPA, EGPA, and MPA, these three AAVs are heterogeneous, and those differences and their specificities influence/modulate therapeutic options and choices. Disease severity is also a factor that should be considered in choosing the best treatment strategy. A given patient's age and comorbidities must also be taken into account to adapt the regimen of choice. The five-factor score (FFS) was devised to evaluate disease prognosis and to adapt the therapeutic strategy accordingly, depending on the entity [2]. However, GPA treatment should not be modified according to the FFS: CS and an immunosuppressant or rituximab should systematically be prescribed for these patients. Adapting MPA and EGPA treatment to the FFS remains debated. Nephrologists published most MPA-patient series and, unsurprisingly, they had renal manifestations that should be treated with CS and an immunosuppressant or rituximab [3–7].

Since the discovery of ANCA, more benign MPA forms, associating, for instance, skin manifestations and arthralgias but no visceral manifestations, have been described. ANCA positivity and informative skin biopsy findings can lead to the diagnosis. For such cases, we were able to demonstrate that CS alone are effective and that cyclophosphamide has no added value [8]. In addition, the results of a recent randomized controlled trial (RCT) showed that azathioprine, combined with CS, could neither lower the AAV remission rate nor prevent relapses [9]. Our group published the only study showing that long-term relapses were more frequent in patients initially treated with CS alone, compared to combination therapy with an immunosuppressant [10].

EGPA treatment is complex. Because of its asthma and/or ear, nose, and throat (ENT) manifestations, which usually precede the vasculitic disease phase and reoccur often over the long term, even when vasculitis remission is obtained, prolonged CS intake is necessary. Consequently, EGPA should be treated according to the patient's FFS. When FFS = 0, we recommend treating EGPA with CS alone; however, when FFS $\geq$ 1, a combined regimen with CS with immunosuppressants is required. That distinction remains a sticking point in international guidelines, further confounded by the fact that some authors cosigned recommendations for and against it [11, 12].

Vasculitis therapy also has to be adapted to the patient's age, renal function, nutritional status, and comorbidities. Notably, lower CS and immunosuppressant doses for systemic necrotizing vasculitis patients $\geq$65 year old improved outcomes because of fewer treatment-associated adverse events (AEs) [9].

Prescribing prophylaxis against infectious complications is another important aspect of AAV therapy, with co-trimoxazole (or pentamidine aerosols in the case of sulfa drug allergies) to avoid *Pneumocystis jirovecii* pneumonia. Immunizations against seasonal flu and invasive pneumococcal infection are strongly recommended [11]. Although some patients suffered EGPA flares after vaccination, the benefit/risk ratio largely favors immunization of vasculitis patients [13]. However, we are now wondering about vaccine efficacy in rituximab-treated patients, whose immune responses produce only low-titer protective antibodies, as previously shown for patients with rheumatoid arthritis or primary immune thrombocytopenia [14–17].

17.3 Remission Induction Therapy

17.3.1 Corticosteroids

Prednisone or prednisolone (1 mg/kg/day) is initially prescribed to obtain AAV remission. When AAV is severe, intravenous (IV) pulses of methylprednisolone (7.5–15 mg/kg/day) can be given for 1–3 days. While expert consensus has been reached for the initial CS dose, experts remain divided on how long CS should be given or their tapering schedules. The European Vasculitis (EUVAS) group and the Vasculitis Clinical Research Consortium (VCRC) recommended rapid CS tapering, with a 25% decrement every week until week 7, at which time a CS dose ~30% of the initial one could be reached [12].

We demonstrated that, during induction therapy for elderly patients, prednisone and cyclophosphamide doses could be at least one-third lower and still achieve remission while limiting AEs [18]. Because CS act rapidly to control vasculitis and asthma flares, inducing clinical remission and eosinophilia normalization, they represent the cornerstone of EGPA treatment. However, long-term CS use is not anodyne and can be responsible for many AEs, especially when dose diminution is not possible because of persistently uncontrolled asthma and/or ENT manifestations. Thus, how long treatment should last becomes more complex; it is addressed below in the section on maintenance therapy.

17.3.2 Immunosuppressants

17.3.2.1 Cyclophosphamide

Cyclophosphamide, either oral or IV, is the most frequently prescribed immunosuppressant to control severe vasculitis [19–21]. The results of different trials that prescribed oral or IV cyclophosphamide to obtain AAV remission were analyzed retrospectively and showed a trend toward more relapses in patients receiving it IV [22]. However, to date, no other drug has yet surpassed cyclophosphamide efficacy against severe vasculitides.

Authors of prospective RCTs designed to compare rituximab to cyclophosphamide, combined with CS to induce AAV remission, concluded that rituximab is not inferior but also not superior to cyclophosphamide [23, 24]. At present, physicians tend to prescribe rituximab more often than cyclophosphamide to treat AAVs because of safety concerns associated with the latter: high doses or prolonged intake leading to sterility and heightened long-term cancer risk [25, 26].

The recommended cyclophosphamide dose of 0.5–0.7 g/m^2 or 15 mg/kg for each infusion should be administered on days 0, 14, and 28, then every 3 weeks until remission is obtained, usually after six such doses. Oral cyclophosphamide (2–3 mg/kg) should be taken for 3–6 months, but it delivers a higher cumulative dose than IV administration. However, it is important to underscore that shortening the treatment duration has limited AEs, thereby making cyclophosphamide a more "acceptable" drug than in the past.

17.3.2.2 Azathioprine and Methotrexate

Azathioprine is not a usual first-line therapeutic choice for AAVs, but it is indicated for maintenance therapy. Methotrexate's indication is the same as that of azathioprine, but it has been used to induce remission of nonsevere GPA without renal involvement [27]. In a prospective 12-month RCT, methotrexate efficacy was comparable to that of oral cyclophosphamide, but its associated relapse rate was higher [27].

17.3.2.3 Mycophenolate Mofetil

A prospective, RCT compared mycophenolate mofetil to cyclophosphamide to induce AAV remission [28]. Although remission rates at 6 months were similar, relapses rate after azathioprine switch as remission regimen were higher within the group of patients who initially received mycophenolate, especially for PR3-ANCA AAV.

17.3.3 Intravenous Immunoglobulins and Therapeutic Plasma Exchanges (TPEs)

17.3.3.1 Intravenous Immunoglobulins (IVIg)

IVIg (2 g/kg/cycle) were given as remission induction therapy, alone or combined with other agents [29–32]. They are thought to be immunomodulating agents that can interact with ANCA. They are contraindicated when severe chronic kidney disease is present. Evaluated prospectively in a RCT, IVIg were shown to have only a transient effect and that relapses could occur. Nowadays, IVIg are mostly used during disease flares, when the effects of other drugs are insufficient. IVIg (0.4–0.5 g/kg/cycle) are also indicated as replacement therapy for hypogammaglobulinemic patients or those with severe infections. In that context, immunoglobulins can alternatively be injected subcutaneously.

17.3.3.2 Therapeutic Plasma Exchanges (TPEs)

TPEs were first used to treat vasculitides in the 1970s. A benefit was shown for two small series of patients with rapidly progressive crescentic glomerulonephritis [33, 34]. The first RCTs, designed to treat all vasculitis forms, failed to demonstrate any improved survival advantage [35]. TPE adjunction to CS and cyclophosphamide for severe vasculitides yielded similar results [31]. However, more recently, TPE efficacy was demonstrated in patients with severe renal insufficiency (creatininemia >500 μmol/L) among a homogeneous subgroup of an AAV population. The results showed that when TPEs were added to oral cyclophosphamide and CS in a prospective RCT, that combination was superior to the arm with pulse methylprednisolone given to counter the severity of renal impairment [36]. However, again, no survival benefit was obtained. The new ongoing PEXIVAS trial was designed to evaluate TPEs, first as a CS-sparing agent, and second, for less severely ill patients, that is, AAV patients with creatininemia clearance <50 mL/min and intraalveolar hemorrhage.

17.4 Targeted Drugs (Biotherapies)

17.4.1 Antitumor Necrosis Factor-Alpha (Anti-TNFα)

The anti-TNFα molecules, infliximab, a chimeric anti-TNFα monoclonal antibody, and etanercept, which blocks the TNF receptor, have been used to treat AAV patients. Infliximab combined with conventional therapy was shown to be effective in an open study: 88% of the patients with acute or persistently active AAVs entered clinical remission [37]. Our group's retrospective evaluation of infliximab in 15 patients with refractory/relapsing systemic necrotizing vasculitides [38] confirmed its only short-term efficacy, with most patients relapsing. The efficacy of etanercept, also combined with conventional cyclophosphamide or methotrexate induction for limited disease, was tested to treat AAVs in the WGET trial: it failed to prevent relapses compared to placebo [39]. More importantly, some severe AEs occurred. Pertinently, etanercept's lack of activity against granulomatous diseases could explain, at least partially, its poor efficacy against AAVs. In our opinion, although infliximab or etanercept might have some indication for potential use, neither should be considered first-line induction or maintenance choices for AAV patients.

17.4.2 Rituximab

This chimeric anti-CD20 IgG1 mouse–human monoclonal antibody, which selectively depletes mature and memory B cells, is now considered one of the best first-line remission induction agents for AAVs, vying for the place long held by cyclophosphamide. Rituximab (MabThera® or Rituxan®) induces B-cell apoptosis, and hence, theoretically abrogates autoreactive antibody production, thereby explaining its reported activity against various autoimmune disorders. However, the specific mechanisms underlying rituximab efficacy in autoimmune disorders remains poorly elucidated. In light of the pleiotropic functions of B cells, therapies targeting them might also exert their efficacy by preventing antigen presentation, T-cell activation, or cytokine production [40].

Rituximab noninferiority to cyclophosphamide as an AAV remission induction agent is clearly established. According to the results of the RAVE trial, which compared oral cyclophosphamide to rituximab for induction, respective remission rates at 6 months were 64% and 53% (statistically not significant) [23]. Consequently, rituximab has revolutionized the standard of care for AAVs and is now recommended as first-line therapy for many GPA and MPA patients [12]. The European Medicines Agency (EMA) and the American Food and Drug Administration (FDA) licenses recommend infusing 375 mg/m^2 body surface area once a week for 4 weeks to induce remission. Empirically, doubling the dose every fortnight (i.e., 1000 mg on days 1 and 15) was advanced; despite having apparently been as effective in a retrospective study, it remains to be fully evaluated [41]. Rituximab's most frequent

AEs are allergic reactions during infusion, infections, and a trend toward lower IgG levels, mainly IgM. Although low immunoglobulin levels can persist for several months or even years, for most patients, such eventualities are not associated with more infections, but some opportunistic infections were reported, including progressive multifocal leukoencephalopathy.

17.4.3 Abatacept

Abatacept limits T-cell activation by blocking the binding of the costimulatory CD28 receptor to its ligand. Therefore, it might have some activity on the pathophysiological mechanisms attributed to AAV onset. So far, only small series of patients with nonsevere relapsing AAVs have been treated with abatacept [42]. To the best of our knowledge, it has not been used to treat severe or refractory AAVs and its long-term impact obviously remains unknown.

17.4.4 EGPA-Specific Agents

Because of EGPA specificities and rarity, most patients with that vasculitis were not enrolled in trials testing remission induction regimens with new targeted biotherapies. However, some experience has been obtained with drugs devoted exclusively to treating EGPA, for example, interferon-alpha, omalizumab, and mepolizumab.

17.4.4.1 Interferon-Alpha (IFNα)

In vitro, IFNα blocks interleukin (IL)-5 secretion and tempers the skewed Th2 profile, characteristic of EGPA pathophysiology, and therefore, might be able to downgrade eosinophilia in blood and tissues. IFNα was used to treat a series of four patients and in prospective open-label studies [43, 44], and an uncontrolled retrospective analysis of 30 patients followed for at least 2 years [45]. Despite some reported remission induction success, high relapse rates and numerous AEs (e.g., depression and neuropathy) were observed during long-term follow-up. The EGPA Consensus Task Force recommended using IFNα only as second- or third-line therapy to treat relapsing/resistant EGPA [11].

17.4.4.2 Omalizumab (Anti-IgE)

Omalizumab (Xolair®), an IgG monoclonal antibody that targets free IgE in blood, blocks the allergic cascade [46]. It is injected subcutaneously every 2 or 4 weeks, with its dose calculated based on the patient's weight and total plasma IgE levels.

Omalizumab has documented efficacy against allergic asthma. That activity led to the hypothesis that it might be beneficial for EGPA patients, especially those whose asthma is severe. However, omalizumab was initiated to treat EGPA with CS-dependent asthma and hypereosinophilia, rarely for ENT or nonsevere vasculitis manifestations, so experience with this agent is essentially based on case reports [47–54]. Although omalizumab indeed controlled most patients' asthma symptoms, some of them suffered severe asthma exacerbations while taking it [47]. Overall, omalizumab was well tolerated, but EGPA flares were observed in three patients [47, 51]. Although omalizumab was prescribed to treat isolated asthma in at least 10 patients who later developed EGPA [55–58], it remains unclear whether the latter is directly attributable to omalizumab or an indirect unmasking of previously unknown EGPA as a consequence of CS weaning. At present, omalizumab's place in the treatment of EGPA is not known but seems likely to be limited to controlling severe CS-dependent asthma.

17.4.4.3 Mepolizumab (Anti-IL-5)

Mepolizumab (Nucala®) is an IgG1 monoclonal antibody that binds free IL-5, which is a major cytokine regulating eosinophil homeostasis [59]. By inhibiting IL-5 functions, it was able to prevent activation, recruitment, and tissue accumulation of eosinophils in asthma patients, and diminish blood and sputum eosinophilia [60]. Approval has been accorded to use mepolizumab as an add-on therapy for the management of severe eosinophilic asthma [61].

Mepolizumab was first tested to induce EGPA remission in small patient series [62–65]. Promising results were obtained, with mepolizumab making it possible to quickly taper CS and control systemic EGPA manifestations. Moreover, the results of a large RCT validated mepolizumab's indication to control EGPA, primarily its asthma manifestations [66]. In that trial, uncontrolled EGPA patients who had received conventional therapy for a median of 5 years were then randomized to receive mepolizumab (300 mg injected subcutaneously once a month) or placebo. One year later, significantly more mepolizumab-treated patients were in remission and relapse free, when asthma/ENT and vasculitis features were considered together, and without active vasculitis for the overwhelming majority of patients. Overall, mepolizumab was able to lower relapse rates by 50% without severe AEs. As a consequence, patients in the mepolizumab arm could have their CS doses tapered. Even though the results of that study suggested that anti-IL-5 was potentially beneficial for EGPA patients, mepolizumab's place remains to be determined, notably in terms of vasculitis manifestations and the most severe forms of the disease which were not clearly assessed by that study's design. Our group will conduct a prospective RCT, testing CS and anti-IL-5 therapy or cyclophosphamide to induce EGPA remission (French protocol PHRCN-17-0415).

17.4.4.4 Rituximab

Information on rituximab's clinical impact on EGPA is only available from low-evidence-based, open-label studies and case reports [67–71]. The main findings of those studies indicated potential advantages, especially for ANCA-positive patients with severe refractory/relapsing EGPA. An ongoing French prospective study is comparing rituximab to immunosuppressants, both combined with CS. Hopefully, its results will contribute to more clearly discerning rituximab's indications in treatment of EGPA and possibly help identify patient characteristics suggesting who would benefit the most from its use.

17.5 Maintenance Therapies

We have known for a long time, at least several decades, that prolongation of AAV remission induction therapy is essential to sustain remissions and prevent relapses. However, the real need for maintenance therapy was challenged by the RAVE trial strategy of withholding treatment until relapse after rituximab-induced remission [23, 72]. Below, we detail different therapeutic options for maintenance, which are mainly dependent on the induction regimen used.

17.5.1 The Conventional Approach

Knowing that 4–5 years postremission onset 40–50% of AAVs relapse, several preventive therapeutic options can be prescribed. Historically, a successful oral cyclophosphamide and CS induction regimen led to gradual CS tapering and total withdrawal, achieved after approximately 2 years. However, that strategy is now considered unacceptable because of its short-term (infections) and long-term (sterility and malignancies) severe AEs.

The CYCAZAREM trial [73] compared oral cyclophosphamide maintenance regimens for 3 or 12 months, then relayed by azathioprine: the two arms had comparable survival and relapse rates. Based on those findings, it is clear that the "lighter" regimen to sustain remission was as effective as the "heavier" one.

Various molecules, for example, azathioprine, methotrexate, or mycophenolate mofetil, have been used to maintain AAV remissions. Azathioprine was compared to methotrexate to maintain remissions induced with conventional CS and pulse cyclophosphamide in an RCT; after a mean follow-up of 29 months, respective relapse rates were 36% versus 33% [74]. It should be noted that almost three quarters of those relapses were observed after azathioprine and methotrexate had been stopped, with 15.1 versus 13.6 relapses/100 patient-years, respectively.

The abilities of azathioprine and mycophenolate mofetil to prevent relapses were also compared. Based on the results of a prospective RCT [75] demonstrating azathioprine superiority to mycophenolate mofetil, the authors concluded that mycophenolate mofetil should not be considered a first-choice therapeutic to sustain AAV remission.

AAV remission maintenance has unquestionably been revolutionized by the advent of rituximab. With 5% versus 28% relapse rates at the month 28 endpoint, MAINRITSAN trial results demonstrated rituximab superiority over azathioprine [76], respectively. Although those rates were further confirmed by the difference between arms after 60 months follow-up [77], relapses still occurred, usually 18–24 months after the last rituximab infusion.

17.5.2 Sustaining Rituximab-Induced Remission

The RAVE trial [23] prospectively compared two arms: CS and oral cyclophosphamide remission induction regimen for 3–6 months, then azathioprine, or CS and rituximab (375 mg/m²/week for 4 consecutive weeks) for an additional 12–15 months, then placebo. Month 18 relapse rates were comparable for the two arms. Sustained complete remissions at 12 and 18 months, respectively, had been obtained by 39% and 33% of the patients receiving cyclophosphamide–azathioprine versus 48% and 39% of those given rituximab–placebo. Based on those observations, after rituximab induction, azathioprine does not contribute to sustaining remission. But, because very high relapse rates were still seen in both arms, the search for an effective remission maintenance regimen is not yet over.

The MAINRITSAN trial results support the notion of using low-dose rituximab infusions every 6 months for 18 months to sustain remission as more reasonable than no treatment [76]. In that prospective RCT, 500 mg of rituximab were infused every 6 months for 18 months. The first infusion was given 3–4 weeks after terminating the cyclophosphamide and CS induction therapy regimen, the second was given 2 weeks later, then every 6 months. When follow-up ended 28 months postrandomization and 10 months after the final rituximab infusion, relapses had been noted in 5% of rituximab recipients versus 28% of azathioprine arm patients. Those patients were then monitored for an additional 60 months: despite relapses in both arms, rituximab remained superior to azathioprine to sustain remissions. At the end of the trial, the protocol stipulated that no further treatment would be given. Although rituximab superiority at sustaining remission was demonstrated, rituximab did not cure AAVs because relapses could occur during the months or years after its final scheduled infusion.

Those findings lead us to pose two questions now: (1) Should patients be given additional rituximab infusions, perhaps at an even lower dose, after 18 months? (2) Could azathioprine help maintain remission?

We are hopeful that our ongoing MAINRITSAN-3 trial will provide at least a partial response to the first question, as it compares, postrandomization, four additional 500 mg rituximab infusions at 6-month intervals to placebo, for patients who had received rituximab infusion(s) (every 6 months or as needed based on trimestrial laboratory results: ANCA titer or reappearance and/or plasma CD19+ B-cell reconstitution) during 18 months. It can readily be envisaged that prognostic factors and predictors of relapses will be used to determine how long treatment(s) should be administered in the not too distant future.

Concerning the second question of using azathioprine to maintain remission, RAVE trial results demonstrated that azathioprine was not better than placebo, and those of the MAINRITSAN trial demonstrated rituximab superiority over azathioprine. Combining those outcomes, we would like to advance that, despite prospective trial observations indicating that 48 months of azathioprine led to fewer relapses, its impact on relapse occurrence is limited [78]. However, because azathioprine's ability to maintain remission is poorer than that of rituximab, azathioprine seems to afford little benefit as a maintenance therapy. Moreover, that conclusion can probably be extended to methotrexate and mycophenolate mofetil, despite the absence of prospective trials testing them. Some vasculitis specialists prefer, once rituximab has induced remission, waiting for relapse to occur before represcribing drugs. In light of the potential severity of new manifestation(s) and possible sequelae (renal function, for example) that cannot be predicted, we feel uncomfortable applying that approach. In our opinion, relapse prevention with sequential rituximab infusions is preferential.

17.5.3 Predicting Relapses

The results of different prospective studies indicated that it is more or less possible to predict relapses and, consequently, to modulate maintenance treatment accordingly. ANCA are predictors of relapses [23, 77]. Patients with antimyeloperoxidase (MPO)-ANCA relapse less frequently than those antiproteinase-3 (PR3)-ANCA positive, who are at high risk of relapse. Based on our long-term analysis of MAINRITSAN trial data showing that, in addition to PR3-ANCA positivity or negativity at diagnosis, patients who were still PR3-ANCA positive 1 year after starting maintenance therapy relapsed more frequently than those who became ANCA negative by that time [77]. ANCA reappearance is also predictive of relapses or AAV flares. The results of one of our prospective trials, designed to evaluate the ability of ANCA titer/reappearance and/or CD19+ B-cell detection or not to predict relapses, indicated those parameters made it possible to adapt when to reinfuse rituximab and meant that AAV patients in remission received fewer rituximab doses (3 infusions [i.e., 1500 mg] vs. 5 [i.e., 2500 mg]) [79]. Moreover, those findings, unlike previously reported observations, indicated that ANCA parameters alone could not reliably predict relapses.

17.5.4 Adapting the Therapeutic Regimen to Disease Severity

In the 1970s, vasculitis outcomes were quite dismal, with only about 10% survival without treatment, but that rate rose to 50% for patients given CS alone [80]. Survival further improved significantly with the adjunction of cyclophosphamide to CS [19]. Although the new biotherapies have dramatically improved treatment efficacy, it cannot be forgotten that conventional regimens markedly improved survival. And with experience and the results of prospective therapeutic trials, we are now able to use those drugs more safely and prudently, sometimes in combination and even devise individually tailored regimen strategies. However, treatment guidelines for severe vasculitides are still lacking because most prospective trials excluded patients with the most severe manifestations.

17.5.4.1 Definitions of Severe and/or Refractory Vasculitis

Life-threatening symptoms or visceral involvement that affect organ function are the hallmarks of severe vasculitis, as previously reported and confirmed by disease severity scores [2, 81, 82]. Although persistent repercussions of those manifestations are not always foreseeable and sometimes cannot be prevented, organ involvement at disease onset must be treated rapidly.

Vasculitis unresponsive to therapy is an evolving concept. When, in 1979, Fauci et al. [19] demonstrated that cyclophosphamide could control vasculitides, the diseases had been considered unresponsive to that era's "gold standard" treatment. Even though progressive improvement of therapeutic strategies over time effectively lowered the number of vasculitides unresponsive to treatments, refractory forms did not completely disappear. For those hard-to-treat cases, new treatment approaches, like newly available therapeutic agents or drug combinations, should be assessed. Refractory AAV is not necessarily the same thing as severe vasculitis. The chronicity of GPA patients' symptoms is well-known, especially those affecting ENT organs and/or the upper respiratory tract. Although not always severe, those clinical manifestations, for example, facial tissue necrosis, should be viewed as progressively destructive, chronic, and unfortunately unresponsive to conventional regimens.

17.5.4.2 What Treatment Options?

For severe AAVs or those failing to respond to conventional drugs, we usually increase the CS dose until control is obtained and that dose is continued for 2–3 weeks, before attempting to taper it again. However, when AAV is severe, more than CS alone are required, and we prescribe at least a combination of CS and one of several available cytotoxic agents. Cyclophosphamide is the standard cytotoxic agent, par excellence. Historically, we administered IV cyclophosphamide (0.5–0.7 g/m^2, every 2–3 weeks) and recommended treating nonresponders with oral cyclophosphamide (2 mg/kg/day). However, since the advent of rituximab, recourse to oral cyclophosphamide is usually reserved only to treat disease unresponsive to IV cyclophosphamide and rituximab [23].

To control AAV unresponsive to combined CS and cyclophosphamide, other drugs can be prescribed.

Because mycophenolate mofetil was found to be noninferior to cyclophosphamide at 6 months for newly diagnosed AAV [28], it is highly unlikely that mycophenolate mofetil could be potent enough to induce remission of severe or refractory AAV. Methotrexate might be a possible treatment option for some predominantly granulomatous nonrenal forms of GPA [27].

In fact, most AAVs unresponsive to conventional regimens do indeed respond to rituximab and that biotherapeutic product can again be active against relapses. But how should we treat the most severe AAV forms that have not yet been recognized as rituximab targets by prospective trials? Based on our clinical experience, those severely ill patients can also be given rituximab but it may take longer to obtain a clinical response. When kidney failure and/or alveolar hemorrhage are signs of severe AAV, adding high CS doses and TPEs might tide things over until the response to rituximab kicks in. But that therapeutic strategy remains theoretical and unconfirmed by prospective trials or large case studies.

For localized and more granulomatous manifestations (e.g., orbital mass, subglottic or tracheal stenoses) of unresponsive AAVs, no therapeutic regimen has yet been codified. For AAVs not responding to immunosuppressants and rituximab (independent of the order of administration), other therapeutic approaches, drugs, and/or local interventions for tracheal manifestations (e.g., dilatation, stents, local injections of CS, or immunosuppressants) should be considered. Experimental approaches could include drug combinations. Radiotherapy for orbital mass is not effective and enucleation was sometimes considered for refractory disease.

Patients with refractory EGPA, despite ongoing immunosuppressant use, predominantly have refractory asthma that requires high-dose CS. Nowadays, a new strategy could be the adjunction of IL-5-targeting therapies, shown in a prospective trial to effectively obtain CS dose reduction and prevent relapses [66].

References

1. Jennette JC, Falk RJ, Bacon PA, et al. 2012 Revised International Chapel Hill Consensus Conference nomenclature of vasculitides. Arthritis Rheum. 2013;65(1):1–11.
2. Guillevin L, Pagnoux C, Seror R, et al. The Five-Factor Score revisited: assessment of prognoses of systemic necrotizing vasculitides based on the French Vasculitis Study Group (FVSG) cohort. Medicine (Baltimore). 2011;90(1):19–27.
3. Serra A, Cameron JS, Turner DR, et al. Vasculitis affecting the kidney: presentation, histopathology and long-term outcome. Q J Med. 1984;53(210):181–207.
4. Savage CO, Winearls CG, Evans DJ, Rees AJ, Lockwood CM. Microscopic polyarteritis: presentation, pathology and prognosis. Q J Med. 1985;56(220):467–83.
5. D'Agati V, Chander P, Nash M, Mancilla-Jimenez R. Idiopathic microscopic polyarteritis nodosa: ultrastructural observations on the renal vascular and glomerular lesions. Am J Kidney Dis. 1986;7(1):95–110.
6. Adu D, Howie AJ, Scott DG, Bacon PA, McGonigle RJ, Micheal J. Polyarteritis and the kidney. Q J Med. 1987;62(239):221–37.
7. Guillevin L, Durand-Gasselin B, Cevallos R, et al. Microscopic polyangiitis: clinical and laboratory findings in eighty-five patients. Arthritis Rheum. 1999;42(3):421–30.
8. Ribi C, Cohen P, Pagnoux C, et al. Treatment of polyarteritis nodosa and microscopic polyangiitis without poor-prognosis factors: a prospective randomized study of one hundred twenty-four patients. Arthritis Rheum. 2010;62(4):1186–97.
9. Puéchal X, Pagnoux C, Baron G, et al. Adding azathioprine to remission-induction glucocorticoids for eosinophilic granulomatosis with polyangiitis (Churg–Strauss), microscopic polyangiitis, or polyarteritis nodosa without poor prognosis factors: a randomized, controlled trial. Arthritis Rheumatol. 2017;69(11):2175–86.
10. Samson M, Puéchal X, Devilliers H, et al. Long-term follow-up of a randomized trial on 118 patients with polyarteritis nodosa or microscopic polyangiitis without poor-prognosis factors. Autoimmun Rev. 2014;13(2):197–205.
11. Groh M, Pagnoux C, Baldini C, et al. Eosinophilic granulomatosis with polyangiitis (Churg–Strauss) (EGPA) Consensus Task Force recommendations for evaluation and management. Eur J Intern Med. 2015;26(7):545–53.
12. Yates M, Watts RA, Bajema IM, et al. EULAR/ERA-EDTA recommendations for the management of ANCA-associated vasculitis. Ann Rheum Dis. 2016;75(9):1583–94.
13. Guillevin L, Guittard T, Bletry O, Godeau P, Rosenthal P. Systemic necrotizing angiitis with asthma: causes and precipitating factors in 43 cases. Lung. 1987;165(1):165–72.
14. Kostianovsky A, Charles P, Alves J-F, et al. Immunogenicity and safety of seasonal and 2009 pandemic A/H1N1 influenza vaccines for patients with autoimmune diseases: a prospective, monocentre trial on 199 patients. Clin Exp Rheumatol. 2012;30(Suppl 70):S83–9.
15. Adler S, Krivine A, Weix J, et al. Protective effect of A/H1N1 vaccination in immune-mediated disease—a prospectively controlled vaccination study. Rheumatology (Oxford). 2012;51(4):695–700.

16. Westra J, van Assen S, Wilting KR, et al. Rituximab impairs immunoglobulin (Ig)M and IgG (subclass) responses after influenza vaccination in rheumatoid arthritis patients. Clin Exp Immunol. 2014;178(1):40–7.
17. Moulis G, Lapeyre-Mestre M, Mahévas M, Montastruc J-L, Sailler L. Need for an improved vaccination rate in primary immune thrombocytopenia patients exposed to rituximab or splenectomy. A nationwide population-based study in France. Am J Hematol. 2015;90(4):301–5.
18. Pagnoux C, Quéméneur T, Ninet J, et al. Treatment of systemic necrotizing vasculitides in patients aged sixty-five years or older: results of a multicenter, open-label, randomized controlled trial of corticosteroid and cyclophosphamide–based induction therapy. Arthritis Rheumatol. 2015;67(4):1117–27.
19. Fauci AS, Katz P, Haynes BF, Wolff SM. Cyclophosphamide therapy of severe systemic necrotizing vasculitis. N Engl J Med. 1979;301(5):235–8.
20. Guillevin L, Cordier JF, Lhote F, et al. A prospective, multicenter, randomized trial comparing steroids and pulse cyclophosphamide versus steroids and oral cyclophosphamide in the treatment of generalized Wegener's granulomatosis. Arthritis Rheum. 1997;40(12):2187–98.
21. de Groot K, Harper L, Jayne DRW, et al. Pulse versus daily oral cyclophosphamide for induction of remission in antineutrophil cytoplasmic antibody-associated vasculitis: a randomized trial. Ann Intern Med. 2009;150(10):670–80.
22. Harper L, Morgan MD, Walsh M, et al. Pulse versus daily oral cyclophosphamide for induction of remission in ANCA-associated vasculitis: long-term follow-up. Ann Rheum Dis. 2012;71(6):955–60.
23. Stone JH, Merkel PA, Spiera R, et al. Rituximab versus cyclophosphamide for ANCA-associated vasculitis. N Engl J Med. 2010;363(3):221–32.
24. Jones RB, Cohen Tervaert JW, Hauser T, et al. Rituximab versus cyclophosphamide in ANCA-associated renal vasculitis. N Engl J Med. 2010;363(3):211–20.
25. Heijl C, Harper L, Flossmann O, et al. Incidence of malignancy in patients treated for antineutrophil cytoplasm antibody-associated vasculitis: follow-up data from European Vasculitis Study Group clinical trials. Ann Rheum Dis. 2011;70(8):1415–21.
26. Le Guenno G, Mahr A, Pagnoux C, Dhote R, Guillevin L, for the French Vasculitis Study Group. Incidence and predictors of urotoxic adverse events in cyclophosphamide-treated patients with systemic necrotizing vasculitides. Arthritis Rheum. 2011;63(5):1435–45.
27. de Groot K, Rasmussen N, Bacon PA, et al. Randomized trial of cyclophosphamide versus methotrexate for induction of remission in early systemic antineutrophil cytoplasmic antibody-associated vasculitis. Arthritis Rheum. 2005;52(8):2461–9.
28. Jones RB, Hiemstra TF, Ballarin J, et al. Mycophenolate mofetil versus cyclophosphamide for remission induction in ANCA-associated vasculitis: a randomised, non-inferiority trial. Ann Rheum Dis. 2019;78(3):399–405.
29. Jayne DR, Davies MJ, Fox CJ, Black CM, Lockwood CM. Treatment of systemic vasculitis with pooled intravenous immunoglobulin. Lancet. 1991;337(8750):1137–9.
30. Richter C, Schnabel A, Csernok E, de Groot K, Reinhold-Keller E, Gross WL. Treatment of anti-neutrophil cytoplasmic antibody (ANCA)-associated systemic vasculitis with high-dose intravenous immunoglobulin. Clin Exp Immunol. 1995;101(1):2–7.
31. Jayne DR, Lockwood CM. Intravenous immunoglobulin as sole therapy for systemic vasculitis. Br J Rheumatol. 1996;35(11):1150–3.
32. Jayne DR, Chapel H, Adu D, et al. Intravenous immunoglobulin for ANCA-associated systemic vasculitis with persistent disease activity. QJM. 2000;93(7):433–9.
33. Pusey CD, Rees AJ, Evans DJ, Peters DK, Lockwood CM. Plasma exchange in focal necrotizing glomerulonephritis without anti-GBM antibodies. Kidney Int. 1991;40(4):757–63.
34. Glöckner WM, Sieberth HG, Wichmann HE, et al. Plasma exchange and immunosuppression in rapidly progressive glomerulonephritis: a controlled, multi-center study. Clin Nephrol. 1988;29(1):1–8.
35. Guillevin L, Cevallos R, Durand-Gasselin B, Lhote F, Jarrousse B, Callard P. Treatment of glomerulonephritis in microscopic polyangiitis and Churg–Strauss syndrome. Indications of plasma exchanges, Meta-analysis of 2 randomized studies on 140 patients, 32 with glomerulonephritis. Ann Med Interne (Paris). 1997;148(3):198–204.

36. Jayne DRW, Gaskin G, Rasmussen N, et al. Randomized trial of plasma exchange or high-dosage methylprednisolone as adjunctive therapy for severe renal vasculitis. J Am Soc Nephrol. 2007;18(7):2180–8.
37. Stone JH, Uhlfelder ML, Hellmann DB, Crook S, Bedocs N-M, Hoffman GS. Etanercept combined with conventional treatment in Wegener's granulomatosis: a six-month open-label trial to evaluate safety. Arthritis Rheum. 2001;44(5):1149–54.
38. Josselin L, Mahr A, Cohen P, et al. Infliximab efficacy and safety against refractory systemic necrotising vasculitides: long-term follow-up of 15 patients. Ann Rheum Dis. 2008;67(9):1343–6.
39. Wegener's Granulomatosis Etanercept Trial (WGET) Research Group. Etanercept plus standard therapy for Wegener's granulomatosis. N Engl J Med. 2005;352(4):351–61.
40. Voswinkel J, Mueller A, Kraemer JA, et al. B lymphocyte maturation in Wegener's granulomatosis: a comparative analysis of VH genes from endonasal lesions. Ann Rheum Dis. 2006;65(7):859–64.
41. Charles P, Néel A, Tieulié N, et al. Rituximab for induction and maintenance treatment of ANCA-associated vasculitides: a multicentre retrospective study on 80 patients. Rheumatology (Oxford). 2014;53(3):532–9.
42. Langford CA, Monach PA, Specks U, et al. An open-label trial of abatacept (CTLA4-Ig) in non-severe relapsing granulomatosis with polyangiitis (Wegener's). Ann Rheum Dis. 2014;73(7):1376–9.
43. Tatsis E, Schnabel A, Gross WL. Interferon-alpha treatment of four patients with the Churg–Strauss syndrome. Ann Intern Med. 1998;129(5):370–4.
44. Metzler C, Csernok E, Gross WL, Hellmich B. Interferon-alpha for maintenance of remission in Churg–Strauss syndrome: a long-term observational study. Clin Exp Rheumatol. 2010;28(Suppl 57):24–30.
45. Seeliger B, Förster M, Happe J, et al. Interferon-α for induction and maintenance of remission in eosinophilic granulomatosis with polyangiitis: a single-center retrospective observational cohort study. J Rheumatol. 2017;44(6):806–14.
46. Soresi S, Togias A. Mechanisms of action of anti-immunoglobulin E therapy. Allergy Asthma Proc. 2006;27(Suppl 1):S15–23.
47. Jachiet M, Samson M, Cottin V, et al. Anti-IgE monoclonal antibody (omalizumab) in refractory and relapsing eosinophilic granulomatosis with polyangiitis (Churg–Strauss): data on seventeen patients. Arthritis Rheumatol. 2016;68(9):2274–82.
48. Detoraki A, Capua LD, Varricchi G, Genovese A, Marone G, Spadaro G. Omalizumab in patients with eosinophilic granulomatosis with polyangiitis: a 36-month follow-up study. J Asthma. 2016;53(2):201–6.
49. Giavina-Bianchi P, Giavina-Bianchi M, Agondi R, Kalil J. Administration of anti-IgE to a Churg–Strauss syndrome patient. Int Arch Allergy Immunol. 2007;144(2):155–8.
50. Pabst S, Tiyerili V, Grohé C. Apparent response to anti-IgE therapy in two patients with refractory "forme fruste" of Churg–Strauss syndrome. Thorax. 2008;63(8):747–8.
51. Lau EMT, Cooper W, Bye PT, Yan K. Difficult asthma and Churg–Strauss-like syndrome: a cautionary tale. Respirology. 2011;16(1):180–1.
52. Iglesias E, Camacho Lovillo M, Delgado Pecellín I, et al. Successful management of Churg–Strauss syndrome using omalizumab as adjuvant immunomodulatory therapy: first documented pediatric case. Pediatr Pulmonol. 2014;49(3):E78–81.
53. Graziani A, Quercia O, Girelli F, et al. Omalizumab treatment in patient with severe asthma and eosinophilic granulomatosis with polyangiitis. A case report. Eur Ann Allergy Clin Immunol. 2014;46(6):226–8.
54. Aguirre-Valencia D, Posso-Osorio I, Bravo J-C, Bonilla-Abadía F, Tobón GJ, Cañas CA. Sequential rituximab and omalizumab for the treatment of eosinophilic granulomatosis with polyangiitis (Churg–Strauss syndrome). Clin Rheumatol. 2017;36(9):2159–62.
55. Nazir S, Tachamo N, Fareedy SB, Khan MS, Lohani S. Omalizumab-associated eosinophilic granulomatosis with polyangiitis (Churg–Strauss syndrome). Ann Allergy Asthma Immunol. 2017;118(3):372–4.

56. Bekçibaşı M, Barutçu S, Çelen MK, Dayan S, Hoşoğlu S. Churg–Strauss syndrome occurring during omalizumab treatment. Eur J Rheumatol. 2015;2(3):129–30.
57. Szwarc D, Veillon F, Moser T, Averous G, De Blay F, Riehm S. Churg–Strauss syndrome under omalizumab treatment: a rare visceral manifestation. J Radiol. 2009;90(11 Pt 1):1737–9.
58. Wechsler ME, Wong DA, Miller MK, Lawrence-Miyasaki L. Churg–Strauss syndrome in patients treated with omalizumab. Chest. 2009;136(2):507–18.
59. Mepolizumab: 240563, anti-IL-5 monoclonal antibody—GlaxoSmithKline, anti-interleukin-5 monoclonal antibody—GlaxoSmithKline, SB 240563. Drugs R D. 2008;9(2):125–30.
60. Leckie MJ, ten Brinke A, Khan J, et al. Effects of an interleukin-5 blocking monoclonal antibody on eosinophils, airway hyper-responsiveness, and the late asthmatic response. Lancet. 2000;356(9248):2144–8.
61. Keating GM. Mepolizumab: first global approval. Drugs. 2015;75(18):2163–9.
62. Kahn J-E, Grandpeix-Guyodo C, Marroun I, et al. Sustained response to mepolizumab in refractory Churg–Strauss syndrome. J Allergy Clin Immunol. 2010;125(1):267–70.
63. Kim S, Marigowda G, Oren E, Israel E, Wechsler ME. Mepolizumab as a steroid-sparing treatment option in patients with Churg–Strauss syndrome. J Allergy Clin Immunol. 2010;125(6):1336–43.
64. Moosig F, Gross WL, Herrmann K, Bremer JP, Hellmich B. Targeting interleukin-5 in refractory and relapsing Churg–Strauss syndrome. Ann Intern Med. 2011;155(5):341–3.
65. Herrmann K, Gross WL, Moosig F. Extended follow-up after stopping mepolizumab in relapsing/refractory Churg–Strauss syndrome. Clin Exp Rheumatol. 2012;30(Suppl 70):S62–5.
66. Wechsler ME, Akuthota P, Jayne D, et al. Mepolizumab or placebo for eosinophilic granulomatosis with polyangiitis. N Engl J Med. 2017;376(20):1921–32.
67. Umezawa N, Kohsaka H, Nanki T, et al. Successful treatment of eosinophilic granulomatosis with polyangiitis (EGPA; formerly Churg–Strauss syndrome) with rituximab in a case refractory to glucocorticoids, cyclophosphamide, and IVIG. Mod Rheumatol. 2014;24(4):685–7.
68. Pepper RJ, Fabre MA, Pavesio C, et al. Rituximab is effective in the treatment of refractory Churg–Strauss syndrome and is associated with diminished T-cell interleukin-5 production. Rheumatology (Oxford). 2008;47(7):1104–5.
69. Thiel J, Hässler F, Salzer U, Voll RE, Venhoff N. Rituximab in the treatment of refractory or relapsing eosinophilic granulomatosis with polyangiitis (Churg–Strauss syndrome). Arthritis Res Ther. 2013;15(5):R133.
70. Mohammad AJ, Hot A, Arndt F, et al. Rituximab for the treatment of eosinophilic granulomatosis with polyangiitis (Churg–Strauss). Ann Rheum Dis. 2016;75(2):396–401.
71. Fanouriakis A, Kougkas N, Vassilopoulos D, Fragouli E, Repa A, Sidiropoulos P. Rituximab for eosinophilic granulomatosis with polyangiitis with severe vasculitic neuropathy: case report and review of current clinical evidence. Semin Arthritis Rheum. 2015;45(1):60–6.
72. Specks U, Merkel PA, Seo P, et al. Efficacy of remission-induction regimens for ANCA-associated vasculitis. N Engl J Med. 2013;369(5):417–27.
73. Jayne D, Rasmussen N, Andrassy K, et al. A Randomized trial of maintenance therapy for vasculitis associated with antineutrophil cytoplasmic autoantibodies. N Engl J Med. 2003;349(1):36–44.
74. Pagnoux C, Mahr A, Hamidou MA, et al. Azathioprine or methotrexate maintenance for ANCA-Associated vasculitis. N Engl J Med. 2008;359(26):2790–803.
75. Hiemstra TF, Walsh M, Mahr A, et al. Mycophenolate mofetil vs azathioprine for remission maintenance in antineutrophil cytoplasmic antibody-associated vasculitis: a randomized controlled trial. JAMA. 2010;304(21):2381–8.
76. Guillevin L, Pagnoux C, Karras A, et al. Rituximab versus azathioprine for maintenance in ANCA-associated vasculitis. N Engl J Med. 2014;371(19):1771–80.
77. Rituximab versus azathioprine to maintain remission of ANCA-associated vasculitides (MAINRITSAN): follow-up at 60 months. ACR meeting. Abstracts. http://acrabstracts.org/abstract/rituximab-versus-azathioprine-to-maintain-remission-of-anca-associated-vasculitides-mainritsan-follow-up-at-60-months/. http://doi.org/10.1136/annrheumdis-2017-212768 or pubmed. PMID: 29724729.

78. Karras A, Pagnoux C, Haubitz M, et al. Randomised controlled trial of prolonged treatment in the remission phase of ANCA-associated vasculitis. Ann Rheum Dis. 2017;76(10):1662–8.
79. Charles P, Terrier B, Cohen P, et al. Comparison of systematic vs individually tailored rituximab regimen to maintain ANCA-associated–vasculitis remission: results of a prospective, randomized–controlled, phase 3 trial [Internet]. ACR Meeting. Abstracts. http://acrabstracts.org/abstract/comparison-of-systematic-vs-individually-tailored-rituximab-regimen-to-maintain-anca-associated-vasculitis-remission-results-of-aprospective-randomized-controlled-phase-3-trial/.
80. Leib ES, Restivo C, Paulus HE. Immunosuppressive and corticosteroid therapy of polyarteritis nodosa. Am J Med. 1979;67(6):941–7.
81. Luqmani RA, Bacon PA, Moots RJ, et al. Birmingham Vasculitis Activity Score (BVAS) in systemic necrotizing vasculitis. QJM. 1994;87(11):671–8.
82. Guillevin L, Lhote F, Gayraud M, et al. Prognostic factors in polyarteritis nodosa and Churg–Strauss syndrome. A prospective study in 342 patients. Medicine (Baltimore). 1996;75(1):17–28.

Index

R. A. Sinico, L. Guillevin (eds.), *Anti-Neutrophil Cytoplasmic Antibody (ANCA) Associated Vasculitis*, Rare Diseases of the Immune System,
https://doi.org/10.1007/978-3-030-02239-6

MIX
Papier aus verantwortungsvollen Quellen
Paper from responsible sources
FSC® C105338

If you have any concerns about our products,
you can contact us on
ProductSafety@springernature.com

In case Publisher is established outside the EU,
the EU authorized representative is:
Springer Nature Customer Service Center GmbH
Europaplatz 3, 69115 Heidelberg, Germany

Printed by Libri Plureos GmbH
in Hamburg, Germany